RETHINK
FOOD

RETHINK FOOD

FOOD

100+ DOCTORS CAN'T BE WRONG

SHUSHANA CASTLE

AMY-LEE GOODMAN

Two Skirts Productions, llc
Houston, Texas

Published by Two Skirts Productions llc
P.O. Box 27202, Houston, TX 77227 USA

This book is intended to be educational and informative. Please do not adjust your diet or medications or begin any type of exercise program without first consulting your physician, especially if you are currently being treated. The authors, publisher, and contributors disclaim all responsibility for any liability or risk that may be associated with the application of any of the contents of this book. We encourage you to share the information from this book with your health care provider before making changes.

The authors, publisher, and contributors disclaim all responsibility for any liability or risk that may be associated with the application of any contents of this book.

Publisher's Cataloging-In-Publication Data

Castle, Shushana, author.
    Rethink food : 100+ doctors can't be wrong / Shushana Castle, Amy-Lee Goodman.

    pages ; cm

    Includes bibliographical references and index.
    Issued also as an ebook.
    ISBN: 978-0-9913588-0-9

    1. Veganism--Health aspects. 2. Nutrition. 3. Health. I. Goodman, Amy-Lee, 1987-   , author. II. Title.

RM236 .C37 2014
613.2/62

ISBN 978-0-9913588-0-9
Rethink Food/100+ Doctors Can't Be Wrong/ Shushana Castle and Amy-Lee Goodman

Includes bibliographical references and index.

Two Skirts Productions llc makes every effort to print this title on recycled, acid free paper.

Copies are printed in the United States of America for US distribution.

For promotional use or special sales, go to www.rethinkfoodbook.com

*Mom, you really are the best there is, ever. I love you
more. Thanks for making me savory fruit'n veggie platters
and scrumptious salads every day. The tradition lives on.
You're a fabulous joke teller, especially when you start
laughing before you finish.*

*My darling Jack, I am truly blessed you are in my life.
Thank you for showering me every day with your
beautiful friendship and loving heart.*

*For Mom, you will forever and always be my hero.
Thank you for having the courage to first rethink
food and inspiring me to be a woman who will.*

*And for Gully, this one is for you.
I will love and miss you always.*

Acknowledgments

First and foremost we want to thank the 100+ extraordinary doctors and experts who not only dedicated their time to sharing their wealth of knowledge but who also inspired *Rethink Food.* You are the pioneering leaders in healthcare and without you this book would not have been possible. To our amazing plant-powered athletes who shared their stories of success and serve as admirable examples of the testament to the human spirit of adventure, endurance, and compassion. It has been an absolute honor and privilege to learn from and work with all of you. Thank you for your commitment to all your patients and your quest for real healthcare answers. We are forever grateful.

Mom, thanks for cooking for us during this book birth. My sweet Samantha, not only are you a brainiac, but wonderfully inventive. Thank you for contributing your creative hands towards the book design cover. To my dear husband who totally pampered me throughout this exciting and exhausting ordeal of composing *Rethink Food,* I am grateful. To Hayden, for your gifted vision for perfection and tough compromise. To Trevor for your beautiful smile, sweetness and great company. You are brilliant. Tap into it. Fielding , you are perfect. To our kind friend Beth Rivera for helping us with the book title and everything else. To Jen Roosth for your brilliance and wonderful humor and Mary Es Beaver for your highly valued input and great friendship.

Dear Amy, we make such a superb writing team. This accomplishment could not have been possible without you and us working together, the way we do. I will miss you. This has been a wonderful journey with you and I will always remember the tough with the fun times we experienced working together. Wow. In some strange way I will somehow miss staying up until 3am going back and forth on emails with you for *Rethink Food.* You have taught me.

Thank you to my amazing family for standing by me every step of this journey. Mom, thank you for pushing me to exceed even my own expectations. Greg, my best friend, for the midnight coffee runs and being one of my biggest cheerleaders. You are the doctor of the future and I am so proud of you. My beautiful Jay, you and your story is inspiring. Thank you for letting me share it. Dad, for your advice, guidance, and much needed lunch dates. You always kept me smiling. To my brilliant power suit Wellesley sisters and Gillian, Sima, and Lissa, thank you for your words of encouragement. I love you all so much.

My dear co-author Shushana, you are an incredible woman that I am beyond blessed and grateful to have as a friend, mentor, and partner. We make such an amazing team and I can't thank you enough for this opportunity. I have loved our long coffee dates and late night working sessions. You have shown me anything is possible, and have made me the writer I am today. I have grown and learned so much from you and will forever cherish this exhilarating experience.

Thank you everyone who helped form the book: Posie Owens, Brittany Bakacs, Lisa Nuss, Toni Knapp, Sue Balcer, Alan Hebel and Ian Koviak for designing our book cover, our agent Steve Harris, Kim Coffman, Edward Sanchez, Aileen Moul and our amazing sounding board of friends and supporters that helped us perfect our literature. We thank you with all of our plant-powered hearts!

Table of Contents

WE AREN'T MEANT TO BE SICK

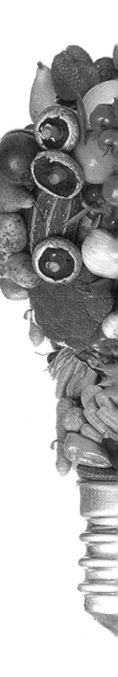

As a global society we speak of disease as something that runs in our families and are conditioned to believe that our health is out of our hands. However, in the history of disease we have never before faced such rampant levels of illnesses from heart disease to cancers, diabetes, Alzheimer's, obesity and numerous autoimmune and degenerative diseases. What is happening to us? Are our genetics to blame or are we unknowingly inflicting these diseases with our lifestyle choices?

Today, healthcare primarily uses band-aids in the form of pills, surgery, and procedures that masquerade as solutions without sincerely addressing the root causes of disease. However, we have been neglecting a vital component of our treatment plan.

Our food choices hold the most profound but overlooked influence on our health. For years we have been eating foods that damage rather than nourish our bodies and the evidence speaks for itself. Today, our woeful obsession with meat and dairy is literally killing us and the science can no longer be ignored.

Our impetus for *Rethink Food* came from simultaneously watching family and friends struggle with today's most common diseases for years and then completely rid themselves of the debilitating symptoms and re-gain their health and vitality upon adopting a whole foods plant-based diet within months.

Amy-Lee grew up as a meat and potatoes girl in Texas. Very involved in ballet and tennis, she carefully counted calories and carbs and thought ordering lean meat was making a healthy choice. But this all changed when Amy-Lee's younger sister, Jessica, was diagnosed with a debilitating case of juvenile rheumatoid arthritis when she was 9 years old. By her late teens, doctors predicted Jessica would be confined to a wheelchair. Although Jessica went through a variety of treatments, from chemotherapy to Enbrel injections twice a day, nothing worked. At 16 years old, she had become a skeleton of her former vibrant and vivacious self. After Amy-Lee's mom read how dairy can contribute to autoimmune diseases in *The China Study* by Dr. T. Colin Campbell, Jessica went off all dairy and animal products. Within 3 months her arthritis had gone into complete remission and has stayed that way ever since. Her doctors could not believe the drastic change and neither could Amy-Lee's family. As Amy-Lee continually researched the connection between diet and health, she could not consciously eat meat and dairy without knowing she was destroying her health. Amy-Lee and her whole family have been vegan and plant-based since 2005.

Shushana, also a vegan since 2005, grew up eating mainly a whole food, plant-based diet with very little meat and dairy. Her mom put bell peppers, cucumbers, and carrots as snacks for her daily lunch as a child, served huge salads and handfuls of raw nuts every night, and had fruit bowls around the house. She was known for eating massive quantities of food every day without gaining a pound. Always interested in nutrition, after reading dozens of books on plant nutrition she became impassioned to spread this knowledge on the overlooked connection between diet and disease. At age 81, Shushana's mother needed eye surgery to improve her deteriorating vision. After she removed meat and dairy from her diet, her vision returned within a few weeks and to her doctor's astonishment she no longer needed surgery. From strangers at the grocery stores, to airports and corporate boardrooms, Shushana realized that most people do not understand how and why some foods can harm us and others can heal us. In order to provide answers to ill friends and family, she began interviewing doctors and found that success stories from going plant-based were not confined to our limited social circle or the United States but are becoming a world- wide phenomenon.

We wrote **Rethink Food** to bring you these renowned physicians, scientists from distinguished universities, and nutritionists from around the world that uncover the entire spectrum of amazing health benefits from a plant-based diet. As these doctors attest, there is a powerful and intimate connection between disease and wellness that is strongly associated with our dietary choices. Challenging the status quo, these doctors substantiate how each and every chronic condition covered is DIET RELATED.

Contrary to popular belief, the following experts tell us why meat and dairy is a disaster for our health and the main cause of the today's leading chronic diseases. For instance, did you know that cow's milk doesn't actually promote strong bones? The truth is high dairy consumption is most associated with high rates of osteoporosis. While we have believed animal protein is good for us, these prominent cardiologists, weight-loss surgeons, and diabetic experts demonstrate how our excessive animal protein consumption is associated with increased risk of obesity, diabetes, kidney failure, heart disease, fatigue, and lower rates of longevity. With all of the misinformation surrounding our children's health, we can finally put to rest the confusion over what to feed our children. Our doctors confirm that nutrient rich plant-based foods best promote our children's healthy growth and development.

From the Ivy Leagues of Harvard, Princeton, Yale, and Cornell to the UK, India, Germany, Italy, Brazil, Mexico, and New Zealand, *Rethink Food's* experts explain how we can reverse heart disease and diabetes, eliminate food allergens and autoimmune diseases, live pain- free from arthritis, prevent Alzheimer's, and even bring cancer into remission. Former Olympic and celebrity trainers as well as former NBA and NHL players demonstrate how we can achieve peak performance powered by plants. Despite genetics, it is clear that a diet based on whole, plant-based foods is most directly linked to health, wellness, fitness, and longevity.

The misinformation surrounding our health is one of today's greatest injustices. Our health is our most valuable investment and prized possession. It is easy to take being healthy for granted until we are faced with a life altering problem. It's time we have real answers to our health problems and put health back into healthcare. The good news is the answer is tastefully simple and on our plates. We need to redefine the relationship between nutrition and disease.

We hope these doctors will inspire and empower you to take simple steps towards great health. Changing what we eat has the power to change our lives. It all begins with the courage to re-think food. Join us!

one

DISEASES: THE NEW NORMAL

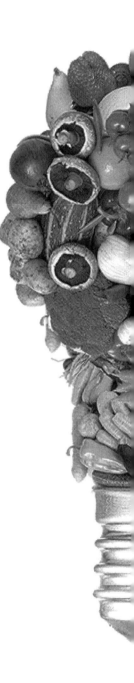

In the past, diseases plaguing our global society were mainly confined to an aging population, as evidenced by their definition as "degenerative" chronic conditions. Yet, today we see them in school-age children. We have accepted the leading chronic conditions such as heart disease, cancer, arthritis, Alzheimer's, and diabetes as the new "normal" and turned to technology, surgery and pills for healing. Yet, we are no further along in our quest for wellness evidenced by our continual rise in disease. The good news is we have the power to change this paradigm.

As a global community, we work hard to eradicate treatable diseases such as malaria and tuberculosis. Why do we treat the leading killers of the world differently when the chronic conditions plaguing the majority of the world's population, whilst preventable in the first place, can be treated with a simple, natural, and cost-effective solution?

We tend to blame poor health on genes, environmental factors, age, and chance, but we are missing the crucial connection between what we eat and how we feel. The following doctors will speak to the fact that our growing diseased population is from our choice to stray from our herbivore roots and eat foods our bodies were never designed to process. Our "evolution" to an omnivore diet coincides with our rise in disease. Simply by returning to our herbivore roots, we can re-establish sound health, wellness, and prevention.

The Limitations and Opportunities of Modern Medicine

Hans A. Diehl, DrHSc, MPH, CNS, FACN

After receiving the distinguished Bower Science Award, Denis Burkitt, MD, known for his legendary medical work that carries his name "the Burkitt Lymphoma", pronounced to an audience of some 600 physicians and guests, that "the greatest medical discovery of the last 20 years is the understanding that our Western Diseases are largely lifestyle-related. Therefore, they must be preventable and potentially reversible."[1]

Spoken more than 20 years ago, these words have taken on a prophetic meaning in that we now know that most of our chronic diseases (then referred to as Western Diseases), currently consuming 75% of our national health care budget, are indeed largely reversible.[2] Since that famous acceptance speech by Dr. Burkitt in 1992 the reversal-of-disease data has been accumulating. We are learning that we must go beyond the mere medical management of the symptoms of these chronic diseases. We can and must do more than settle for treating the symptoms of diseases, such as coronary heart disease, type 2 diabetes, essential hypertension, obesity, depression, and erectile dysfunction. But the cure is not dispensed in the form of a pill or procedure. As valuable as these high-tech modalities may be in improving the quality of life, they don't provide a cure. The cure is dispensed most often in the form of a more low-tech approach implementing a whole food, plant-based diet coupled with a consistent exercise program.

The Limitations of Modern Medicine

The accomplishments of modern medicine have been prodigious. We have seen the development of proton accelerators that can zap cancers, surgical robots that can be employed in performing coronary bypass surgeries, and advances in molecular biology and genetics that can open doors to amazing new worlds. And yet, these advances in high-tech medicine to take care of acute and episodic diseases have not altered the advances of our modern killer diseases. Rarely found some 100 years ago, these chronic diseases, also referred to as 'degenerative diseases', are now accounting for 70% of deaths.[3]

This term 'degenerative disease', is really a misnomer. For years, people fatalistically accepted the idea that coronary heart diseases, stroke, cancer, diabetes, diverticulosis, arthritis and other ailments were 'diseases of old age' and therefore to be expected. The fact that an increasing number of younger people are now suffering from them refutes this, as does their increase in near epidemic proportions despite everything science can do.

The statistics are convincing. Cardiovascular disease (coronary heart disease and stroke) and cancers of the breast, prostate, colon, and lungs are now claiming every third and fourth American life, respectively. In the 1900s fewer than 10% of deaths in the United States were attributed to cardiovascular disease and now it is the number one killer.[4] In spite of newer and refined forms of insulin and a plethora of bioengineered medications, the incidence rate of the common form of diabetes has gone up 700% since World War II, and especially since 1975 when diabetes began to "inexorably advance, doubling every 15 years.[5] The chance of becoming a diabetic in America for a new born baby is now 1 in 3.[6] And we have no medical cure."[7]

Concurrently, we have seen an enormous rise in the prevalence of excess weight, making it necessary for manufacturers to super-size everything from shirts to pants and from gurneys to coffins.[8] Modern epidemiology is unraveling the mystery: most of these modern killer diseases are lifestyle-related. Let's take a look at the world's number one killer, heart disease, and its underlying disease process—atherosclerosis to better understand the diet- disease relationship.

Atherosclerosis: An Insidious Killer

We were born with clean, flexible arteries, and they should stay that way throughout our lives. The arteries of most Americans, however, are clogged with cholesterol, fats, and calcium.[9] This narrowing process can even be seen in autopsies of American teenagers.[10]

Atherosclerosis-related diseases, however, are not a "natural" way to go. Atherosclerosis only became more apparent in Japan some 20 years after World War II with the import of the rich Western diet laced with meat, eggs and dairy products. We have seen similar trends more recently in China in response to the Western lifestyle involving dietary affluence. Research has consistently demonstrated that these atherosclerotic plaques can be created and promoted by consuming a diet high in saturated and trans fats and high in cholesterol. But they can also be prevented, arrested and reversed by removing these dietary stimuli.[11,12]

Opportunities of Modern Medicine

The renowned Framingham Heart Study, initiated in 1949 and still running after more than 60 years, found that 63- 80% of all major coronary events before the age of 65 could be prevented if Americans simplified their diet to lower their cholesterol to less than 180 mg and their systolic blood pressure to less than 125, and quit smoking.[13]

Dean Ornish, MD, convincingly evidenced that a plant-based whole food diet coupled with exercise and stress management could reverse not only the atherosclerotic plaques in coronary patients but also indolent prostate cancer.[14] Caldwell Esselstyn, MD, at the Cleveland Clinic, showed that of his "walking dead" cardiac patients, 74% were still alive after 20 years following adopting a simple plant-based diet that reversed their atherosclerotic plaques.[15] Neal Barnard, MD, has demonstrated that a diet devoid of animal products was very effective in reversing diabetes. Of his diabetic patients, 71% were off their oral medications within 4 weeks and with normal blood sugar levels.[16] Intensive educationally-centered lifestyle intervention programs, such as offered at the Pritikin Longevity Center (with over 75,000 graduates) as well as the CHIP program (Complete Health Improvement Program) offered by the Lifestyle Medicine Institute (with over 65,000 graduates from its community-based intervention program), have seen their patients reverse their chronic conditions by markedly improving their dietary and lifestyle habits.[17,18]

Outlook

Consider this: In the 1900s, Americans got 70% of their protein from *plant foods*.[19] Today, they get 70% of their protein from *animal products*,[19] high in *saturated fat*, cholesterol, trans fat, and devoid of fiber. And it is these *saturated* and *trans fats* found in meat, eggs and dairy when augmented by the trans fats found as hydrogenated fats in processed foods that stimulate the cholesterol production by the liver, thus becoming the foremost contributor to the circulating cholesterol levels in the blood.

The greatest health benefits are likely to accrue from efforts to improve the health habits of people instead of further medicalization. The research data is coming in every day stronger: the road to better health and longer life is reducing the amount of fats and oils, cholesterol, sugars and salt, alcohol and caffeine and eating more whole grains, legumes, fruits, and vegetables, and some nuts and seeds, and drinking plenty of water. Many mistakenly have been sold on the idea that medical care is synonymous with health care. With more than 70% of our well-being determined by lifestyle factors, medical care actually has little impact on health. Promoting health, therefore, has to do with treating the causes of chronic disease so as to facilitate their prevention, arrest and reversal. We have to go beyond the mere relief of symptoms and palliative treatments, as helpful as they may be at the time. We know how to create many of our common chronic diseases, and we know how to reverse them: it's healthy by choice, not by chance!

Hans Diehl, DrHSC, MPH, FACN, CNS, *is the founder of CHIP and the Lifestyle Medicine Institute in Loma Linda, California. His pioneering efforts with Nathan Pritikin and Dr. Denis Burkitt have shown that many of today's killer diseases can be powerfully influenced through adapting simple lifestyle changes. Dr. Diehl is a best-selling author, researcher, and top-ranking motivator. More than 30 articles published in medical and scientific journals show the efficacy of this lifestyle medicine approach to the chronic diseases. Currently, Dr. Diehl is the Clinical Professor of Preventive Medicine at Loma Linda University, School of Medicine.*

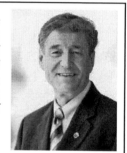

Wheat-Eaters or Meat-Eaters?

Juliet Gellatley BSc, Dip CNM, Dip DM, FNTP, NTCC

What is Our Natural Diet? Are Humans Evolutionarily Adapted to Eat Animals, Plants, or Both?

One of the most pervasive myths surrounding a whole foods plant-based diet is the belief that humans are naturally meant to eat meat and dairy; that we are evolutionarily adapted to eat and thrive on dead flesh or the milk of other species. Humans belong to the primate family. Our closest living relatives, chimpanzees and gorillas, live on a diet of foods overwhelmingly derived from plants. Of all the living primates, humans are the only ones to eat large animals. We ignore our evolutionary past at our peril, and it shows with the growing epidemics of killer diseases such as cancer, heart disease, obesity, and diabetes now occurring in almost every corner of the planet.

Back To Our Roots and Meat-Eating Beginnings

Our Stone Age predecessors ate three times the amount of plant foods that we do– about nine servings daily of fruits and vegetables, compared to the UK average of three. Today we consume just a fraction of the antioxidants, calcium, iron, and other nutrients that our ancestors ate every day. Fruits, green leafy parts of plants, shoots, seeds, nuts, roots, and tubers are the fundamental components of the primate eating pattern. Our anatomical structure indicates that these foods should be the foods that humans eat too.

Scavenging meat began in the last two million years with the advent of Homo erectus, who lived until 300,000 years ago.[1] The earliest evidence for hunting technology in the form of hafted spear points, currently dates back to about 500,000 years ago.[2] However, this species still largely consumed plant-based foods. Even as human beings became omnivorous when climatic changes destroyed food sources in certain regions, very little meat was eaten in comparison to today's excessive consumption patterns. In evolutionary terms, the length of time that humans have been omnivorous is a very short period but has had drastic health consequences.

Cues from the Body: We're Wheat-Eaters, Not Meat-Eaters

Basic anatomical comparisons show that people have much more in common with herbivores than carnivores or even omnivores. Humans' natural inability to efficiently and effectively process meat is seen throughout the design of our digestive system. For example, let's look at a human's mouth. The jaw and throat opening is too narrow for anything but relatively small pieces of food; we are unable to swallow food whole and must chew them finely and mix them with saliva before food will slide down the esophagus. By contrast, carnivorous animals such as cats tear off whole chunks and swallow them almost immediately.

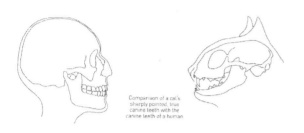

Comparison of a cat's sharply pointed, true canine teeth with the canine teeth of a human

Our jaws can open and close as well as move forwards, backwards and side-to-side. This is ideal for biting off pieces of plant matter and then grinding them down with our flat molars. In contrast, carnivores' lower jaws have very limited side-to-side motion. They are fixed only to open and close, which adds strength and stability to their powerful bite. Unlike these carnivorous animals' canine teeth, our teeth are not sharp blades and are not designed for processing meat. In fact, our blunted teeth are much better suited for eating starches, fruits, and vegetables.

From top to bottom, the human digestive system is evolved to efficiently process plant foods. Our digestion is aided by the salivary enzyme amylase, which solely aids in breaking down complex carbohydrates from plant foods into simple sugars. As there are no carbohydrates in meat, true carnivores do not need this enzyme and their salivary glands do not produce amylase.

The stomach juices of meat-eating animals are highly acidic. They have to be so that they can break down the large quantities of muscle and bone materials they eat. By contrast, our stomach has much lower concentrations of stomach acid as it takes less acid to digest starches, vegetables, and fruits. Weight for weight, plant protein requires half the amount of hydrochloric acid to digest it, compared to animal protein. It is also digested in half the time. This is why vegans and vegetarians have fewer peptic ulcers than meat-eaters.

You Got Guts

The human intestine is long and coiled, much like that of (other) herbivores. This makes digestion slow, allowing time to break down and absorb the nutrients from plant foods. In contrast, the intestine of a carnivore-- such as a cat-- is short, straight, and tubular. This means that flesh can be digested rapidly, and the remnants excreted quickly, before they putrefy (rot).

The difference in transit times (time taken for food to make its way from the mouth to the anus) between humans and carnivores are the primary anatomical difference. Humans – even those on a high fiber diet – have an average transit time of almost 41 hours. In stark contrast, the average transit time in a pure carnivore such as the mink is just 2.4 hours![3] This means when people eat meat, the meat has plenty of time to putrefy (rot) and produce cancer-causing agents.

Cholesterol Calamity

Meat-eating animals have an unlimited capacity to process and excrete cholesterol from their bodies. For example, you could feed a cat egg yolk all day long, and the cat would excrete all of it-- never suffering from a build up of cholesterol. On the other hand, people's livers (like other plant-eating animals) have a very limited capacity for cholesterol removal. Most people have great difficulty eliminating the amounts of cholesterol that they take in from eating animal products. We were made to consume plant foods containing no cholesterol; therefore we have never needed a highly efficient cholesterol-eliminating system.

But Surely Milk is Natural?

All 4,500 species of mammals produce milk for their young. Only humans continue to drink milk after weaning – and not even their mother's milk, but milk from another species. Nature never prepared us for this. This is why three quarters of the world's population are lactose intolerant. Most humans (95% of Asians; 75% of Afro-Caribbeans; 50% of Mediterraneans; and 10% of Northern Europeans) lose the ability to break down the sugar in milk, lactose, after weaning.[4] In fact, our species has been drinking cows' milk for only 6,000 years.[5] In evolutionary terms this is a blink of an eye. Still cows' milk is marketed as pure, essential, and natural for humans. Cow's milk is natural for calves, but it is certainly not natural for human babies. The 2 have very different needs, and the varying composition of the milk reflects this difference. For example, if not breast fed, our babies must not be given cows' milk but rather a formula that closely mirrors human milk.

Humans are naturally completely plant-based and were never meant to eat meat or dairy. Our bodies are simply not designed to consume flesh. By continuing to eat against our nature we put our health in serious peril. The sooner we ditch the 'meat maketh man' myth and exclude animal products from our diets the better.

Juliet Gellatley, BSc, Dip CNM, Dip DM, FNTP, NTCC *has a degree in zoology and is a qualified nutritional therapist. She is the founder & director of Viva!, Viva! Health in the UK, and Viva! Poland. She has given hundreds of public talks and is the author of several books, guides and reports.*

Juliet@viva.org.uk www.viva.org.uk www.vivahealth.org.uk

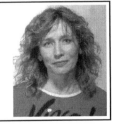

Eating the SAD Diet

Zarin Azar, MD

Einstein once wrote: "Nothing will benefit human health and increase chances of survival for life on earth as much as the evolution to a vegetarian diet." After almost one hundred years, never more than before in recent human history is the necessity and immediacy of this proclamation more evident. Our health is quickly deteriorating.

When I first came to the United States over 30 years ago, I was fascinated with the American way of eating-- especially fast foods-- that my daily diet changed to hamburgers, chickens, pizzas, eggs, and occasional bacon with breakfast and cold cuts. They tasted great. They were affordable and fast. More importantly, according to advertisements, I was sure I was providing my body with the most nutritious food in the form of animal products. I could not have been farther from the truth.

I did not know that my diet high in animal products deprived my body of antioxidants, vitamins, anti-cancer and anti-inflammatory phytochemicals, enzymes, vitamins and minerals, essential fatty acids, fiber, and many other important ingredients which only are found in plants. My animal-based diet was inflammatory and acid forming-- deteriorating my body, causing rapid aging, and an array of diseases. I started to gain weight and feel tired and fatigued. My mood started to change. My brain was foggy and my body felt heavier and heavier. More importantly I did not even know it was not normal to feel that way. After getting bigger and sicker every day for 2 to 3 years, I finally decided this was not how I wanted to treat my body and my mind. As I learned about the importance of diet and lifestyle on health, I was surprised that this pivotal issue was not more pronounced in my medical education and training.

As I changed my diet, my weight started to normalize, my energy increased, my fatigue and depressed mood improved, and my heart burn and stomach problems disappeared. I felt much lighter and better physically and emotionally after I changed to a plant- based diet.

Thousands of scientific studies prove that the best and the most health promoting diet is plant-based and devoid of animal products.

Man on Fire

Animal products are inflammatory because they produce Tri-methylamine. L-Carnitine in red meat and choline in egg is metabolized by intestinal bacteria to produce Tri- methylamine which after oxidation in the liver forms TMAO. TMAO's contribution to atherosclerosis and other inflammatory conditions like cancer and high cholesterol is well known. TMAO producing bacteria does not exist in vegan's intestinal tract.[2]

Two of the most damaging components of animal products are saturated and trans fats. Saturated fats are found in butter, meat and other animal products. The high saturated fat content in animal products contributes to heart disease, Alzheimer disease, and cancers including breast and prostate. Recent studies prove that as far as heart disease is concerned, consumption of 1 egg a day is the equivalent of smoking 5 cigarettes a day for 15 years.[1]

There is a link between consumption of saturated fat found in animal products and cognitive diseases of the brain such as dementia and Alzheimer's disease. Studies show that consumption of 25 grams of saturated fats increases the risk of Alzheimer's twofold.[3,4] This is because saturated fats in animal products clump together and form deposits in the wall of blood vessels along with cholesterol and proteins. They increase the body's natural production of cholesterol by increasing production of acetate during metabolism. These deposited plaques clog the smaller and then larger arteries of different organs including the heart and brain. This clogging of the arteries, known as atherosclerosis, causes micro infarction, meaning that part of the heart or brain tissue dies due to the lack of blood flow. This phenomenon is a contributing factor to dementia and Alzheimer disease, which is why meat eaters have 3 times more dementia than vegetarians.[4]

> **Keep the Weight Off with Propionate!**
>
> A high consumption of fiber, which animal products are devoid of, is paramount in preventing obesity, constipation, health of gastrointestinal tract and colon cancer. Propionate which has an anti-obesity effect is made by bacteria in our intestinal tract from fiber. Animal products do not have fiber so Propionate is found only in the intestines of vegetarians and vegans. The lack of propionate is a contributing factor to obesity.[5]

Additionally about 50% of the trans fats in our diet actually come directly from animal products like cheese, milk, and yogurt. Trans fats contribute to arterial damage in our organs. Since our brain, kidneys, and pelvis are highly vascular, trans fats from animal products contribute to conditions such as coronary artery disease, kidney disease, infertility and impotence.[6]

The majority of the diseases afflicting human societies today can be cured by a shift to a plant-based diet. As a gastroenterologist whose first line of therapy for her patients is a plant-based diet, I experience and observe this transformation every single day. Many gastrointestinal diseases like persistent acid reflux disease, gastritis, ulcers, irritable bowel syndrome, constipation, diarrhea, hemorrhoidal diseases, diverticular disease, fatty liver, and many other hepatic diseases, can potentially completely heal or improve significantly with a change of diet. Even an unlikely disease as inflammatory bowel disease is healed or improved by omission of animal products from the diet and the switch to a whole food, plant-based diet.

Our human bodies are amazing at self-healing-- we only need to assist them with a natural, whole foods, plant-based diet and a healthy life style to use this innate property, saving us billions of dollars on pharmaceuticals, wasteful studies, and procedures. The power of our own healing is in our hands.

Zarin Azar, MD, *received her MD and completed her Internal Medicine internship and residency from the University of Texas Medical Branch in Galveston. She completed her specialty training in Gastroenterology and Hepatology at UC Irvine. Dr. Azar is a proud member of the National Health Association and the Physicians Committee for Responsible Medicine among others. She maintains a widely popular educational website in Farsi on healthy lifestyles at* www.zarinazar.com.

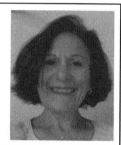

two

WHAT'S MISSING IN MEDICAL SCHOOL?

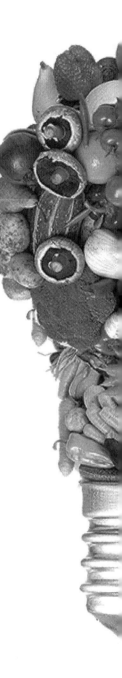

"The doctor of the future will give no medicine, but will interest his patient in the care of the human frame, in diet, and in the cause and prevention of disease."

- Thomas Edison

We look to our doctors as authorities on health, but they may be as confused and misinformed as we are. Think about this: in the 1950's doctors promoted cigarettes as a healthy activity and even a useful mechanism with which to open our lungs. Today this "good health" advice seems ridiculous. Yet, we will probably look back years from now and say the same thing about our doctors promoting animal based foods!

Unfortunately, most doctors do not know the relationship between diet and health. This is not our doctors' fault. The problem stems from education. There is very little focus on preventative care throughout medical school and training- putting patient care constantly on the defense. It is time we play offense with disease.

Our current approach of pills, procedures, surgery, and technology pays the companies but it is costing us our health. The following doctors speak out on this disease-centered paradigm and shockingly, how doctors are only given a brief overview of nutrition in medical school. From recent medical school graduates to renowned physicians, not much has changed in terms of education over the last 40 years. Optimistically, these doctors acknowledge our medical education system needs to change. The answers to our leading health woes are not at the bottom of a pill bottle, but on the end of our fork.

The Health Care Paradigm Shift

James F. Loomis Jr., MD

always thought I led a pretty healthy lifestyle. My diet consisted mainly of whole grains, low-fat dairy products, lean meat, and plenty of fruits and vegetables, just like I had been taught. I allowed myself the occasional cheeseburger and fries (on a whole grain bun!) or bowl of ice cream, but only in "moderation." In the summer 2011, I had my yearly physical and much to my astonishment (and disappointment), my LDL (bad) cholesterol and triglycerides were high, my HDL (good) cholesterol was low, and I had borderline elevations in my blood sugar and blood pressure. I had metabolic syndrome.

Metabolic syndrome is a combination of medical conditions noted by 3 of the 5 following conditions: 1) a waist circumference greater than 40 inches in men or 35 inches in women 2) triglycerides above 150 mg/dl, 3) HDL (good) cholesterol below 40 mg/dl in men or 50 mg/dl in women 4) blood pressure equal to or greater than 130/85 or already on medication for high blood pressure 5) a fasting blood sugar greater than or equal to 100 mg/dl).

The presence of metabolic syndrome markedly increases one's risk for heart disease and type 2 diabetes and now affects more that 25% of the population in the US.[1]

My primary care doctor spoke about starting me on a statin, which I routinely use to treat my own patients. Statins work by reducing production of cholesterol in the liver, but come with several side effects, including inflammation of the liver and muscles. I was reluctant to take the medication, because I realized that it really didn't address the underlying lifestyle causes of my problems.

A short time later, I stumbled across the documentary *"Forks Over Knives."* After reviewing some of the medical research, I realized it would be unconscionable for me not to try a whole-food, plant-based diet for three months and then answer three questions: 1) How hard was it to shop, prepare meals, and eat out? 2) How did it affect my energy level and mood? 3) At the end of 3 months, how did it affect my numbers (weight, blood sugar, blood pressure, and cholesterol)?

At the end of 3 months, the results were nothing short of miraculous. I found that shopping for and preparing healthy, complete, flavorful meals was not nearly as difficult as I had anticipated. Many restaurants were more than willing to prepare a plant-based meal with advance notice. More amazing were the mental and physical changes that occurred. My mood and energy markedly improved. Despite only a minimal change in physical activity, I lost 25lbs, my cholesterol dropped from 240 to 150, and my blood sugars and blood pressure were now in the normal range. Since then, I have lost almost 60 lbs total, and have completed five half-marathons and several triathlons, including a half-Ironman.

The Problem with a Disease-Centered Approach to Medicine

These changes have led me to completely rethink my views on what it means to be healthy. I have come to realize how our current health-care system is part of the problem and is contributing to the epidemic of obesity, type 2 diabetes, and other chronic diseases we are seeing in today's society. Almost all of the chronic diseases I was trained to treat are directly or indirectly, related to living a lifestyle in dissonance with the one we are designed to lead. Yet we define the optimal treatment of diseases as reaching a certain number with prescription medication(s), and then we are satisfied that we have done a good job. In reality, we are far from optimal treatment, as this approach is just putting a band-aid on the symptoms rather than addressing the true cause of the problem.

Our Food Disconnect

We have also adapted a reductionist approach to nutrition. Over the last 200 years or so, advances in science have allowed us to take food apart and discover what it is made of— nutrients like vitamins, minerals, fatty acids, carbohydrates, and protein. This reductionist approach allows us to think we can take food apart and put all the good stuff in a pill, and somehow that is better than food itself. We can re-engineer food and manipulate the fat, salt, or sugar content of food to sell more products. This has led to a huge industry of vitamins and supplements meant to replace the vitamins and nutrients that were stripped from the whole foods in the first place. It shows a lot of hubris to think that taking fiber and antioxidants pills is somehow healthier than eating a sweet potato. The whole message of "healthy eating" has been subverted by the food industry and its often times cozy relationship with the government agencies designed to oversee them. It is no wonder people are confused about what to eat!

Transformation

Since the profound transformation that I have personally experienced over the last 2 years, it is very clear to me that the food we eat, combined with regular physical activity, is the most powerful medicine we have. I have shared this message with my patients and those who have embraced it have had the same astounding results. Oftentimes they have been able to stop the medications they were taking. Even with their success, there is often resistance from their other physicians, who treat their cholesterol or diabetes, about the wisdom of stopping medications. This paradigm of treatment, as opposed to a paradigm of true prevention, is ingrained in most medical professionals.

However, following a lifestyle that is concordant with the one we are supposed to lead can have profound effects on our individual health, the health of our society, as well as the health of our planet. The growing awareness of the benefits as voiced through some of its champions such as the noted Caldwell Esselstyn, M.D. and T. Colin Campbell, Ph.D, as well as through like-minded health care professionals (such as myself), can play an extremely important and transformative role in helping individuals overcome industry and government obstacles and reap the truly amazing health benefits of achieving true "wellness."

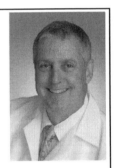

James F. Loomis Jr., MD, *graduated from the University of Arkansas Medical School, and completed his residency in internal medicine at Barnes Hospital in St. Louis, Missouri. He is Board Certified in internal medicine and is on the clinical faculty of the Department of Internal Medicine at Washington University School of Medicine. Loomis has also completed the certification program in Plant-Based Nutrition from Cornell University. In addition, Dr. Loomis received a MBA from the Olin School of Business at Washington University in St. Louis. Dr. Loomis served as the team internist for the St. Louis Rams football team and the St. Louis Cardinals baseball team. He is currently Director of Prevention and Wellness at St. Luke's Hospital in Chesterfield, Missouri and serves as Corporate Medical Director for InfoTech, Inc. He has completed numerous half-marathons and triathlons, including a half-Ironman. Loomis lives with his partner, Elise, and has three sons—Jimmy, William, and Bobby.*

There is a Lack of Nutritional Education

Mark McCabe, MD

It probably wasn't until the end of the 20ᵗʰcentury that medical education began incorporating nutrition into its curriculum. Even then, the subject of nutrition was often given scant attention—usually eclipsed by the "more important" hard sciences. At some point in the history of modern medicine there was a profound shift away from prevention and towards the development of more sophisticated technologies of diagnosis and cure. This shift mirrored our country's military and industrial might after WWII. Through science and technology and the sheer intellectual willpower of man, it was assumed that disease could be eradicated in the same way an enemy could be vanquished on the battlefield. Human illness became viewed as the stage on which man could flaunt his biomedical greatness against the scourges of both acute and chronic disease. To some extent, modern medicine was right. Many of the life-threatening illness that had ravaged the world, especially infectious diseases, really seemed within our control. There was even talk in the mid-twentieth century of the eradication of *all* disease.

In our zeal to conquer, we lost sight of the true meaning of the age-old adage that an ounce of prevention is worth a pound of cure. Nutrition and the role of diet in health is a perfect example. Most of the modern chronic diseases that afflict millions such as diabetes, heart disease, certain cancers, etc arise out of a lack of mindfulness about our food choices. Today, many people thoughtlessly consume processed foods, dairy products and animal proteins that are by-products of the corporate food industry. Synthetic hormones, pesticides, toxic fillers, and antibiotics are awash in our meat and dairy supplies, applied with the goal of maximizing yield, not the health of the consumer. The refined foods we live on have been stripped of their fiber and nutrients and are manufactured with salt, sugar, and fat to enhance taste and increase the addictive quality of these foods. The unfortunate consequence of this however, is a new list of diseases that is ravaging our population and bankrupting our economy.

This gets back to why nutrition has been so neglected in medical education. Medical educators realize that prevention is not a widely used practice, so nutrition in general gets pushed aside as insignificant, or not the doctor's role. The problem with this approach is that it sends a message that diet and health are areas of specialty concern, and somehow not integral to the doctor-patient relationship. Nothing could be further from the truth. The role of primary care includes primary prevention in addition to diagnosis and treatment of both acute and chronic problems.

In my practice as a primary care internist, I see so many illnesses that are clearly the result of people not taking a critical or questioning view of their relationship to the food they eat. For example, the dairy industry has touted its products as "good for the bones." While this has been a very successful advertising campaign going back at least 100 years, it is entirely false. Countries with the highest dairy consumption, such as the United States, Sweden, and England, also have the highest rates of bone disease.

The consequences of a century of misinformation are profound and affect the health of millions. Even the medical problems that are not so life threatening —such as irritable bowel syndrome and persistent dyspepsia, erectile dysfunction, skin problems, bone and joint health, diverticular disease, migraine headaches, cognitive clarity, and one's general sense of wellbeing—all have some root in the choices we make about what and how we eat.

I believe the tide is shifting as more and more people have access to industry-free information thanks to the internet and projects like *Rethink Food, Forks Over Knives,* and the work of individuals such as Drs. T. Colin Campbell, Caldwell Esselstyn, Dean Ornish, Neal Barnard, and others.

I recommend that people start thinking about a "plant-based diet, with the core foods they consume being vegetables, fruits, legumes, and whole grains. I tell my patients that the extent to which they can approximate a vegan diet is the extent to which they will be able to reverse their chronic disease or decrease their reliance on medications. The simple lifestyle choices they make start having important payoff in their lives. Weight comes down, sleep improves, vitality increases, and mood even begins to shift.

As physicians, we can use all the science and pharmacologic therapy we want to try to cure diabetes and reverse heart disease, obesity and arthritis. But until doctors and patients understand the connection between the food they eat and the diseases they develop, we as physicians (especially in the primary care setting) are never going to make significant headway in improving the quality of life and overall wellness of our patients. Change has to start with knowledge, and in this case self-knowledge is the beginning of taking control of one's health through awareness of what one eats.

Mark McCabe, MD, *received his medical degree from the Pritzker School of Medicine at the University of Chicago. He is board certified in Internal Medicine and completed his internship and residency at the University of Washington. He earned his BA degree in philosophy from Yale, and studied pre-med and molecular, chemical, and developmental biology at the University of Colorado.. He is a member of the Physician's Committee for Responsible Medicine, and American College of Physicians. Before attending medical school, he worked as a professional firefighter for 7 years.*

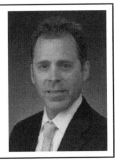

Pioneering the Science of Food as Medicine

Joel Kahn, MD

During the 1980s when I completed medical school and cardiology fellowship there was no discussion about nutrition and health in the halls of academic medical centers. In 1987 a friend, handed me a copy of *A Diet for a New America* by John Robbins and the case presented for the health, environmental and ethical reasons to select a vegetarian lifestyle made a powerful impact on me and pushed me more and more to completely plant- based. In 1990, the year I began the practice of cardiology, Dr. Dean Ornish and colleagues published the Lifestyle Heart Study demonstrating reversal of advanced heart atherosclerosis in heart patients with terrible blockages using a vegan and low fat diet. No one had ever lectured me about reversing heart disease by lifestyle during my 7 year span of training to be a heart specialist and I was hooked. From that point on it was vegan for me and a recommendation to read Dr. Ornish's book for all my patients. This expanded to the work of Dr. Colin Campbell, Dr. Caldwell Esselstyn, Dr. Neal Barnard, Dr. David Jenkins, Dr. Brian Clements, and other pioneers in the science of food is medicine.

* Please read Dr. Kahn's Pills vs Plants? in the For Men Only chapter

A Physician's Duty: Understanding Nutrition in the Aetiology of Disease

Aryan Tavakkoli MB BS, MRCP (UK)

Here's a word of warning: Doctors in general possess very little knowledge about nutrition. In fact, the knowledge we do have can sometimes cause more harm than good. From time to time I hear of someone who is advised by her doctor that little Johnny is low in iron and therefore needs to eat more meat. Mom dutifully makes sure that he eats more pork chops and sausages, because the doctor said it is good for him. Women with iron deficiency can also be at the receiving end of this advice, despite the fact that any benefit from obtaining iron through eating meat would be offset by the numerous detrimental effects of consuming animal protein. I shudder at the thought of the harm we can cause our patients through our own ignorance.

I certainly don't recall learning about the importance of nutrition in the aetiology (cause) or prevention of disease. Nutrition wasn't exactly considered a 'hardcore' medical topic in my medical school, compared to the cutting edge areas of genetics and molecular biology, which is reflective of why many doctors know very little about nutrition let alone healthy nutrition. The problem is our patients think we do.

Diet and Risk Factors for Disease

According to the World Health Organisation (WHO),[1] diet is second only to tobacco as a potentially preventable cause of cancer, accounting for up to 30% of cancers in industrialized countries. *Thirty percent!* The cancer most commonly associated with meat consumption is colorectal cancer, but breast cancer, prostate cancer, and other cancers have also been found to be linked to dietary factors.[2-5] Furthermore, in their 2004 paper on "Global Strategy on Diet, Physical Activity and Health"[6], WHO states that "Overall, 2.7 million deaths (per year) are attributable to low fruit and vegetable intake."

When observing the clinical management of patients with conditions such as stroke, cancer, and heart disease, rarely do I see the patient's diet being addressed. The management almost always focuses on pharmaceutical intervention. In overlooking the vital role that diet plays in the aetiology of disease, we overlook a valuable tool in aiding our patients' recovery.

It is important to note that food does not only have the capacity to act as a disease *causing* agent, but can also be a valuable mode of therapy to treat or prevent disease by acting as a disease-modifying agent, providing anti-inflammatory effects, cancer protective effects, or other beneficial actions that reduce the risk of developing a disease, or even reverse a disease process. For example, there is clear evidence that consuming a plant-based diet confers multiple health benefits to individuals, including a lower risk of developing diseases commonly diagnosed in industrialized countries, such as cancer, cardiovascular, disease and diabetes.[7-9]

Physician, Know Thyself

Once physicians understand the essential role of healthy nutrition in the prevention and treatment of disease, we will have tapped into a powerful means of guiding our patients towards better health. It is our responsibility as physicians to accept the deficiencies in our knowledge in any area, including nutrition, and it is up to us to educate ourselves where our medical training has failed to educate us. We would serve our patients well by utilizing in our clinical practice, the knowledge that food can be implicated in the aetiology of disease, and the fact that it can be used to complement current medical therapies in the prevention and treatment of disease.

The pioneering work of organizations such as the Physicians' Committee for Responsible Medicine, and other health professionals successfully incorporating a plant-based diet into the management plan of patients, will surely lead the way to a new and better understanding in the prevention and management of disease. May we all be well nourished, healthy and happy!

Aryan Tavakkoli MB BS, MRCP (UK), FRACP, MBAcC, Dip. Phyt., S.A.C. Dip. Vegetarian and Vegan Nutrition (Distinction) *is a specialist in respiratory medicine in the UK. Dr. Tavakkoli has written and spoken widely on the topic of diet and its effect on both personal and planetary health. She has lectured in New Zealand and Australia, given interviews for numerous local and national radio shows and newspapers, and been a guest speaker at national rallies. Her talks and publications on these topics, as well as other important information regarding the vegan lifestyle, may be viewed on her website Vegsense.net and on her YouTube channel: aryan tavakkoli*

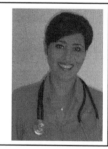

What Are Our Future Doctors Learning?

Gregory Goodman, MD and Jeremy Krell, D.M.D.

In an age of connectivity, we are surprisingly disconnected. It is essential that we revisit the primitive building blocks of prevention and the foundation of general health and wellness— our diet.

Dr. Goodman: As a recent 2013 medical school graduate, I was surprised that in my 4 years of training, I received little education on wellness and prevention. After 2 years of pre-clinical training ended, I quickly picked up on key patterns being taught: memorize the facts, diagnose the disease, and use evidence-based treatment methodologies.

Surprising but true, most physicians receive less than 15 hours of nutrition instruction in medical school. For example, the medical nutrition course objectives taught are: diet patterns and nutrition intake, nutrition counseling for patients with chronic disease, clinical risk associated with nutrient deficiency or excess, the basic science of nutrition as it relates to clinical disorders, and role of non-physicians in nutrition care. While on the surface this seems to be a perfectly great way to teach nutrition to medical students and to understand nutrition as it relates to disease, in my estimation, we are missing the big picture and one of the largest opportunities in health care.

It is an intriguing time to be entering the health care sector, as there is an inherent need to bring prevention, nutrition, and general wellness to the forefront. What if we taught physicians how to keep patients healthy and used nutrition and wellness programs to prevent diseases instead of additional units of care?

When I started my rotations in the clinical setting, there wasn't talk of how to prevent disease or the role of diet when interacting with a patient. Instead, as students we are taught a disease-management approach to medicine. A typical clinical example is a patient recently diagnosed with diabetes. The doctor uses evidence-based medicine to place the patient on standard medical therapy which is prescriptions to lower blood sugar, and tells the patient to eliminate sugar. According to the doctor, he has done his best as he was trained to diagnosis and treat. It is now the patient's job to "manage" his diabetes by keeping his sugars under control. Although this looks like a sufficient outcome by helping the patient control their diabetes, large epidemiological intervention studies indicate we can do much better by, in many cases, reversing the patient's diabetes on a plant-based diet. Yet the patient leaves without this knowledge because as physicians we are taught about disease management, not prevention.

Having adopted and greatly benefited from a plant-based diet for over 7 years, I hope to inspire other young physicians to be leaders and innovators in offering plant nutrition as treatment for their patients. With the rising costs of healthcare, we should be looking at integrating new ways to achieve excellent outcomes in a cost-effective manner. This requires a system that is open and ready for change, one that trains medical students about nutrition as it relates to prevention and wellness.

Dr. Krell: As a vegan for 3 years now, I made the switch due to gastrointestinal health, familial hypercholesterolemia, and dairy and egg allergies. Since changing my diet, I have been without pain, and my immune system is more apt to protect me.

Similar to the education medical students receive, there is limited focus on how plant-based diets can improve oral health. The nutrition instruction future dentists learn primarily focuses on limiting sugary (namely, sucrose containing) and acidic food and drinks as these are considered the most detrimental to oral health. Teeth will suffer the effects of decalcification in highly acidic environments so frequent dietary and hygiene measures must be taken to avoid long-term injury.

However, the microbiology, nutrition, and oral health courses focusing on nutrition and oral health, dietary standards and guidelines, and protein and vegetarianism, to name a few, indicate a positive step in the right direction. On a national scale, the USDA's decision to replace "Meat" with "Protein" on their MyPlate dietary guidelines also indicates an encouraging move by recognizing and incorporating plant-based protein sources. Hopefully the future of medicine and dentistry will focus more prominently on prevention in sickness and instill the core principles of dietary choices in health care students to apply within their clinical practices.

Whether physicians or patients, we must exercise our voices to ensure that the health care revolution begins with wellness, nutrition, and prevention.

Gregory Goodman, MD *received his B.S. from Brandeis University and recently graduated from Tufts University Medical School in 2013. Dr. Goodman served as the Chief Development Officer of a medical clinic in partnership with iFundAfrica that has since treated 8,000 patients at their Zemero clinic in Ethiopia. Dr. Goodman is specializing in internal medicine with a focus on improving quality patient care and prevention.*

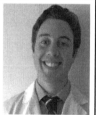

Jeremy N. Krell, D.M.D. *received his B.S. degree from Brandeis University, and was awarded the Dr. Ralph Berenberg '65 prize for excellence in leadership within the dental community. Dr. Krell graduated from Tufts University School of Dental Medicine in 2013. As an entrepreneur across a wide variety of different industries, he is tailoring his career to health enterprise management and innovation.*

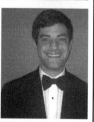

The Science Is On Our Side

Peggy Carlson, MD

In the late 1960s and early 1970s, the most common question that nutrition studies set out to answer was whether or not vegetarian diets were nutritionally adequate. Research proved the answer is a resounding "*yes.*" So science moved on to the next step.

Thousands of studies, becoming progressively more rigorous in their scientific design over time,[1] conclude that vegetarian diets have positive health benefits for a number of chronic diseases. Many factors have been proposed as possible explanations for the positive health effects of a vegetarian diet. These include increased intake of fiber, antioxidants, phytochemicals, unsaturated fats, potassium, and fruits and vegetables. The positive effects may also be attributed to a lower incidence of obesity among vegetarians, as well as lower intakes of saturated fat, cholesterol, meat, animal protein, and heme iron from animals. It is most likely a combination of factors, some perhaps not yet even discovered that work in concert to produce a symphony of health benefits.[2]

As a physician, it is my hope that all health care providers and others learn to benefit from the power of a vegetarian plate and choose to make vegetarian meals their dining preference. A transition from meat-based to vegetarian eating, on both individual and societal levels, will take time and effort, especially given such imbedded impediments as a culture of meat-eating, fear of change, easy availability of meat-based fast-foods, the powerful meat and dairy industries, and lack of public knowledge about the benefits of eating vegetarian. A vegetarian diet is a tasty and powerful tool in both preventing and treating disease and I hope many of you will choose to embark on this journey toward better health.

Peggy Carlson, MD *is board-certified in emergency medicine and has practiced medicine for nearly 30 years. She has been vegetarian for about 45 years and vegan for nearly 25 of those years. She authored a section in* The Clinical Practice of Emergency Medicine, *and edited and wrote several chapters in* The Complete Vegetarian; The Essential Guide To Good Health.

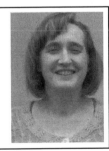

A Whole Food, Plant-Based Diet:
The Next Blockbuster Drug of the Year

Dana S. Simpler, MD

Today the research is clear and overwhelming: from large epidemiologic studies such as the EPIC study in Europe and Dr. T. Colin Campbell's *The China Study* to the numerous microscopy studies showing profound changes in cancer cells – animal products promotes disease and plant products can reduce or eliminate these diseases. I've always loved simple cures, and the simplicity of healing disease with whole, plant- based foods is fantastic. It fills me with incredible joy when I'm able to say "You don't have diabetes anymore" or "We can cancel that carotid artery surgery." With all this amazing data and my own patient success stories, it is baffling to me that there are so few doctors promoting plant-based cures.

Since doctors receive practically no nutritional education during or after medical school it is understandable that there is a level of ignorance among doctors. While treating patients with pills and procedures is very lucrative whereas discussing diet is time consuming and is not reimbursable, shouldn't doctors have an obligation to learn about ALL the ways to cure illness and not just the ones that make money for drug companies and hospitals? I believe we do.

The China Study, by T. Colin Campbell, PhD, was my introduction to the health benefits of a plant-based diet. That book changed the way I practice medicine, and launched me on journey to re-educate myself on medical nutrition. I've discovered an enormous wealth of scientific information from conferences such as the American Institute for Cancer Research for PhD nutritionists, Dr. Michael Greger's, www.nutritionfacts.org, Dr. Joel Fuhrman's website, www.drfuhrman.com, and Dr. John McDougall's website, www.Drmcdougall.com that unequivocally supports a whole food, plant- based diet as exceptionally healthy. Despite the obstacles within the medical community, I have met numerous other plant- based physicians and I look forward to raising awareness among physicians about the powerful dietary recommendations they can offer to heal their patients. In fact, if the health benefits of a plant- based diet could be put in a pill – it would become the blockbuster drug of the decade!

Dana S. Simpler, MD *is board certified in Internal Medicine and has been in private practice since 1987 in Baltimore, MD. Dr. Simpler received her medical degree from the University of Maryland Medical School. She is the director of Carefirst Medical Home and Medicare Medical Home. She is an active member of the Physician's Committee for Responsible Medicine (PCRM) and has been featured on local TV stations including the program "The Woman's Doctor" on WBAL TV.*

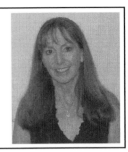

three

A WALK THROUGH THE BODY

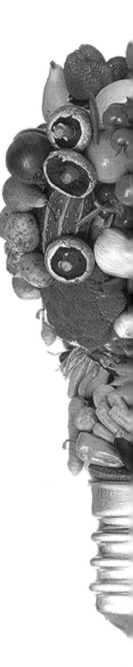

Imagine putting a drop of poison into a glass of clean water. The poison completely pollutes the water- changing each sip from refreshing to lethal. Knowing its potential for harm, we wouldn't consciously drink the toxic water.

Every bite of meat and dairy is akin to a drop of poison that our bloodstream carries throughout our bodies - affecting each and every system from our respiratory, immune and endocrine to our musculoskeletal. Meat and dairy create oxidative stress and produce free radicals that can wreak havoc on every part of our body. The following chapter walks us through this process- showing the full range of damages from animal based foods and conversely the complete and restorative benefits of plant foods.

Although we tend to treat each body system as separate, it is a completely interconnected and intricate machine. Every food choice we make has a profound effect on our internal environment- cleansing it with essential antioxidant promoting nutrients or destroying it with poisonous toxins that lead to disease. It is amazing how easy dietary changes can address the entire spectrum of health and wellness.

See a Healthier You

Lee Duffner, MD

"Eat your carrots; they are good for your eyes!" This advice was common in the United States growing up because American missionaries in developing countries had noted improvement in the vision of malnourished children when carrots—(a vegetable that can be grown almost anywhere outside of the polar areas)-- were added to the diets of children with impaired vision.

Carrots are rich in Vitamin A, a deficiency of which can lead to ulceration, dryness, and even perforation of the cornea of the eye and cause night blindness.

Over 50 years ago, Dr. Frederick Stocker studied a diet of rice, sugar, fruit, and fruit juices and found that such a diet would lower both blood pressure and the pressure of the aqueous fluid inside of the eye. Elevated aqueous fluid pressure is associated with glaucoma, an eye disease that can slowly cause permanent loss of vision.

Currently, the Age-Related Eye Disease Study, a very large evaluation of elderly patients which began years ago at Harvard University and is still ongoing, shows that large amounts of antioxidant vitamins (including those that are in most vegan diets) when combined with supplemental zinc in pill form, deters the development of macular degeneration-- a blinding condition-- in many of the elderly.

In fact, when polled, several nationally known authorities observing the effects of these diets on the visual system, as well as the body as a whole, find no adverse effects but only benefits on the visual system.

Lee Duffner, MD *is a graduate of Marquette University School of Medicine (now known as the Medical School of Wisconsin). He completed his internship at Stanford University and residency in ophthalmology at the Boscom Palmer Eye Institute of the University of Miami School of Medicine where he currently is a Voluntary Professor of Ophthalmology. Dr. Duffner is also a clinical correspondent for the American Academy of Ophthalmology*

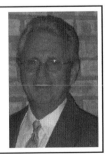

A Plant-Based Diet and Periodontal Disease

Sahara Adams LeSage, DDS, FDSD, PhD

Sugar is not the only food that affects our teeth and gums. The onset and subsequent healing of periodontal disease is influenced by the inflammatory nature of our food choices. Whereas saturated fats and cholesterol found in animal-based products promote inflammation, findings indicate that increased consumption of antioxidants from fruits and vegetables help ameliorate periodontal disease[1] as they remove these inflammatory triggers.

Periodontal disease is an inflammatory disease that takes many forms, from the common chronic periodontitis to the rare acute necrotizing ulcerative gingivitis. The best course of action is to eliminate inflammatory triggers is by eating organic foods, rich in polyunsaturated fats, antioxidant micronutrients like fruits, vegetables, and nuts which calm the microenvironments by removing free radical oxygen.

Saturated fats, found in most animal-based foods, can cause inflammation and susceptibility to disease whereas polyunsaturated fats can decrease inflammation. These free radicals lead to imbalanced redox reactions which set off a cascade of biochemical effects resulting in oxidative stress and immuno-suppression. A biochemical study showed that healthier periodontal tissue is associated with decreased oxidative stress within cells. Oxidative stress is the pressure that is put inside the cell versus the pressure outside the cell. In biochemical terms, it is the imbalance between oxidants and antioxidants. This imbalance leads to a reduction in re-dox signaling, reduced molecular control, and finally damage within the tissues cells and tissue such as gum tissue or cardiac tissue. Nutritional antioxidants in the diet scavenge reactive oxygen species and remove the inflammatory reactions. A study of malnourished populations and Vitamin C intake shows a direct correlation between these factors and periodontal disease.[2]

Removing circulating cholesterol decreases inflammation, plaque formation and hardening inside the arteries. A well known study showed how polysaturated fats in oat bran can remove circulating cholesterol by binding irreversibly to the bile acids during digestion and passing the bile acids in our waste. Oat bran stopped the bile acids from being reabsorbed and stored in the gall bladder. Once the body realizes that the bile acids are not being reabsorbed, it pulls the cholesterol out of the circulating blood to make new bile acids, and thereby decreases the circulating cholesterol in the blood. The total cholesterol is absorbed from the yellow part of the egg and 1 yolk is 300 milligrams, which is more than the human body needs in 1 day. When we eat even 1 egg yolk, we are lining our arterial walls with cholesterol and hardening their arteries. Cholesterol bound to oat bran is a perfect example of how eating the proper polyunsaturated foods can lead to healing inside the body tissues for periodontal disease.

Saturated fat and excess cholesterol are associated with obesity, an important component of periodontal disease risk assessment. Obesity influences the production of pro-inflammatory cytokines in the adipose (fat) tissue. This destructive inflammation increases pocket depth, or how much bone is lost around the tooth and how loose the tooth feels. As plant-based diets are low-fat, the weight loss that normally results from adoption of a vegan diet would tend to ameliorate and in some cases appear to actually heal gingival tissue by removing inflammatory foods and the triggers that lead to immune-suppression and disease. Those with diabetes mellitus are also more susceptible to periodontal disease.

There is a growing body of research on the positive effects of dietary changes on periodontal disease. For example, a Swiss study of adults in a Stone Age environment, one in which diet was restricted to simple sugars and foods rich in antioxidants, and in which oral hygiene was poor, resulted in decreased gingival bleeding and decreased probing. Even though the hygiene was poor, (i.e. the subjects were not allowed to use toothbrushes or fluoride or pastes to imitate the Stone Age conditions) the gums healed.[3] This startling finding is attributable to the diet's lack of complex refined carbohydrates and saturated fats. The absence of these pro-inflammatory foods, along with the presence of foods rich in polyunsaturated fats and antioxidant micronutrients, allows the body to heal itself.

Avoiding periodontal disease is imperative as inflammation in our gums can significantly affect other organs. When the bacterium that has multiplied in the mouth circulates through the blood to the heart, kidneys, and retina it can lead to health problems like bacterial endocarditis, kidney failure, and eye diseases. The smallest of the blood vessels in the body can become clogged with bacteria and over a few short months even contribute to organ failure. Biochemically removing inflammatory triggers from the body decreases the immune suppression that leads to disease periodontal disease, improving overall health on a cellular level.

Sahara Adams LeSage, B.S., D.D.S., F.D.S.D, PhD., *received her dental degree from the University of Texas and a PhD in biochemistry from Texas A&M University. Dr. Adams has presented at numerous conferences across the country and is the co-author and contributor to a number of scientific articles and films.*

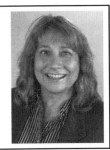

The Effects of Dairy and Meat Consumption on the Ear, Nose, and Throat

Ashmit Gupta, MD, MPH

Do you suffer from constant sinuses? How many times have you been forced to live on medications with only temporary relief? Ear, nose and throat congestion and inflammation are some of the most uncomfortable and frequent health problems in our society affecting nearly 30 million people per year in the United States and costing an estimated annual health care cost of $5.8 billion.[1]Inflammation of the ear, which includes outer and middle ear infections, is among the most prevalent medical condition for children and adults. Nearly 80% of children suffer from ear infections before they turn 3.

While the causes of these conditions are multi-factorial, most people do not realize that dietary considerations are paramount in the susceptibility and development. Scientific and anecdotal evidence has found that the intake of animal products such as dairy and meat can contribute to the development of ear, nose, and throat problems.

Sneezing on the Truth

Milk allergies are frequently associated with chronic sinus problems (rhinitis and sinusitis) which include stuffy noses, nasal congestion, sneezing, post-nasal drip and itching from inflammation or infection of the mucosa of the nasal passages.. A study in the American Journal of Rhinology and Allergy found that 14% of chronic nasal polyposis patients tested positive for cow's milk allergy compared to zero of the tested healthy subjects.[2] There are 2 main proteins in cow's milk that can cause an allergic reaction: casein and whey. Casein is the solid part (curd) of milk while whey is in the liquid part of milk. These proteins are found in milk and many processed foods.

Sinusitis, which is the blockage of nasal drainage pathways, is also affected by the milk allergen casein. Casein in milk has also been shown to be associated with the increase in mucus thickness which can therefore lead to blockages of the sinus openings and eventually to an increase in sinus infection and sinus pressure symptoms.[3] Blockages of the sinus openings and interruptions of this clearance can lead to sinus infections.[4]

Within the scientific and medical community, there is a controversy on this subject between those who believe in the association between milk consumption and thickened mucus and those who do not. As a practicing pediatric and adult otolaryngologist, I see the connection between dairy intake and thicker mucus on a daily basis. Adult patients who have suffered from recurrent and chronic sinusitis and have allergic and sinus symptoms have seen significant changes and improvement in these symptoms when dairy is removed from the diet. Children who have chronic congestion and rhinorrhea and are deemed to have chronic sinusitis or chronic adenoiditis can frequently have improvements in symptoms from the simple reduction of dairy consumption. The correlation between milk and mucus is one of the reasons it is recommended to minimize dairy intake such as ice cream after undergoing tonsillectomy and/ or adenoidectomy.

Generally a child suffering from an upper respiratory infection will also suffer from an ear infection as the membrane that exists in the nasal and sinus passages is inflamed throughout the system. Cow milk allergy is the most common food hypersensitivity in children and ear infections are one of the most common reasons for a child to be brought to the pediatrician. A study in Acta Otolaryngologica found a correlation between cow milk allergy and recurrent ear infections in childhood.[5] Because of the inflammation caused by cow milk allergy, there is additional blockage of drainage from the middle ear and recurrent ear infections occur. In the study, 54 milk allergic children and 204 control schoolchildren were tested and followed and the findings revealed that cow milk allergy in infancy even when properly treated led to significantly more recurrent infections.

Acid Reflux

Acid Reflux is another consequence of consuming dairy products that affects our ear, nose, and throat in pediatric and adult patients. Esophageal reflux disease results from a movement of gastric contents back into the esophagus. Specifically among children, reflex can contribute to a chronic cough. A study in Gut and Liver found a correlation between cow milk allergy and severe reflux disease in infancy.[6] In some cases, elimination of cow milk resulted in a complete resolution of symptoms.

To treat acid reflux, it is advised to remove all dietary irritants including caffeine, tobacco, alcohol, as well as foods such as milk that can cause inflammation of the digestive and upper digestive tract. Consumption of fried foods and high fat and processed meats should also be reduced as frequent consumption has been shown to be correlated to reflux disease but has also been shown to be correlated to laryngeal cancer. In a study in the American Journal of Epidemiology, fried and processed meats were positively correlated with laryngeal cancer with a 95% confidence interval.[7]

The correlation between the intake of animal products such as dairy and meats and certain ear, nose and throat conditions confirms what has been known for years in the lay and medical worlds that our diets as human beings has a significant impact on our health and disease state. Years of eating the wrong foods can contribute to illness but simple adjustments of these dietary practices can lead us down a new path to health and wellness.

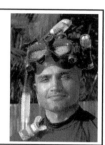

Ashmit Gupta, MD, MPH *is an Adjunct Associate Professor of Otolaryngology in the Department of Otolaryngology-Head and Neck Surgery in the University of Pennsylvania Health System. He is board -certified in otolaryngology. He has presented at numerous national conferences and has authored fifteen articles in the fields of rhinology and sinus disease, laryngology, facial plastics, and sleep medicine.*

Just Breathe: Improving Lung Function with a Plant-Based Diet

Martin M. Root, MS, Ph.D. & Ellen Lawrence

Lung function is not something people think much about. Breathing is something the body does automatically, so what could go wrong? You may not have guessed that pulmonary diseases are the third leading cause of death in the United States. The most common form of pulmonary disease is Chronic Obstructive Pulmonary Disease, or COPD. COPD is characterized by chronic bronchitis, emphysema, the production of large amounts of mucus, and decreased lung capacity. COPD is generally irreversible. Imagine trying to make dinner, do laundry, and run up and down the stairs while breathing through a straw. The disease gets progressively worse as time passes and can eventually lead to death from suffocation.

While lung function declines naturally with age, environmental and genetic factors accelerate the decline through producing oxidative stress. While a small loss in lung function may go unnoticed, gradually reduced lung function is also related to a reduction in quality of life. Even though it may seem obvious, it must be stated that smoking is the single strongest risk factor related to lung function decline and COPD. If you smoke, it is time to stop. However, smoking is not the only factor related to lung function decline. Environmental pollution at home and in the workplace, genetics, asthma, second hand smoke, and respiratory infections are all related to pulmonary disease. In the developing world, indoor pollution from cooking fires can be especially dangerous and lead to the development and progression of COPD. A recent study found that 2.1 million deaths per year worldwide from cardiopulmonary disease and lung cancer can be attributed to environmental pollution.[1] Do not underestimate your need for protection.

So what can you do? The most obvious answer is to not smoke and avoid environmental pollutions. How about what we eat? Can a healthy diet improve our ability to breathe? When comparing a traditional diet of red meat, processed meat, potatoes, boiled vegetables, and added fat to a more cosmopolitan diet with a higher intake of vegetables, wine, and rice, those who consumed a traditional diet had lower lung function as measured by forced expiratory volume in one second (FEV1). They also had a higher prevalence of COPD.[2] Another study found that among smokers, consumption of a traditional Japanese diet reduced the risk of COPD and breathlessness symptoms. One of the dietary factors isolated in the study was isoflavones, which are found in soy products.[3] Isoflavones act as antioxidants and anti-inflammatory agents.

When considering how a plant-based diet might improve health, one might first think about the cardiovascular system. The heart and blood vessels, after all, do pump and provide blood to your entire body. The blood contains nutrients that provide the cells with building blocks to stay healthy, electrolytes which help the cells communicate, and white blood cells which fight off infection. Simpler than this, the blood contains oxygen; it takes only a few minutes for cells in the body to die once deprived of oxygen. Since the pulmonary, or respiratory, system is responsible for removing carbon dioxide from the blood and replacing it with oxygen, keeping it healthy with the right diet is essential.

Breathing seems so simple, yet it is a complicated process to get oxygen from the air into our body and into our cells. Air flows down our mucus-covered windpipe into tubes that get progressively smaller until it arrives in the pulmonary alveoli. The pulmonary alveoli are small thin sacks covered in tiny blood vessels, called capillaries. The walls of the capillaries are so thin that oxygen can pass through into the blood and be exchanged for the outgoing carbon dioxide. Additionally, secretions from the cells along the airway have antimicrobial properties that serve as a key component of the immune system. The movement of air through the lungs allows for speech and coughing and sneezing that helps remove irritating particles of mucus.

A plant-based diet rich in antioxidants and anti-inflammatory foods reduces the loss of lung function that can come from age, environmental pollutants, genetics, and respiratory infections. Body processes are powered by oxidation reactions where the transfer of electrons provides the energy necessary to get work done. These necessary reactions in our cells that utilize the same oxygen we inhale create free radicals through the transfer of electrons as a by-product of their chemical work. These toxic and reactive free radicals can also be created through damage done to the cell by environmental toxins. While the term free radical sounds like a punk band from the 1980s, they are actually molecules that are missing an electron from their outer ring. This missing electron makes the molecule very unstable and allows it to float around the cell doing damage to proteins, lipids, and DNA. Damage to the DNA can cause cells to become mutated, while damage to proteins causes enzymes to work inefficiently as the protein itself begins to break down. This damage leads the body to mount an inflammatory response. While short-term inflammation protects the body in such common features as bruises and fevers, long-term inflammation causes damage to the cells and tissues of the body, including the blood vessels and the lungs. Free radical damage and chronic inflammation both cause tissue damage and increase the rate at which a disease such as COPD progresses. Antioxidants, specifically those found in fruits and vegetables protect the lungs by removing free radicals and preventing damage, thereby reducing the risk and progression of disease.

Over a 4 year time period, researchers found that individuals who consumed more vitamin C-rich foods-- mostly fruits and vegetables-- lost less FEV1 when compared to other individuals. The researchers also found that among individuals who quit smoking within the 4 year time period, consumption of these antioxidants reduced the loss of FEV1 over time. These antioxidants included vitamin E, beta-cryptoxanthin (gives orange juice its orange color), vitamin C, and all fruits and vegetables.[4] Another research study compared the intake of antioxidants vitamin C and vitamin E with lung function. It was found that hard fruits, specifically apples, reduced the rate at which FEV1 decreased over the 4 year time period. Interestingly enough, this association was unrelated to the vitamin C content of the apples and appeared instead to relate to the other antioxidants found in the apple.[5] Common antioxidants include vitamin C, vitamin E, and the pigments found in fruits and vegetables that allow them to be colorful, especially the yellow and orange colors of the carotenoids.

Exciting new research on flavonoids, non-nutrient antioxidants found in fruits and vegetables, and lung cancer continues to back up the benefits of a plant-based diet and lung function. Research has shown that the flavonoids are able to protect the cells of the lungs from developing mutations that lead to lung cancer. A 2008 study that matched recently diagnosed lung cancer individuals with other smokers without lung cancer of the same demographic and geographic location, found that those with the highest intake of epicatechin, catechin, quercetin, and kaempferol-- 4 flavonoid components-- were at the lowest risk of lung cancer among smokers.[6]

Which foods contain these healthful flavonoids? Epicatechin and catechin are closely related and can be found in tea, cocoa, seeds, and the skins of dark red fruit such as black grapes, apples, cherries, pears, and raspberries. Quercetin is also found in the skin of dark fruits like red grapes, blueberries, red apples, red cherries, and blackberries, while kaempferol can be found in tea, broccoli, grapefruit, cabbage, kale, beans, leaks, tomatoes, strawberries, and brussels sprouts. Apparently, even smokers who consume a plant-based diet are able to protect themselves somewhat.

A plant-based diet also provides anti-inflammatory agents including dietary fiber, fruits and vegetables, and nuts and seeds. A large study of 71,365 women and 40,215 men examined dietary fiber patterns and COPD, chronic bronchitis, and emphysema. The researchers concluded that the higher an individual's intake of fiber, the more that individual lowers their risk of COPD. This is especially true for women who showed a greater reduction in risk of COPD with fiber consumption, specifically cereal fiber. A diet high in whole grains as well as other cereal fiber reduced the risk of COPD. While increased intake of fiber also reduced COPD risk in men, the result was less significant.[7] Since a diet high in whole grains, fruits, vegetables, beans, and legumes provides the body with plenty of dietary fiber, a plant-based diet is beneficial in preventing lung function decline.

This connection between consumption of fiber and healthy lung function, backed by several other studies, is interesting in that the effects are indirect—no fiber ever touches the lungs.[8] The explanation for this effect may be again related to inflammation. Detailed research has shown that when diets high in fiber are consumed, a number of blood markers of inflammation decrease.

It is hard to recommend nutritional changes without addressing physical activity. Exercising has huge benefits for both the muscles that move the diaphragm up and down, and those that move carbon dioxide out of and oxygen into the muscles. The muscles of the rib cage and diaphragm can become weak with time, thus reducing the ability of the lungs to move air in and out of the lungs; aerobic activity forces air in and out of the lungs and causes the diaphragm to work. Physical activity not only strengthens the heart and other muscles of the body, but also tends to have an anti-inflammatory effect.

The combination of a smoke-free life, a plant-based diet, and plenty of exercise improves lung function and provides protection against lung related diseases.

Martin Root, MS, Ph.D, *worked as a research technician and research support specialist at Cornell University for 22 years after receiving his BS degree in Biochemistry. His earned his MS is in Environmental Toxicology and his Ph.D. is in Nutrition, both from Cornell. He worked for 16 years with T. Colin Campbell on an epidemiologic project in China that has since become known as the China Study. He spent 12 years with startup company, BioSignia, Inc., developing statistical models of chronic disease onset for the use by health professionals in communicating risk and preventive strategies. Since 2008 he has been teaching and doing research at Appalachian State University where he directs the Graduate Program in Nutrition. He currently lives in Boone, NC with his wife Constance of over forty years. They have three children and seven grandchildren.*

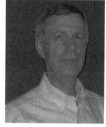

Ellen Lawrence *is a graduate student in the Graduate Program in Nutrition, Department of Nutrition and Health Care Management, College of Health Sciences, Appalachian State University received her BS in Social Work from Saint Louis University and her BS in Food Nutrition and Dietetics at Illinois State University. She is currently pursuing her MS in Nutrition. She is interested in Nutrition Education and Wellness and looks forward to starting her career in dietetics.*

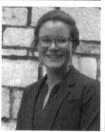

The Impact of Nutrition on Our Hormones

Alireza Falahati-Nini, MD, FCAE

It is important to view our body as whole when considering solutions and treatment for disease. Let's take the endocrine system as an example to examine how diet affects the functioning of an entire system.

The endocrine system is a network of glands that produce hormones that serve as messengers between various organ systems within the body. The communications between different sections of our brain and between our brain and our entire body takes place on a constant basis, thanks to our endocrine system. Our endocrine system also regulates important functions such as human reproduction and the metabolism of glucose (sugar) and other nutrients. A disruption of any part of our endocrine system can lead to a "domino effect," causing a disruption and failure of multiple systems spontaneously. For example, long term exposure to toxins such as excess animal fat and animal protein can affect our immune system and impede our endocrine system, thus leading to common chronic conditions such as cardiovascular disease, cancer, diabetes, osteoporosis, and hyperlipidemia.

The health of our endocrine system depends on the intake of healthy nutrients and absence of various toxins in our diet over an extended period of time. A diet high in saturated fat, cholesterol, and animal protein adds unnecessary amounts of nutrients that our body does not need, such as cholesterol and fat. It also limits "clean" plant-based nutrients that are rich in antioxidants, micronutrients, and desperately needed for proper functioning of our body. **Every meal should be**

Gain Better Control of your Insulin on a Plant-Based Diet

We know that insulin resistance syndrome is one of the main underlying causes of some of the common medical conditions such as premature coronary heart disease, Polycystic Ovary Syndrome, hypogonadism and potentially infertility.

The amount of evidence showing the correlation between a vegan diet and prevention of insulin resistance is overwhelming.[8] A plant-based diet has higher fiber content, higher antioxidant content as well as potentially higher Phytoestrogen content that help control insulin levels. By comparison, a diet containing animal products has higher salt, cholesterol, and fat content, leading to higher insulin levels and resistance. For example, in a study of 203 overweight adolescents the group with a higher intake of skim milk, whey protein and casein (found in dairy products) was found to gain more weight and have higher insulin levels.

considered as an opportunity to take a step towards better health, and this is definitely not possible with a diet rich in animal fat and protein and low in dietary fiber.
A plant-based diet-- defined as a regimen that encourages whole, plant-based foods and
discourages meats, dairy products, and eggs as well as refined and processed foods-- has
been shown to have a very positive impact on various aspects of the endocrine system.
This is in addition to the significantly positive impact it has on cardiovascular health
and on the long-term health of different organ systems.

Diet's Role in Endocrine System Diseases

There is large body of evidence supporting the intuitive philosophy towards diet and
nutrition. Let's review the benefits of a whole food plant-based diet on the endocrine
system by exploring type 2 diabetes, prostate health, osteoporosis, and mood changes.

Type II Diabetes Mellitus (Type 2 DM) is a complex metabolic condition that is usually
associated with additional cardiovascular conditions such as obesity, hypertension, and
hyperlipidemia. Medical literature refers to type 2 DM as "a lifestyle disease". A study of 60,903 patients[2] showed that patients on a plant-based diet were already at a significantly lower risk of developing type 2 diabetes when compared to an omnivore control group. Out of every type of dietary group, vegans, on average, have lower BMIs; this helps to protect them against obesity, which in turn protects against type 2 diabetes. [7]

It is established that changes in diet and exercise habits have a very positive impact on prevention and treatment of type 2 diabetes. Multiple large and small studies have clearly indicated that plant- based nutrition has a superior impact on reduction in Hemoglobin A1c (HbA1c), a marker of the average blood sugar levels over the past few months, blood pressure, and LDL (bad) cholesterol. In one international study,[1] 291 overweight patients (BMI above 25) with type 2 diabetes were randomized to either follow a low-fat vegan diet-- with weekly group support and work cafeteria options available-- or

Life-Long Health Starts in Young Children

The pre-pubertal health status of children is critical in terms of impact on future health. There is a strong body of evidence that obese children are much more likely to struggle with their weight throughout adulthood and are more likely to develop metabolic problems such as type 2 diabetes, hyperlipidemia and coronary heart disease at much younger ages.[3,4] A study of 90 pre-pubertal children[6] compared the impact of vegetarian diet with that of an omnivorous diet and concluded that a vegetarian diet is less likely to cause obesity. Patients on vegetarian diet were found to have a lower leptin level as well a higher concentration of soluble leptin receptors and adiponectin, explaining the lower rate of obesity and healthier eating habits in children on vegetarian diet.

to make no dietary changes for 18 weeks. The daily caloric intake in both groups was matched. At the end of 18 weeks, the group on a plant-based diet had lost significant weight and their total and LDL cholesterol had greatly dropped.

A plant-based diet not only improves glycemic control and has a direct impact on how our body metabolizes sugar (glucose metabolism), but it also improves the control of our blood sugar levels (glycemic control) by positively affecting weight and insulin resistance. By lowering blood pressure and reducing LDL cholesterol levels, a plant-based diet also reduces the risk of cardiovascular disease, the ultimate objective of any diabetic care plan.

Osteoporosis was for decades speculated to be more prevalent in vegans than non-vegetarians who generally consume larger quantities of dairy products. However, recent evidence conflicts with this common belief that we need calcium from dairy for strong bones. As the research builds, it is increasingly clear that the net acid load of the typical Western diet has the potential to negatively influence many aspects of human health, most notably osteoporosis.

Compared to a typical high- animal protein diet, a plant-based diet can be beneficial to bone health and bone quality by better maintaining bone strength. A plant-based diet contains higher levels of certain antioxidants such as carotenoids-- serum carotenoids are used as bio-markers for fruit and vegetable consumption. For example, a study of 59 post-menopausal[5] women clearly showed lower concentrations of serum carotenoids (lycopene, -cryptoxanthin, -carotene, and zeaxanthin) in women with osteoporosis than in post-menopausal women without osteoporosis.

Breast and Prostate Health: A vegan diet is known to contain much higher phytoestrogen content than an omnivorous diet. Phytoestrogens, which are only found in plants and are essentially hormone imitators, bind to "estrogen receptor" (ER) alpha and beta.[8] As the phytoestrogens affinity for ER-beta is higher than the estradiol, they are anti-proliferative and inhibit tyrosine and other protein kinases, which play a key role in tumor development in female breast tissue.

Is Constipation Connected to Breast Cancer?

A common complaint among those who consume a high animal protein/fat diet is constipation. Our gastrointestinal tract is another major part of our endocrine system, which is in charge of secretion of hormones. These hormones are in charge of food processing, digestion, and the metabolism of glucose, protein, and fat, as well as excretion of excess hormones. One great example is the female hormone estrogen, excreted via our bile into the small intestine. Chronic constipation increases the risk of breast cancer; because as the rate of digestion in our small and large intestine slows down, many of the toxins and hormones (in this case estrogen) that are meant to be excreted will be reabsorbed and returned into the blood stream, causing high levels of estrogen, unwanted hormones, and other toxins in the blood.

They also inhibit the production of the androgen 5-alpha dihydrotestosterone, a potent byproduct of Testosterone known to cause prostate enlargement and increase the risk of prostate cancer. As phytoestrogens are only found in plants, it is logical to conclude that a vegan diet can potentially reduce the risk of breast cancer, prostate hypertrophy, and prostate cancer.

Boost Your Mood on Plant-Based Diet

The interaction between our endocrine system and mood is very close. Meat- and dairy-heavy diets are high in arachidonic acid (AA) compared to vegetarian diets. Research shows that a high intake of AA promotes changes in the brain that can disturb mood.[9] A recent study investigated the impact of restricting meat, fish, and poultry on mood. Even those who ate fish, which contains eicosapentaenoic acid (EPA) and docosahexae-noic acid (DHA)-- fats that oppose the negative effects of arachidonic acid-- reported worse moods than vegetarians. Since forms of autoimmune thyroid disease, adrenal disorders as well as sexual function and infertility, are closely linked to a person's mental health, this study suggests an indirect beneficial effect of a plant-based diet on, not only a person's mental health, but also on his or her entire endocrine system.

The fact that a plant-based diet has multiple advantages over an omnivorous diet is common sense. In addition to the multiple benefits from a cardiovascular, neuro-logical, psychological, and renal standpoint, there is a growing body of evidence that a plant-based diet has significantly positive impacts on glucose metabolism, weight, bone health, adrenal and pituitary health, and sexual health over the short- and long-term.

Alireza Falahati-Nini, MD, FCAE *is a Mayo Clinic Trained Endocrinologist with expertise in Osteoporosis and Nutrition. He is published in Journal of Clinical Investigation (JCI), American Heart Journal, American Journal of Cardiology and Clinical Chemistry, etc. He is the current President of the Rocky Mountain Chapter of American Association of Clinical Endocrinologists and the founder of Utah Endocrinology Associates. He is a Member of Mayo Clinic Alumni and is an active Consultant at St. Mark's Hospital in Salt Lake City, Utah.*

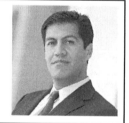

Plant-Based Nutrition and the Musculoskeletal System

Jimmy H. Conway, MD

Falsely believing I was a prisoner of my genes, I knew with certainty that I was destined to get heart disease. My father, who is 82 years old, has had countless cardiac procedures over the past 25 years including cardiac bypass, numerous cardiac stents, angioplasties, and blockages removed from his carotid arteries (the vessels that carry oxygen to the brain) as well as a bypass and stents in his femoral artery (the artery in the leg). Both of my grandfathers, as well as numerous uncles, died of heart attacks. My paternal grandmother died of complications from a stroke. At best I could prolong the inevitable by eating "right" and trying to maintain my weight.

I had no idea what eating "right" really meant, though. I thought eating lean meat was healthy, when in reality cholesterol is in the lean portion of the meat. I thought if a little olive oil was healthy, then a whole lot would be healthier. This is also known in orthopedics as the "bigger hammer theory;" if a little hammer is good then a bigger hammer is better, and if a little hammer does not work, use a bigger hammer! The reality was that I did not have any education on nutrition in medical school. Being a busy orthopedic surgeon, I did not see the need to educate myself. The old saying, "When the pupil is ready, the teacher will appear," is very true in my case.

At the age of 53 I needed cardiac bypass surgery. I had an 85% blockage of my left Anterior Descending coronary artery, an 80% blockage farther downstream, and a 70% blockage of my right Main coronary artery. My cardiologist thought the blockage was too significant to stent and recommended bypass surgery, which would entail cracking my chest open.

As fate would have it, prior to my arteriogram (the test that determined my blockage) a partner of mine recommended I read the book *The China Study* by T. Colin Campbell, PhD. I had never heard or read anything like it. In it, Dr. Campbell referenced another book-- *Prevent and Reverse Heart Disease* by Caldwell Esselstyn, Jr., MD, which I also promptly read. In addition, I did some research on the statistics related to coronary bypass surgery. In a 2005 study in the American Journal of Cardiology there was close to a 45% failure rate of bypass procedures after 12 to 18 months.[1] Armed with the information contained in these two books, along with the statistical information I found, I decided to cancel my bypass surgery. Instead my wife and I adopted a whole food, plant-based diet. Within 6 months I had a normal stress test, my total cholesterol was down from 494 to 115 (HDL 64 and LDL 15), and my triglycerides fell from over 3,200 to 175. I felt better than I had in years. At this point I knew this "diet" was working to improve my health, but I wanted more information. The more I learned the more I saw the connection between food and its effects on the body, in particular the musculoskeletal system.

As an orthopedic surgeon, I primarily treat patients who develop shoulder-related issues. The orthopedic community has known for years that rotator cuff tears start in the area of the rotator cuff that has the poorest blood supply.[2] In addition, most tendonopathies—in which the tendon attached to the bone begins to deteriorate-- occur in areas of the tendon which have the poorest blood supply. Studies show that children who eat the Standard American Diet (the SAD diet) have fatty streaks in their arteries by age 15.[3] This is the beginning of atherosclerosis, or arterial plaque. Arterial plaque has been described as a pimple on the arterial wall. These do not just occur in coronary arteries but throughout the body and can significantly affect the muscles and tendons of the body. This, in turn, hinders our body's ability to heal even minor injuries to tendons and muscles. Food can significantly alter our body's response to injury and aging.

The average age of a person with an asymptomatic rotator cuff tear is 58.7 years of age;[4] the average age of a male that has a Myocardial Infarction for the first time (otherwise known as a heart attack) is 56 years of age.[5] Is this similar age range just a coincidence, or might the same underlying pathology be the cause? We do not know the exact cause of rotator cuff tears, but we do know that they start in the area with the poorest blood flow. Just as erectile dysfunction is now being called "the canary in the coal mine" regarding vascular disease, I think tendonopathies are canaries of vascular disease as well and are ultimately due to poor nutrition. I think most of the degenerative conditions I treat as an orthopedic surgeon are diet-related and can significantly be reversed by adopting a whole foods, no-added oil, plant-based diet.

I see the effects of our poor American diet every day, whether it is in the office or in surgery. Most patients seek orthopedic treatment for degenerative or inflammatory problems that primarily result from lifestyle choices either by inactivity, diet, or overuse. I have performed thousands of surgeries, and I see what our diet does to tendons, muscles, bones, and bursas. I have seen bone so weak it would not hold an anchor or screw; I have seen tendons so degenerated it would not hold suture or a stitch; and I have seen the inside of the shoulder joint so inflamed that the normal white capsule is brilliant red. I believe most of these conditions could be significantly improved-- if not prevented-- by dietary changes.

The Effing F's of Nutrition

There are foods that *fight* inflammation and foods that *feed* inflammation. We are either feeding or fighting the inflammation in our bodies with our *fingers*, our *feet* and our *forks*-- with our fingers by the way we snack, with our feet by how much we exercise, and with our forks by what we eat. Our snacks must be a whole food. We need 30 minutes of moderate exercise a day and we need to eat more whole plant foods with little to no processed food.

The best way to illustrate these effects is to describe two fictitious athletes, Tiger Tim and Cruciferous Carl. While these particular examples are fictional, the science behind what I will describe is very real. Tiger Tim is a typical American soccer player who eats the SAD diet. Cruciferous Carl is also a typical American soccer player, but he eats a whole food, no-added oil, plant based diet.

Both athletes heard they can improve their performance with beet juice-- beet juice and other high nitrate containing foods increase nitric oxide production which is essential to increasing blood flow in exercise. Nitric Oxide makes the production of ATP, our body's energy molecule, 16% more efficient.[6] It also decreases oxygen requirements by 19%.[7] Nitric Oxide production is critically important for the body to heal itself. When our arteries are more relaxed, blood flow increases. Dietary fat (both plant and animal) is shown to affect our blood vessels' ability to relax. The SAD diet gets at least 30% or more of its calories from fat. This amount of fat impedes our body's ability to heal by affecting nitric oxide production. Nitric Oxide production in our arteries occurs in the inner lining of the artery otherwise known as the endothelium-- fat blocks this production. It takes 4 to 6 hours after a high fat meal for the endothelial nitric oxide production to return to baseline.[8]

What does this have to do with our two athletes? If Tiger Tim is eating a SAD diet, his arteries are not going to respond to the addition of the dietary nitrates the same as Cruciferous Carl's will-- nor will Tiger Tim's muscles respond the same to training. The burn felt in the muscle when exercising is due to lactic acid production; however, *delayed* onset muscle soreness is an inflammatory condition.[9] Food contributes significantly to inflammation, either by *feeding* inflammation or *fighting* it. Inflammation also occurs in response to arachodonic acid production. Arachodonic acid is a product from linoleic acid, the essential omega-6 fatty acid. The SAD diet contains entirely too much omega-6 fatty acid as well as too many saturated and trans fats, all of which promote inflammation. After the same amount of time in any given training program, Tiger Tim's muscles will have significantly more delayed onset muscle soreness and inflammation compared to Cruciferous Carl's muscles.

The inflammation in Tiger Tim's muscles is not just due to the Omega-6 fatty acids, but also to the animal flesh he eats. The meat, whether it is chicken, beef, or pork, has bacterial endotoxins which cause an intense inflammatory response.[10] By not eating meat, Cruciferous Carl is not exposed to the endotoxemia that Tiger Tim experiences each time he eats meat; Cruciferous Carl can thus train more intensely. Tiger Tim's arterial walls would also be stiffer than Cruciferous Carl's because of the effects of a chemical that is produced by acenitobacter bacteria during fermentation in his gut; acenitobacter bacteria inhabit the gut of meat eaters, but are not prevalent in the gut of a vegan. This bacterium produces a gas called TMA, trimethylamine. Tiger Tim's liver converts this TMA into TMAO, trimethylamine-N-oxide which stiffens arterial walls, impeding blood flow among other health problems.[11] This stiffness would also hamper the effects of dietary nitrates.

If Tiger Tim drinks dairy, his bones will also be weaker than those of Cruciferous Carl because of the acidity of the protein in dairy.[12] Contrary to what is advertised milk does NOT build strong bones, but in fact weakens them. It has been shown that people with back pain have more clogged lumbar arteries than people with no history of back pain; the greater the blockage, the worse the degeneration in the disc.[13] If we can reverse heart disease-- which numerous doctors have now proven-- back pain might be reversed by the same whole food, no-added oil, plant-based diet. Dairy is also a significant contributor to saturated fat which, as stated earlier, increases inflammation among other things.

We either feed the inflammation and degeneration or we fight it, and I have chosen to fight it. My wife and I give seminars that teach the science of plant-based nutrition, how to begin making changes, and hopefully establishing a community of like-minded people. We have seen such a positive response to our whole food plant-based message that our seminars, which were initially held quarterly, are now being given monthly. The demand is continuing to grow as more and more people are feeling empowered to have control over their own health.

Jimmy H. Conway, M.D. *graduated from the University of Oklahoma Medical School in 1983. He completed his orthopedic residency in San Antonio, TX. Dr. Conway joined Oklahoma Sports Science and Orthopedics is a board certified orthopedic surgeon. He is a member of the American College of Orthopedic Surgeons. Dr. Conway is a member of the American Society for Nutrition.*

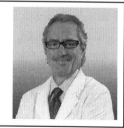

Got Carbs?

Daniel J. Chartrand, MD

As a family physician, one of the most common complaints I hear is fatigue-- the "I don't have any energy, I am tired all the time, I don't feel rested" kind of fatigue. Usually the patient is frustrated; they have tried everything they know to do. They will try to sleep more, eat more, and drink coffee or another form of caffeine. When they finally come to my office we do the complete work-up. I perform a thorough exam and look for signs of congestive heart failure, anemia, and neuropathy among others; I check blood work for blood counts, vitamin B12, thyroid dysfunction, Addison's disease, as well as kidney and liver disease. Only about 2% of the time a cause is found. What about the other 98%? The advice I routinely give follows as such: try to sleep less, try to exercise more, and try to eat better. The first two recommendations are easy to understand, but the third is generally less intuitive for most. What does it mean to eat better?

Nutrition is usually where I start when treating fatigue. Most patients roll their eyes and tell me they already eat "healthy" by getting plenty of protein and taking a number of supplemental vitamins to round off their diet. However, instead of worrying about the micronutrients such as vitamins and minerals (which a balanced modern diet adequately provides but do not produce energy), I focus on the macronutrients: fat, protein, and carbohydrates. Macronutrients are the only way to make energy.

A calorie is the measure of energy that can be obtained from each macronutrient. To make energy, each macronutrient shares a common pathway of metabolism in the mitochondria of every cell. The macronutrients are all metabolized to the same molecule, Acetyl Coenzyme A or Acetyl CoA for short. Acetyl CoA is turned into cellular energy called adenosine triphosphate (ATP). Think of ATP as gasoline for a cell; it is the power behind muscle contractions and neuron signals. Protein and carbohydrates are similar in that they each have the potential to produce four calories for every gram of weight. The energy in fat, though, is more compact and thus produces nine calories for every gram of weight.

What is the Best Way to Make Energy Efficiently and Decrease Fatigue?

It would seem that fat would give us the most energy; however, only certain cells are equipped to use fat efficiently. Ketosis is the process by which the body's cells use fat as their primary energy source. Some cells thrive in this environment, but many others do not. For example, the human heart which is in a state of constant energy demand uses fat as its preferred fuel. The cardiac muscles are well-equipped for this grueling task and use the triglycerides in the blood for fuel (there is a low amount of cholesterol and triglycerides in the blood at all times. The disease state of atherosclerosis or hardening of the arteries is thought to be caused by an increased amount of triglycerides and cholesterol in the blood over time).

The human brain's neurons prefer to use glucose for cellular energy. Most triglycerides (fat in the blood stream) are bound to protein in the blood and cannot easily enter the brain. It takes days for the brain's neurons to turn on the intercellular machinery that converts fat to energy. The process of ketosis is associated with "brain fog," and many patients describe a decrease in mental functions when they deprive themselves of glucose and rely on fat alone for their calories. The problem is that fat is more difficult to digest. The intestines and their cell membrane walls are water-based and fat is an oil. As we well know, oil and water do not mix. Fat in the food we eat then must be dissolved in bile acids to be absorbed across the intestine walls. Most of the fat can make it across, but there is always some left behind. This can cause bloating, pain, and diarrhea. Fat in the intestine also slows digestion. It causes the stomach to slow its release of nutrients to the intestine.

Protein is an important macronutrient, but it is also not the most efficient source of calories or energy. Amino acids are the building blocks of protein. We can think of amino acids in terms of tiny Legos™ making up a larger Lego™ structure: protein. In order to make the transport across the intestine wall into the bloodstream, proteins must be broken down into the tiny amino acids. Because proteins are so complex, hundreds of chemical reactions must take place just to break them apart-- similar to taking apart a Lego™ model. While the human body can make or synthesize 13[2] of the 20 amino acids, there are 9 essential amino acids that must be obtained from our diet. Various studies have shown that the adult human requires as little as 20 grams of protein per day to fulfill the processes of the body.[1] Any leftover amino acids are left to the "protein pool," an intercellular storage space. The protein pool can contribute to cellular energy, but there is some inefficiency.

Protein produces waste when it is converted to energy. Ammonia and urea are produced and must be cleared by the liver and the kidney. Protein can also have other effects on the body, like making us tired. This is why we can experience fatigue or 'food coma' after a large high protein meal.

In comparison to fats and protein, the human body is adapted to use carbohydrates efficiently. Carbohydrate is the generic term for a molecule containing a carbon chain. It can be a simple sugar like glucose or a complex starch such as those found in whole wheat. When we eat carbohydrates, digestive enzymes in the saliva begin to breakdown the sugars immediately. In the intestine, these sugars easily cross the cell membranes and are quickly sent to the liver where they are converted to glycogen. The liver stores the glycogen and then releases glycogen into the blood stream as needed. The process of converting carbohydrates to the Acetyl CoA is more efficient compared to that of the other macronutrients. There are no nitrogen by-products, and the great majority of cells use carbohydrates as their preferred energy source, specifically the brain and the muscles.

The biggest distinction amongst macronutrients is the delivery system the human body uses to move them to the cells during times of need. If fatigue is broken down in simplest terms: cells are in need of more fuel to make more energy. It makes sense then that carbohydrates are superior. When cells are actively making energy, they draw glycogen out of the blood stream and into themselves. As the glycogen content of the blood decreases, the liver releases its stored glycogen into the blood stream to keep a constant supply chain moving. This system is not available to proteins. The "protein pool" is an intercellular space and cannot be shared between cells. For example, if a person is walking up a flight of stairs and the muscles of the legs have used up all of their amino acids for energy production, the amino acids in the cells of the arms, for instance, cannot travel to the leg muscles for use. The protein pool can only hold a limited source of energy, and its supply chain is inefficient.

Fat can be more easily mobilized, but cholesterol and triglycerides contained in fat can have negative consequences. During times of need, fat tissue releases triglycerides into the blood stream for use by other tissues. This is how the heart muscles receive their constant supply of energy. During times of starvation, when there is no glycogen to be released by the liver, all cells are dependent upon triglycerides or their protein pool for energy. The increase in blood triglyceride levels over a long time period can increase the risk for certain cardiovascular diseases. The cells that can use fat/triglycerides efficiently will do well, but other cells will need to convert over to the ketosis stage of energy production and become less efficient. As the body uses protein and fat, keto-acids, ammonia, and urea are produced. In a person with normal liver and kidney function, this is not a big deal in the short term, but can lead to trouble in the long term. For example, a higher protein load increases the rate of kidney function decline and will eventually lead to kidney failure.[2]

Nature can give us a few examples of animal macronutrient digestion and energy use. The king of beasts, the African lion, is on a carbohydrate-restricted diet. It consumes muscle protein and fat exclusively. Its energy is produced by the breakdown of proteins into acetyl CoA. The lion has short bursts of energy, but spends the great majority of its time lying around. Its majesty has a relatively short reign, though: the average life span of a lion in the wild is 10 to 15 years. Contrast this with the African plains zebra.

The zebra, a food source of the lion, is a vegetarian. It eats plant carbohydrates, and its energy is derived from glucose. Zebras spend the majority of their days in motion. They sleep sparingly and in the wild live about 25 years. The American bald eagle also consumes a carb-restricted diet, consuming wild salmon rich in protein and omega-3 fats, it lives 15 to 25 years in the wild. By comparison, the macaw eats fruits, leaves, and nuts and lives 3 to 4 times longer than a bald eagle-- up to 60 years in the wild.

There are human examples, too. Endurance athletes with tremendous stamina and energy eat a high carb diet before competitions. They will eat pounds of pasta in the mornings prior to marathons. All of these carbs are stored in the liver as glycogen and released for their use in the muscles. During their runs they choose glucose gels and carbohydrate sports drinks-- not protein smoothies-- to give them energy.

So where does this leave the fatigued patient? In my clinic, when I have ruled out the usual suspects of fatigue, I encourage patients to make their bodies' energy production more efficient. I ask them to limit and severely decrease their fat intake because it slows digestion, encourages ketosis, and contributes to their cholesterol as well as limit their protein because it increases waste, decreases efficiency, can promote fatigue, and is not needed. Since our bodies are designed to process carbohydrates, I ask them to eat more carbohydrates.

The western world has bastardized carbs into the doughnut, the candy, and the sugary soft drink. These are not real foods but rather a concoction of chemicals designed to ensnare human senses. Carbohydrates are not bad for humans, they are merely misunderstood. Carbohydrates come from plants. It is the starch of the potato, the grain of wheat, the pulp of an orange, and the kernel of a bean. I prefer a plant-based diet consisting of 90% REAL carbohydrate calories: oatmeal, brown rice, corn, potatoes, beans, and fresh fruits and vegetables. This means a very limited amount of protein, nuts, and plant oils. I have found with this approach that the majority of patients after 5 to 6 hours of sleep they are wide awake and full of energy. They have an increase in stamina and exercise tolerance and report feeling younger. While energy levels cannot be measured like blood glucose or quantified like a 5 kilometer run, the results speak for themselves.

Daniel J. Chartrand, MD *is a family physician in private practice in McKinney, Texas. He graduated from Saint Louis University School of Medicine and after completing his Family Medicine Residency at the University of Texas Southwestern, he worked as an emergency room physician for five years. Dr. Chartrand helps patients regain their health with food and exercise.* www.harmonyfamilyhealth.com

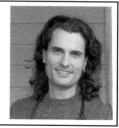

Gut as a Gateway to Autoimmune Disease

Roger L. Greenlaw, MD, FACP/G, ABIHM

Is there a relationship between what we eat and developing an autoimmune disease such as Crohn's, Celiac, or Multiple Sclerosis? New research supports the theory that changes in our diet as well as antibiotics alter our intestinal environment (flora) and our gastrointestinal tract function in ways that are influencing our current epidemic of autoimmune disease.

Our gut processes food intake, breakdown, digestion, and absorption in the upper gastrointestinal tract, specifically the esophagus, stomach and small intestine. In the upper tract everything is absorbed without much attention to potential health or harm, sending whatever is taken in as 'Texas Crude' via the portal vein from the small intestine to the liver 'refinery' for processing before distribution to the body. The liver absorbs this digestive mix of nutrients, drugs, chemicals, poisons, toxins, etc. which are sorted and sent to appropriate areas of the body for further processing as nutrients, foreign substances, toxins, and waste.

Less well known are the functions of the lower tract, or colon in recycling water while preventing the re-absorption of waste that is being held for elimination. The lower bowel dehydrates waste (absorbs water), firming our stool for later elimination, while recycling water to help maintain hydration. If these processes work as intended we are nourished, protected from absorption of harmful material and our waste is eliminated.

Newer research reveals that the colon's single layer of protective lining cells, called *enterocytes*, are not able to nourish themselves from the blood stream like other body cells. Rather these cells get their nutrients from the waste stream.[1] Most of the fuel comes from absorption of (Butyric Acid) Butyrate, produced by the digestion of fiber by the good bacteria that live in the colon.

Fiber, which humans have no enzymes to digest, was previously thought to be only good for softening stool. Now fiber is understood to be food for the colon or *prebiotics. Prebiotics* are digested downstream in the colon by good bacteria called *probiotics*, which produce nutrients absorbed by the enterocytes. This fiber digestion provides basic food for the colon lining cells.

Just like animals have skeletons for body support, a plant's skeleton is fiber. Fiber is only found in foods made from plants. There is no fiber in meat, eggs, dairy products or any other food that comes from animals. It plays a vital role in maintaining a healthy digestive system by: slowing gastric emptying, increasing satiety, decreasing abdominal fat, lowering body weight, nourishing the gut lining cells to prevent leaky gut, balancing the immune system, decreasing the risk of autoimmune disease, and supporting good bacteria. Dietary fiber contributes to the prevention of a range of disorders and diseases, including coronary heart disease, stroke, hypertension, diabetes, obesity, and gastrointestinal disorders.[2]

When the right mix of probiotics are absent from the bowels and/or fiber is absent from the diet, the enterocytes in the colon are undernourished. Enterocytes are held tightly together to prevent re-absorption of waste by 'tight junctions' which are anatomic and electrochemical connections between these cells. When these tight junctions malfunction due to nutritional deficiencies it allows what is called a 'leaky gut'.[3]

Our immune system guards the linings of our gut because the outside world literally passes through us. About 70% of our immune system cells are packed in the deep layers of our gut to protect against invasion or absorption of unhealthy material. When tight junctions are dysfunctional due to inadequate production of the cellular nutrient 'butyrate', then material such as sloughed enterocytes, bacterial cell parts, food particles and chemicals may come in contact with immune cells through weak (leaky) tight junctions. These are materials that the immune cells should never see. When the immune cells detect foreign material, an inflammatory process is set in motion to destroy the material. If the material is part of our lining cells, our normal bacteria, components of our diet, or chemicals that are just passing through, then 'friendly fire' can occur and a chronic disease can be set in motion.

When we eat meat, eggs and dairy laden meals with little or no fiber, and processed grains with greatly reduced fiber, we do not properly nourish our colon and that can lead to a leaky gut and subsequent autoimmune problems. When we eat a healthy diet, with 30 or more grams of fiber per day, we feed our good bacteria, which in turn release butyrate from their digestion of fiber that nourishes our enterocytes to maintain healthy tight junctions, preventing inappropriate activation of our gut's immune active cells, preventing a setup for autoimmune disease, allergy and chronic inflammation.

Patients with chronic disease often ask "What can *I* do to help treat my disease? Too often medical professionals state, "There is nothing you can do, just take your medication and call me if problems arise". Not only is there a great deal that patients can do for themselves, but most of what can be done to prevent, arrest and reverse these lifestyle related diseases of western culture can *only be done* by them. It is now clear that a whole foods, plant based diet combined with daily exercise, stress management skills and human connection (social support) can prevent, arrest and often reverse lifestyle related chronic diseases.[4] Self-care is the new primary care.

Roger L. Greenlaw, MD, FACP/G, ABIHM *attended the University of Missouri Medical School, Columbia, Missouri where he completed his internal medicine residency. He completed his Fellowship in Gastroenterology, Yale University School of Medicine. Dr. Greenlaw was Clinical Professor Emeritus of Medicine at the University of Illinois College of Medicine-Rockford. He has been widely published in numerous journals, a frequent speaker at lifestyle health conferences been awarded numerous teaching honors. Dr. Greenlaw is currently a consultant for lifestyle medicine solutions for personal, community, and corporate health.*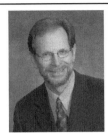

four

PLANT-POWERED ATHLETES

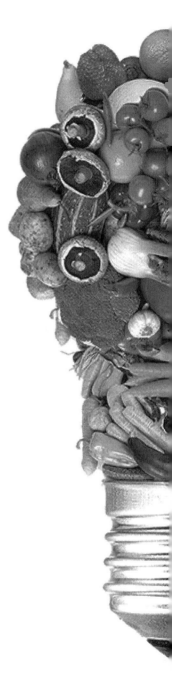

"Where do you get your protein from?" is the first question most of us are confronted with when we tell people we don't eat meat or dairy. Just like we are obsessed with our calcium intake, our society is similarly laser focused on the amount of protein we are consuming, especially for athletes wanting to build muscle. We are led to believe that protein from animals is our best source of protein and a cornerstone for good nutrition.

In order to build muscle and stand at the top of the podium, we need to feed our body right. We have mistakenly believed for too long that building muscle requires whey protein post-work out shakes, and lean meat meals. Animal protein is directly connected to inflammation that sets the stage for chronic disease. In fact, casein- the primary protein in cow's milk is so predictive of cancer that researchers found they could turn cancer on and off simply by altering the casein intake! Athletes, casein is found in most of our bodybuilding materials and all milk and cheese.

Although many of us think we are fueling our body with the right foods to get the gold, most of us are setting up our bodies for long term disease. As the following accomplished and world renowned athletes from former NBA star John Salley to Olympic sports doctors Scott Stoll will demonstrate, we don't need animal protein to win. Rather, our bodies successfully thrive both on and off the field on plant power.

Can Plants Take You to the Top of the Podium?

Scott Stoll, MD

Remarkably, some of the top athletes in the world have unhealthy diets filled with sugar, processed foods, excessive animal product consumption, and a paucity of plant-based foods. As I travel with college and Olympic level teams, I am constantly shocked by the dietary habits of top athletes. Plates piled high with meat, eggs, pancakes and syrup, bread, pizza, fast food, and Snickers bars as protein bars. In the short term-- often because of superior physiology and disciplined workouts-- they do not feel any of the negative effects of their diet, creating a false sense of "health" security. I often discuss with them that it is important to occasionally look to the horizon of life, beyond their athletic goals and dreams, and consider the long-term implications of their diet.

In the athletic world, food is often relegated to a couple of rudimentary paradigms:

1. Sufficient calories are needed to maintain rigorous exercise regimens and avoid weight loss

2. Protein is king and carbohydrates are required for glycogen stores to improve endurance and must be consumed in large quantities

3. If you are missing anything, take a supplement.

As a physician working with athletes at every level from PeeWee sports to Olympic gold medalists-- as well as during my own Olympic career-- I fully understand that these ideas are hardwired into belief systems that are very difficult to overcome. I know bodybuilders who eat boxes of Pop Tarts to help maintain their weight. However, there is a growing group of intelligent athletes who recognize that food is more intricate than macronutrients, the body far more complex than caloric balance and weight, and that the food we eat now affects both our present and future. Theoretically and scientifically it is becoming more apparent that a diet rich in plant-based foods provides the greatest opportunity to optimize the function of an athlete's body.

Let's explore recovery and the future implications of an athlete's diet which are often missed in preparation for the big game or competition.

Recovery:

A diverse plant-based diet, carefully constructed to meet an athlete's needs, possesses the necessary micronutrient profile to mitigate the inevitable damage that occurs during workout and competition. In the hours and days that follow a workout, the body is in a recovery and regenerative mode that is either hindered or helped by nutrition. The ability of the body to fully recover before the next workout determines the quality of the next workout, and this trend applied over months can make or break the preparation for a competition. A plant-based diet provides the greatest opportunity to maximize training times due in large part to decreased soreness and recovery times, improved strength, and less perceived fatigue during exercise.

During a high level workout the body is often pushed to its maximum capacity. In the muscle, micro-tears occur, connective tissue is stretched, and hypoxic damage from oxygen deficiencies all lead to the production of free radicals (unstable atoms that rip through cells seeking an electron for stability). Free radicals are used by the immune system to help digest damaged tissue in the first 24 hours and are often associated with the sensation of delayed onset of muscle soreness or DOMS.[1] The delayed soreness and underlying tissue damage will ultimately limit workout progressions[2] and potentially contribute to overuse injuries.[3] Decades of research on strenuous exercise reveal that with increased intensity of exercise there is a rise in systemic inflammation and DNA damage.[4,5] The body attempts to combat this damage through its antioxidant systems, like glutathione, that are significantly depleted after an intense physical effort for up to two weeks.[6,7,8] These antioxidant systems are replenished by the micronutrients found in whole, plant-based foods.

Micronutrients, obtained from whole foods, possess a comprehensive array of antioxidants/ phytochemicals, vitamins, and minerals that work in symphony to repair damaged cells. The first 24 hours of recovery may be the most important period to help your body overcome the local and systemic effects of an intense workout, decrease soreness, and prepare for the next workout or competition. Supplemental antioxidants, isolated and independent of a whole food, have not been found to be helpful and in some cases are potentially harmful.[9]

Several progressive studies have actually used whole food based sources to investigate the effect on oxidative stress and recovery. A group of Polish rowers was given a pure chokeberry extract during a 1 month workout period. Compared to the placebo group, the rowers consuming the antioxidant rich chokeberry extract demonstrated a significant decrease in free radical damage and lower levels of antioxidant enzymes-- due to fewer free radicals-- in the first 24 hours.[10] Another study utilized cherry juice over an 8 day time period in a group of athletes asked to perform a bicep exercise designed to induce muscle damage and soreness. The placebo group exhibited a 22% loss in strength in the first 24 hours and peak in pain at 48 hours compared to a 4% loss of strength in the cherry group and peak muscle pain at 24 hours.[11] The improved recovery time and decreased pain have been corroborated by several other studies using plant-based interventions.[12,13]

Additionally intense workouts and competition stress the body and can suppress the immune system.[14] Common infectious diseases can derail the best training schedule, devastate a long awaited competition, and spread through a team in a matter of days. I have worked with teams that have missed competitions due to infections. After an intense workout the immune cells involved in fighting infections are suppressed and athletes are at an increased risk of infection for one to two weeks.[15,16] Dietary components including sugar, excessive protein via acidosis and alteration of the probiotic gut environment, alcohol, and saturated fats can further impair immune function. In contrast, plant based foods enhance immune function, alkalinize the body, and contain fiber that nourishes beneficial gut bacteria.[17] The prevention found in a plant-based diet can yield significant benefits in athletic wellness.

Don't Plant Seeds of Disease

Unhealthy dietary patterns and habits established during athletic years combined with decreased activity can lead to an increased risk of disease, such as heart disease, later in life.[18] If the athlete's diet of excess-- a diet higher in meat, fat, and sugars-- spills over into post athletic life, they will significantly increase their risk for a host of degenerative diseases.[19]

Most of these chronic diseases develop slowly over decades before the physical manifestations are evident. Heart disease may take 10 to 20 years to develop from of a diet rich in meats, sugars, fats, and stress.[20] Many cancers also have incubation periods of 10 to 20 and are the result of an unhealthy lifestyle overlaid onto susceptible genes.[21]

Return on Investment

A wise investment is one that returns the maximum amount in both the short and long term. An athlete's diet should be constructed with this principle in mind. We need to capitalize on the benefits of antioxidant/phytochemical-rich foods designed to reduce inflammation, repair DNA, build bone and muscle, repair and maintain cartilage and soft tissue, improve immunity and recovery time.[22] We can then reap the future rewards of a strong, vibrant, healthy body that supports continued physical activities and opens the door to opportunity.

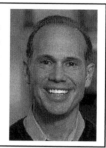

Scott Stoll, MD *is a member of the Whole Foods Medical Scientific Advisory Board, Plantrician Advisory Board, Future of Health Now advisory board, team physician at Lehigh University, and department chairman of Physical Medicine and Rehabilitation at Coordinated Health. Dr. Stoll is the co-founder of the North American Plant Based Nutrition Healthcare Conference. Dr. Stoll is the author of "Alive! A Physician's Biblical and Scientific Guide to Nutrition". He was a member of the 1994 Olympic Bobsled team and now serves as a physician for the United States Bobsled and Skeleton team. Dr. Stoll resides with his wife and six children in Bethlehem, Pennsylvania. For more information:* FullyAliveToday.com.

Sports, Athletic Performance, Protein and Vegan Diets

David Musnick, MD

As a Sports Medicine Doctor I frequently get asked if vegan diets are good for athletes. The answer: Absolutely! Vegan diets include healthy carbohydrates, good for muscle glycogen and having energy to exercise. However, the biggest question is whether vegan athletes can get enough protein. **Any plant- based athlete can get enough protein to be at the top of their game**.

Here are some recommendations as to how:

- Make sure your breakfast has at least 20 grams of protein to start your day. Make a protein smoothie with soy, hemp or pea based protein powder and soy milks.

- Have nuts and seeds for snacks.

- Eat a variety of beans, legumes and whole grains.

Read Dr. Musnick's "Minimize Toxins with a Plant-Based Diet" in the Processed People Chapter

Vegan Athletes: An Oxymoron?

Matthew Ruscigno, MPH, RD

For too long the term "vegan athlete" has been treated like an oxymoron. Where could they possibly get their protein? Athletes should have the best diets in the world; their performance depends on it. Fortunately whole food, plant based diets do not sacrifice performance, and a plethora of athletes are proving this every day. You can not only get all of the nutrients you need from plant foods to excel in any discipline, but there are also benefits to eating a plant-based vegan diet.

How Do They Do It? Getting the Nutrition You Need From Plants

Once we get into the science of nutrition it is not hard to see that vegan diets are adequate, and beneficial for athletic endeavors. When sports nutrition is discussed, all too often the fact that fruits and vegetables are the most nutritionally dense foods available is completely forgotten. When I do nutrient analyses on vegan athletes often their Recommended Daily Allowances for the major nutrients show up in the vicinity of 300%-- well above average. This is because they are eating vast amounts of nutrient-rich foods like vegetables, fruits, whole grains, legumes, nuts, and seeds.

Protein

Let's have a serious talk about protein requirements for athletes and put some myths to rest for good. Protein, put simply, is a combination of amino acids. These amino acids have specific roles in our bodies, from metabolism to muscle development. Nine of them are absolutely essential to our basic functions which means they must come from food. When you hear about one protein source being better than another, it is in reference to the amino acid makeup. Fortunately, all whole plant foods contain protein and all of the essential amino acids. Getting enough protein is not an issue for vegan athletes.

There is No Such Thing as Incomplete Protein

The phrase 'incomplete protein' is misleading, and health professionals and vegans should stop using it. Combining proteins was popularized in the 1970's, and even though it has been deemed unnecessary for decades, the idea lives on. It is true: some animal foods contain all of the amino acids in the exact amounts we need per serving. If you ate only eggs and nothing else, in the exact number of calories you needed every day, you would not get an amino acid deficiency. However, do the same with lentils and you may not get enough methionine. Like many myths, the idea that one source of protein is 'complete' is based on a truth.

But, guess what? No one eats like this! Saying a protein is incomplete ignores the big picture and is often used by pseudo-health professionals as a critique of plant-based diets.

It is unnecessary to "combine proteins" because our bodies pool amino acids and uses them as needed-- regardless of the perceived completeness of the source. We eat a variety of foods, most of which have some protein, and at the end of the day, we get all of the amino acids we need. It is that simple!

How Much Protein Do You Need?

It is true that athletes need more protein than the average person. Conservative recommendations are that vegans increase their protein consumption by 10%. But achieving this small amount with plant foods is easy. Firstly, athletes also need more carbohydrates and fat -- the overall caloric needs are much higher since we burn more energy while training. Because we are eating more calories, we are automatically consuming more protein. As your caloric needs go up from the exercise, your intake of protein grams goes up too.

It is important to remember that protein, and therefore the essential amino acids, is in every whole food. Lentils and soymilk are over 30% protein, and "high carb" foods contain a fair amount of protein such as whole-wheat pasta (15%) and brown rice (8%). Even bananas and other fruit contain protein! If you are eating enough for your activity level and consuming a variety of whole foods, you can get all the protein you need.

Calculate Your Protein Intake

There are a few different ways to make protein recommendations. One is by grams based on your body weight. The Dietary Reference Intake (DRI), for the 'average person,' is 0.8 grams of protein per kilogram of body weight or 0.36 grams per pound of body weight. This is useful for calculating the number of grams of protein most people need for each day.

Caloric Density

Getting enough calories is one of the most important considerations for vegan athletes. When you combine the high metabolism of athletes with the high-fiber diet of plants, caloric needs may go up more than expected. Athletes need to take this into consideration.

Healthy fats like walnuts, almonds, and avocado can and should be a part of a vegan athlete's healthy diet. Additionally, simple carbohydrates from fruits make for an excellent fuel source.

While other athletes look to refined sugar and carbohydrate products for quick energy, eat whole fruit with confidence! A popular breakfast I suggest to my athletes is 4 mashed bananas, 1 to 2 tablespoons of almond butter, and 1 diced apple. It is both nutrient-dense and calorically-dense and keeps you full for your long days of working and training. In addition, keep fruit in your locker and eat it as soon as you are done working out to replace the glycogen you worked off and to start repairing damaged cells.

Benefits of Vegan Foods for Training

When you go to a supported sporting event like a marathon or a bicycle race you will notice that most of the food offered to the competitors is plant-based. Easily digestible carbohydrate-rich foods that have some protein are the best foods to be eaten during workouts.

For recovery, plant foods are high in phytochemicals and antioxidants that repair damaged cells after a hard workout. The highest concentrations of these beneficial components are found in berries, cacao, fruits, tea, and wine especially, but in smaller amounts in nearly every single plant food. These phytochemicals and antioxidants are only found in plant foods. Therefore every type of athlete could benefit from eating a plant-based recovery meal.

Many athletes are only concerned about the immediate benefits of food and supplements, but they, like everyone, need to consider the long-term effect of what we eat. Eating the best foods for your training is also beneficial for your long-term health as those who eat more fruits and vegetables, statistically have lower rates of every major chronic disease. As athletes we are role models and promoting healthy food is an important part of what we do.

A Rise in Vegan Athletes

From Ultra Running to MMA Fighting and Track Cycling, there is a considerable rise in vegan athletes as more and more individuals recognize the benefits of eating plant-based to achieve better results.

Ultra Running

One of the most dominant ultra runners of all time (and vegan) is Scott Jurek. The author of *Eat and Run,* Scott won the Western States 100-- one of the most competitive and challenging 100-mile running races-- seven times in a row. He has the second best distance in a 24 hour race of all Americans of all-time. He is also a two-time winner and the previous course record holder for the grueling 135-mile Badwater Ultramarathon, a run through Death Valley in the summer where temperatures can reach 130 degrees Fahrenheit.

At the 2011 Javalina Jundred, a 100-mile trail running race, the third place elite runner was Jay Smithberger, who holds one of the top 10 fastest 100-mile times ever recorded at 13 hours and 49 minutes. Also running was Catra Corbett, a vegan of nearly 2 decades who has run over ninety 100-mile races-- that is 9 thousand miles of running, excluding all of her training miles and shorter races.

Mixed Martial Artists

Mixed Martial Artist (MMA) Mac Dazig has long been both a successful fighter and proponent of veganism. He makes it very clear that his diet is about ethics and equally clear in the ring that his masculinity is not sacrificed. He has successfully defended the King of the Cage Lightweight Championship 4 times. Jake Shields is another lifelong vegetarian and now vegan that holds numerous championship belts and was ranked in the top 10 in the world amongst middleweight fighters.

Strength Athletes

In the summer of 2013 a group of vegan bodybuilders and trainers attended the Naturally Fit Super Show in Austin, Texas, as the Plant Built Vegan Muscle Team. Their team won 9 first place awards and 18 podium awards, including four overall championships. Former bodybuilder Patrik Baboumiam competes in strongman events that include log lifting, deadlifting, and bench pressing. He has squatted 600 pounds, bench pressed 440 pounds, and holds the current "keg lift" world record. Although a vegetarian for many years, Patrik went vegan the same year he won Germany's Strongest Man competition in 2011.

Track Cycling

Less popular than the Tour de France, but equally demanding, is track racing. These athletes compete on a circular, banked velodrome and reach speeds near 50 miles per hour. In order to win they have to be able to sprint which takes significant muscle strength. Jack Lindquist, a former Olympic hopeful and vegan of 10 years, requires special pants to fit his giant quad muscles. Zak Kovalcik of Portland, Oregon is a vegan of over a decade and the reigning Omnium National Champion in the United States.

How To Make It Work For You

Making big changes in your life is never easy. Simply start by making vegetables the focus of your plate, complemented with whole grains and beans and eliminating animal protein. Sometimes we lapse, but what is most important is getting back out there, both in training and in healthy eating. Do your best and don't give up!

Read All About It!

- Day in the Life of Vegan Athletes Web Series, www.truelovehealth.com

- "Vegetarian Sports Nutrition" by Enette Larson-Meyer

- "Eat and Run" by Scott Jurek

- "No Meat Athlete" by Matt Frazier and Matthew Ruscigno

- "Vegan For Life" by Ginny Messina and Jack Norris

- "Plant-powered Diet" by Sharon Palmer

- "Finding Ultra" by Rich Roll

Matthew Ruscigno, MPH, RD *is a Registered Dietitian and a vegan of over 17 years. He is the past Chair of the Vegetarian Nutrition Dietary Practice Group of the Academy of Nutrition and Dietetics. He is the co-author of "No Meat Athlete" with Matt Frazier and "Appetite for Reduction" with Isa Moskowitz. An athlete himself, Matt has completed numerous marathons, ultra races and triathlons including the Norseman, considered the hardest Ironman in the world and is a three-time finisher of the Furnace Creek 508, a 500-mile non-stop bike race through Death Valley deemed the 8th hardest race in the world. He writes at* www.truelovehealth.com.

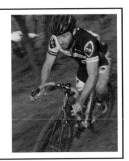

Where Do You Get Your Protein?

Ellen Cutler, DO

Many people are obsessed with protein intake. Although protein is certainly an essential nutrient which plays many key roles in the way the body functions, this concern about protein is misplaced and we do not need huge quantities of it.

Too many people today eat animal products to secure their protein needs. Although animal based foods are high in protein, people who eat meat and dairy tend to have more heart disease, cancer, osteoporosis, and kidney disease. To our benefit, plants have enough protein to keep us healthy and all of the amino acids in proper balance for ideal human growth. As antioxidants, enzymes, vitamins, and minerals are abundant in vegetables, plant-based diets reduce the likelihood of chronic diseases.

Most important of all is digesting the protein we are eating. Problems losing weight can be related to the toxicity created from eating high amounts of animal protein. The liver simply cannot process large amounts of animal protein, causing people to become endemic, lethargic, and a have a slower metabolism. The liver plays a particularly important role in the elimination of toxic waste by filtering toxins from the blood. If this filtering process becomes overburdened or breaks down, toxins begin assaulting liver cells, causing damage and scarring which can lead to liver failure.

When we eat plant-based food that our bodies can readily digest, we minimize toxicity, curb cravings, and reduce inflammation. Vegetarian sources of protein include legumes, grains, nuts, and seeds. Soy is considered a complete protein source possessing all the essential amino acids. Quinoa and amaranth are particularly high in protein, as are beans and legumes and blue-green algae and spirulina. According to the Vegetarian Resource Group, a cup of soybeans 29 grams of protein, a cup of lentils has 18 grams of protein and a 4-oz. serving of tofu has 11 grams of protein.[1] Even a cup of spinach has 5 grams of protein, and a cup of oatmeal has 6 grams. I absolutely encourage everyone to try a vegan approach to brighten your life and optimize your well being.

Ellen Cutler DO, *is a passionate advocate of natural health and healing and a raw vegan. Author of Clearing the Way to Health and Wellness and MicroMiracles: Discover the Healing Power of Enzymes. She is the developer of the Ellen Cutler Method, (incorporating enzyme therapy with nutritional counseling, detoxification, and the identification and correction of food and other sensitivities)*

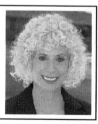

John Salley

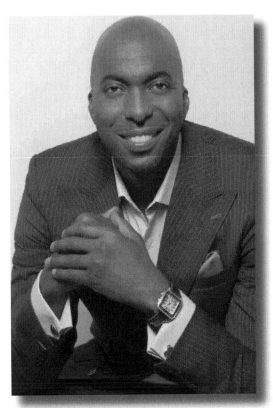

As a father, athlete, entrepreneur, actor, talk show host, and philanthropist I always take the time to choose high value nutrition foods for each meal. I am one of the first NBA players to win four championships with three different teams. My positions were a power forward and center for the Detroit Pistons, Miami Heat, Toronto Raptors, the Chicago Bulls, Los Angeles Lakers, and the Panathinaikos BC.

I was a teammate on the Bulls 72 win record breaking season along with my teammates Michael Jordan, Scottie Pippen, and Toni Kukoc. After I retired, for many years I was grateful to be a host on Fox Sports and share my love of basketball.

I embrace a raw vegan diet lifestyle and believe plant nutrition gives me excellent endurance and vitality that I experience daily. Educating societies on the benefits of good nutrition and healthy eating habits is an integral part of my life and is very rewarding to me.

I have spoken in front of Congress asking members to increase vegetarian options in meal plans served in public schools and represent the Child Nutrition Act. My dear father was stricken with diabetes which led me to join and support the fight against diabetes. I watched him experience the hardship with the disease and I am determined to expand the education about food choices that can reverse diabetes and other diseases.

Teaching people to be their best and go plant-based gives me great fulfillment and I love sharing with others the knowledge of plant foods for optimal nutrition and health. (*Photo Credit: www.3cubedstudios.com*)

Georges Laraque

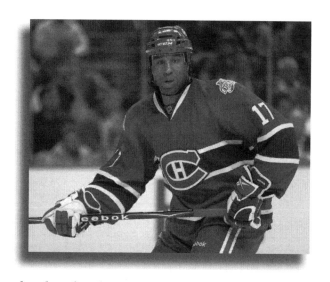

If someone had told me 10 years ago that I would be vegan, I would have thought they were crazy. Like the majority, I thought I would lose my strength and muscle mass. In 2009, however, I did become vegan for ethical reasons after watching *Earthlings*. It was a life changing experience, and the only regret I have is that I did not adopt veganism twenty years earlier!

I realized my childhood dream when I joined the NHL in 1997 and played hockey for the next 13 years until 2010. I was one of the biggest players in the NHL- 6'3" and 260 lbs. My role on my team was an enforcer, meaning I was a fighter hired to protect the smaller players on my team. I did not know much about nutrition, but, in my mind, as a fighter, I needed to eat meat to retain my strength. And I was eating a lot of it.

Before switching my diet, I went to a heart institute to test my blood, my heart, my cholesterol, etc. At that time, I was taking meds for high blood pressure and asthma. Four months after going plant-based, these conditions disappeared, I no longer needed medication, and my test scores had dramatically improved. I was stronger and healthier without any supplements.

I spent my last year in the NHL as a vegan. Unfortunately, I was diagnosed with 2 herniated disks and had to be released. Against my doctors' push for surgery and rest, I decided to run everything from 90km relays to marathons. I was in the best shape of my life all due to my new plant-powered lifestyle. I am certain if I had started this diet in the beginning of my career, I could have played 20 years instead of 13.

Moving on from the NHL, I help people change their diet and witness the positive changes in their lives every day through 2 raw vegan restaurants "Crudessence" and "Rise Kombucha" and lecturing at conferences around the world. I now live my life at a 100% rather than surviving at 75%.

Steph Davis

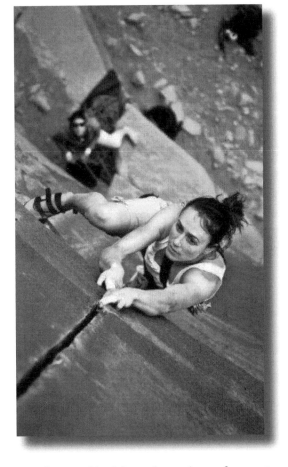

initially switched to a vegan diet (without refined sugar or flour) in 2002 as a year-long mission to find the best nutrition plan as a rock climber, base jumper, and wing suit pilot. As a climber for 22 years, I have made first ascents in Pakistan, Patagonia, Baffin Island, and Kyrgyzstan. I was the first person to free solo Castleton's North Face and base jump from the summit. I am the second woman to free climb El Capitan in a day and the first woman to free climb the Salathe Wall on El Cap.

Although veganism was largely dismissed by climbers at that time, I quickly found that I was performing much better on the rock and in the mountains. I needed less food, which matters when you have to carry your food in a backpack or up a vertical wall. After learning about factory farming, it cemented my commitment to the vegan diet.

I am the author of 2 books *High Infatuation* and *Learning to Fly* and also have a training business in Utah. To learn more about climbing, jumping, the outdoors, simple living and vegan recipes, visit my blog at www.highinfatuation.com.

Damien Mander

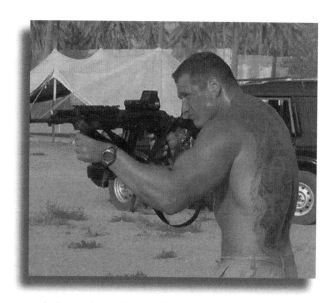

served as a Special Operations Sniper and Clearance Diver in the Australian Defense Force for 12 years. After on the frontlines of the Iraq war as a private contractor, I left the army and went to Africa; it is here that I came face-to-face with the wildlife poaching. I founded the International Anti-Poaching Foundation in 2009, (www.iapf.org.) which focuses on ranger training, operations, and integrating modern technology for conservation in Southern Africa. IAPF's work has since been featured in the media such as National Geographic Magazine, 60 Minutes, Discovery Network, TEDx, Animal Planet, Carte Blanch, Al Jazeera, ABC, Forbes, The Sunday Times, and the UK Daily Telegraph.

During the time I founded IAPF I shifted to veganism, and it has been one of the most significant positive shifts in my life. A plant-based diet provides clarity of mind, energy, determination, and added strength to go out onto the frontlines and defend wildlife. The environmental benefits of this shift towards veganism compliment the life I have chosen.

Christine "Peanut" Vardaros

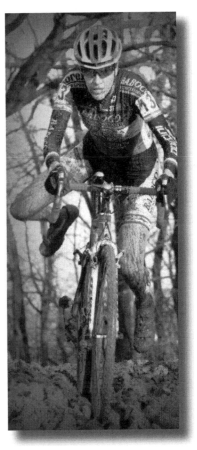

Over my 10 plus years as a pro cyclist, I have won numerous international events; podium'd at many others; and represented my country as a US National Team member in over 30 World Cups, as well as in a few World Championships. Thanks to my vegan diet I am still successfully racing at the top professional level at age 43 – not bad for a gal who eats grass!

Although I had been vegetarian 10 years prior, I became vegan in 2000 for sporting advantages as I upgraded to professional ranks. It became very clear that I was able to recover incredibly well after hard workouts or races. In addition, my breathing dramatically improved, my genetic asthma had all but disappeared, and I am rarely ever sick. I even have more energy than when I was vegetarian years ago. Combining these benefits adds up to more days of training or racing, giving me a serious sporting advantage. The ethical ramifications keep me 100% plant-powered as I even pick sponsors that match my lifestyle.

I contribute as a journalist to magazines and sites like VegNews magazine, CYCLOCROSS magazine, and CyclingNews.com. Follow my adventures on ChristineVardaros.blogspot.com and on my Facebook fanpage. (*Photo Credit: R. Roegiers*).

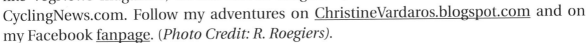

Andy Lally

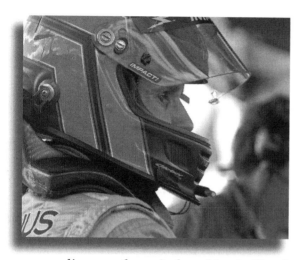

I have been racing cars for 20 years. About 10 years ago, I made the switch to a vegetarian diet and then transitioned to fully vegan. This last decade has been the most successful of my career. I attribute much of my success to being strong inside the car both mentally and physically. I have been fortunate to win the Rolex 24 Hours of Daytona 4 times now, as well as an additional 3 Championships and other long distance race wins. These long races are grueling on the mind and body. You have to be extremely fit in order to push your heart rate as high as it will go while enduring the constant g-force and high cockpit temperatures of a race car.

I went vegan for ethical reasons. Since I was not fully educated on the health benefits of a plant-based diet, I was actually worried how my body would react when I made the transition. While the first couple of weeks were tricky because of the will power it takes to break bad habits, it was easy once I was over that hump, and I quickly started to feel better. My 10k runs were faster, and my mountain bike races for cardio conditioning produced better results. As a practicing martial artist in Brazilian Jiu Jitsu, I always feel I have an edge on my opponents when it comes to cardio during a long match. Ethics aside, I would never go back to my old eating habits after seeing how well my performance has been while vegan.

Ellen Jaffe Jones

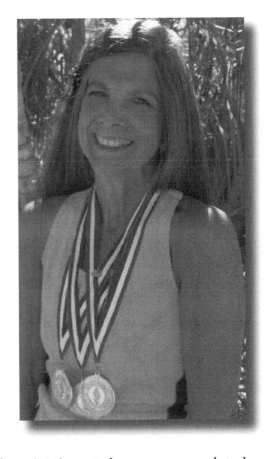

Given my family history of cancer, diabetes, osteoporosis, and Alzheimer's, my doctors are shocked to find I am on no medication at my age. When I was 28, I had a life threatening colon blockage. Rather than taking medications for the rest of my life, I searched for other answers. I read *Don't Forget Fibre in Your Diet* by Denis Burkitt, *Diet for a Small Planet* by Frances Moore Lappe, and *The McDougal Plan* by Dr. McDougal. Switching to a low-fat, plant-based diet, I lost weight and felt amazing. Each time I added back in dairy or fish, I had a major health problem.

As I switched my diet, I started running and placed in 58 5K races for my age group since 2006. In 2010, I ran my first marathon and was the 5th oldest female to finish. In 2013 I placed 7th in the United States at the 2013 National Senior Games in my age group (W60-64) in the 1500 meters. I completely credit my 1500 meters success to a vegan diet by keeping pain and inflammation at a minimum. The publisher of the "Running Journal," says that vegan or not, it is rare for anyone with sprint times to have ever completed a marathon.

I am the author of *Eat Vegan on $4 a Day- A Plan for the Budget-Conscious Cook*, and *Kitchen Divided- Vegan Dishes for Semi-Vegan Households.* I am currently writing 2 more books under contract with a publisher. I am a certified personal trainer (Aerobics and Fitness Association of America) and a certified running coach (Road Runners Club of America) and vegan lifestyle coach in the Bradenton/Sarasota, Florida area.

Fiona Oakes

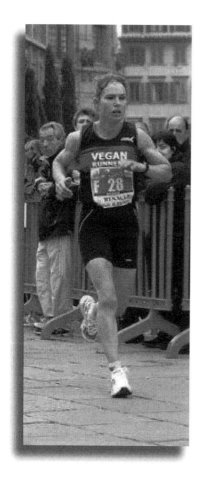

A vegan since age 6 for ethical reasons, I began running marathons to prove that plant-powered athletes can excel in the most challenging of events.

Fifteen years later I have placed in the top 20 in some of the biggest races in the world – Berlin and London, top 10s in Amsterdam, Moscow, Nottingham, Adelaide, along with 6 marathon victories and 5 course records. I have challenged myself to some of the toughest foot races including the Marathon des Sables in 2012 and the North Pole Marathon. The Marathon des Sables race is 7 days of self-sufficiency in the Sahara Desert running roughly a marathon a day with one 'double' marathon stage. The North Pole Marathon tests supreme endurance and physical and mental abilities, as it involves running in temperatures of negative 30 degrees Fahrenheit on the Polar Ice Cap. I not only completed this race, but broke the course record by over 44 minutes in the worst conditions both underfoot and temperature-wise the race had ever seen finishing third overall.

My diet is plain and simple, as I don't have the time or money for 'fancy' extras and supplements. My training consists of running between 80 to 100 miles a week. I base my training, as I do the rest of my life, on discipline, dedication and devotion. This is important since athletic performance is not just about physical conditioning but also mental conditioning. Currently, I am trying to become the fastest woman to run a marathon on every Continent (plus the Polar Ice Cap). I am confident I can do it solely on plant-power.

five

INFLAMMATION: WE CAN'T PUT A BAND-AID ON IT

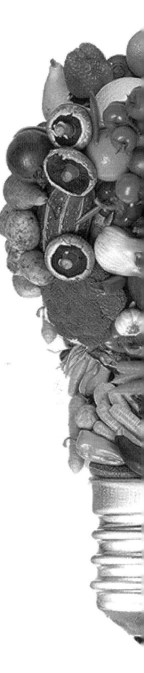

Inflammation is the genesis of every chronic disease. Our body is constantly striving to achieve a perfect pH balance at all times. Humans function in a slightly alkaline pH state which is absolutely critical for good health.

The following experts discuss how acidity in meat and dairy upsets our body's internal pH balance which leads to a pro-inflammatory state, thus laying the foundation for disease. This prolonged state of a highly acidic environment is referred to as low grade metabolic acidosis, which can lead to kidney stones, autoimmune conditions such as Crohn's disease, arthritis, loss of bone mass (osteoporosis) and bone fractures, loss in lean muscle, increase in our waistlines, and the ideal environment for cancer to flourish.

We can think of inflammation as an internal fire. Animal-based foods act as gasoline- changing our gut flora causing the intestinal lining of our gut (endothelial), tissue to become inflamed. It is well established that a single meal high in animal fat can stimulate an inflammatory reaction that harm our arteries, making them stiff as a result.[1] In the 5 to 6 hours it takes for our body to combat this inflammation, it is already time for our next meal. This cycle produces a chronic state of low grade inflammation, one meal at a time. By contrast, plant-based foods are alkaline forming, anti-inflammatory, and antioxidant rich. They function as firefighters, keeping inflammation at bay. Every bite we take will either fuel or put out our internal fire.

Inflammation: Putting Out the Internal Fire

Jay T. Sutliffe, PhD, RD

Lifestyle and food choices have a significant impact on our body's level of inflammation and subsequently the resulting chronic conditions that develop. We have the opportunity and the power to alter, reverse, and prevent many of these conditions by making simple changes at every meal we eat.

Chronic inflammation plays an important role in the development of most of our major lifestyle diseases including atherosclerosis, heart disease, diabetes, and cancers. Think of it as an internal fire taking place within your bloodstream. If we catch the inflammation early enough, we can predict and prevent these conditions from occurring.

Often chronic inflammation goes unnoticed for a long period of time unless it is an obvious pain such as arthritis or joint pain. However, with biomarkers, we can better identify the inflammatory process.

Currently we have found that C-reactive protein (CRP), which is made in the liver, is produced in response to an inflammatory condition in the body.[1] We can think of it as an alarm system where the body detects that there is an invasion or internal dysfunction. While in the past we used homocysteine to look at inflammation levels, CRP is more sensitive. CRP is a measure of acute, or sudden, inflammatory processes within the vascular system in the blood stream.

What Causes Inflammation?

The body is constantly fighting to maintain homeostasis, or balance. For example, in order for our body to maintain certain blood glucose levels, it must also regulate insulin and glucagon hormone levels. This is why type 2 diabetes is also well proven to be connected to inflammation.[2]

Animal protein (meat and dairy) causes an inflammatory response and actually causes CRP levels to rise. One widely proven connection between inflammation and disease is cardiovascular disease. Using the CRP levels, we can actually predict the likelihood of having a cardiovascular event. As the arteries narrow with more and more inflammation, there is continually less passage for the blood flow in the arterial system.[3]

When we bring an onslaught of animal protein into the body, it overloads the body because it is such a concentrated food source. Our bodies do not get a choice to say, "I will deal with that later" -- which is often what we humans do when we have a problem. The body cannot pause, so it has to either: use the food coming in, store it, or get it out of the body.

Animal protein intake causes an overload of nitrogen in the body. Our bodies need to be in a positive nitrogen balance, and the amino acids bring nitrogen into the body. The body has to find a way to deal with the excess nitrogen in a relatively short period of time. We under-emphasize the role of nitrogen in the body as excess causes the kidneys and other organs stress and may initiate the disease process.

Animal-based protein, being highly acidic, also disturbs our body's pH. In order to buffer this acid our body uses calcium, which is leached from the bones, to restore balance. This acidic condition is what initiates the pro-inflammatory response. The antioxidants and minerals from fruits and vegetables attempt to "put out" the fire animal protein creates.

Plant-Based Diets Can Lower Inflammation

I have conducted observational studies, where I have seen the role diet plays in the inflammatory process. We have brought participants into controlled settings for 2 to 3 weeks where we reduce their stress, put them on exercise programs, introduce them to physicians, and monitor them daily. We give them a completely plant-based diet with very minimal processing of the foods. What we have found is that when people consume plant- based foods, the inflammatory response in the body plummets. From our preliminary data, it appears that plant-based diets, which are high in omega 3s and antioxidants, can reduce inflammation in a short period of time. On average, participants are bringing their inflammation levels down dramatically in 17 to 18 days and even more effectively than with medications. [5]

The Western diet, typically very high in processed foods and omega 6 foods and low in omega 3 foods and micronutrients, sets the foundation for a pro-inflammatory condition. Although fish is high in omega 3s, the fish get these nutrients from the green leafy vegetables in the sea (algae). It is better to go straight to the source rather than through animal protein.

It is just as important to completely take out pro-inflammatory foods, which include animal products, processed plant-foods, and simple sugars. Taking out animal protein and replacing it with plant protein will dramatically reduce your inflammation.

Focusing on the Wrong Nutrients: Protein

Protein is the most overrated nutrient. Your protein needs are going to be determined partially by whether or not you are taking in adequate amounts of carbohydrates. If you are eating adequate carbohydrates, then all of your protein can go to build tissue, make enzymes, grow hair, and rebuild your skin and body. The rate of protein consumption and obsession, however, is way beyond where it needs to be.

When your body does not get enough carbohydrates, it can use protein for a fuel source by stripping off the nitrogen. Chemically, if you take the nitrogen off of the protein molecule, it looks like carbohydrate. The body will take a high protein diet and start stripping the nitrogen to use it as a carbohydrate source.

Protein is used to compensate for not just energy but for blood sugar levels as well. Too many people think protein can be used to "fix" their blood sugar levels. However, they are using protein the way fiber is meant to be used. Although protein can buffer fluctuations in blood sugar levels, fiber better controls and regulates blood sugar levels, giving you long-term energy without fluctuations.[6,7] Essentially we are promoting the wrong nutrient, protein, when we should be promoting fiber found in whole plant-foods.

In conclusion, in an effort to prevent or reduce inflammation, the tried and true approach is to consume a wide variety of whole plant foods in as natural a state as possible.

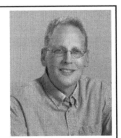

Jay T. Sutliffe, PhD, RD, *is an associate clinical professor in the Health Sciences Department at Northern Arizona University. He holds degrees in Food & Nutrition/Dietetics, Health Education and Public Health, and is also a Registered Dietitian with over 25 years of experience. Together with his wife Chloe they have owned & operated 2 whole foods restaurants/health food store operations and have a passion to assist people of all ages in living an abundant life.*

Acid Trip

Juliet Gellatley, BSc, Dip CNM, Dip DM, FNTP, NTCC

Our body is a finely-tuned organism that works best under certain conditions. We are designed to maintain a stable balance between acid and alkalis in the blood between the slightly alkaline levels of 7.35-7.45. Everything we eat or drink is either acid or alkali forming. and either maintains or upsets this balance. When the acid-alkaline balance in our blood is not stable we put ourselves at risk for developing health conditions, as many illnesses such as cancer thrive and grow in highly acidic conditions.

Animal protein is highly acidic and disrupts our body's stable balance. Since animal based products contain high sulphur content, it turns into sulphuric acid in the body. All animal products are similarly acidifying, flooding the body with acid, which can cause a permanent state of acid overload.[1,2,3] When food is acidic, the body needs to employ one of its buffer systems – namely the skeleton – to neutralize the acid by releasing calcium. Both calcium and acid are then excreted in urine, and only a fraction of the used calcium can be returned to the bones. High acid diets can cause heart disease, obesity, certain cancers, gallstones, kidney stones, bone weaknesses, and other chronic diseases.

We are constantly told that dairy products contain calcium that the body uses to neutralize acid in the blood. While this is true, dairy also contains animal protein, and the acid this creates largely outweighs the alkalis formed by the calcium. The overall effect creates a highly acidic internal environment which uses more calcium to neutralize the acid than the dairy products can provide.[2,3,4] This is one of the major reasons why dairy consuming nations have higher rates of osteoporosis (brittle bones) than those who eat lower amounts.[5]

By contrast, most vegetables, many fruits (including citrus), and nuts and seeds are all alkali-producing foods.[2,6,7] Potassium and magnesium are mainly contained in plant foods and, together with calcium, determine alkaline load. Although some fruits such as lemons and oranges are acidic outside the body, they are alkaline-forming when we digest them. Some grains such as millet, quinoa, spelt, wild rice, and buckwheat are also alkalizing, or are in the 'neutral' zone; some are mildly acidic.[3]

While it is almost impossible to eat only alkaline foods, we need some acidifying foods to maintain a healthy balance. The ideal ratio is around 70:30 of alkalising foods to acidic-producing foods but it is best to steer away completely from animal products – meat, fish and dairy.

A whole food, plant-based diet is not only more alkalising, but it also provide the whole 'package' of goodies needed for a healthy body. It includes vitamins A, C, K, and the B group as well as important minerals – calcium (enough for our daily needs), magnesium, potassium, selenium, boron, iron, copper and zinc. By avoiding animal based products, we feed our body the nutrients it needs and create an environment that lowers our risk for future health problems.

Juliet Gellatley, BSc, Dip CNM, Dip DM, FNTP, NTCC *has a degree in zoology and is a qualified nutritional therapist. She is the founder & director of Viva! and Viva! Health in the UK, and is also the founder of Viva! Poland. She has given hundreds of public talks and is the author of several books, guides, and reports.* Juliet@viva.org.uk www.viva.org.uk www.vivahealth. org.uk

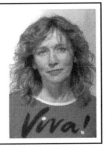

Evolution: Seeing the Light

Dexter Shurney, MD, MBA, MPH

During my time as a practicing general surgeon I became disenchanted with how I and those around me were spending our time and effort caring for patients. The problem was that most of what we were doing was taking care of problems that were largely preventable. Wouldn't it be better to spend our time working to prevent these conditions and ailments on the front-end to avoid all the unnecessary pain and suffering, not to mention the costs?

Preventive medicine is definitely a step in the right direction, but the term is often being misused. For instance, much time is spent on screening efforts with the hope of catching illnesses at an earlier stage in the disease process. Although this is good, such screening doesn't actually prevent the disease from occurring.

Diet Has The Power To Address The Root-Cause Of Illness— True Prevention At The Highest Level

The data on plant- based diets is overwhelming positive and remarkable. The human body has a great capacity to heal itself when provided the right building blocks, or nutrients to work with. Meat and dairy products are largely devoid of most of the essential elements the body needs to repair itself and to sustain optimal health. The essential elements found to be so helpful in this regard are the phyto-nutrients, vitamins, minerals, and fiber which are only found in plant-based, whole foods. In addition to lacking these essential necessary elements, meat and dairy products are also high in harmful saturated fats and cholesterol. **In total, it's a deadly combination to good health.** Given America's preference for an animal-based rather than a plant-based diet, is there any wonder that so many Americans suffer the ill-effects of diet?

Because I suffered from hypertension, hypercholesterolemia, and pre-diabetes (I have a long family history of Type-2 diabetes and coronary heart disease), I decided to try this lifestyle approach and became a vegetarian. Although I was told being vegan would be most effective, I decided to try being vegetarian first and my experiment worked. Within a few months my blood pressure and glucose levels were well within the normal range. I no longer required my diuretic for hypertension and my dose of Lipitor had been cut by more than half. Excited by my success, I decided to take the full plunge and see what would happen to my numbers if I became a complete vegan. On a vegan diet I was able to get off all medications, including Lipitor!

For my patients willing to try, I have seen remarkable results without exception. Since first witnessing the power of a vegan diet on myself, I now highly recommend this diet to all my patients. As a physician and based on the studies I know, it would be negligent on my part not to do so.

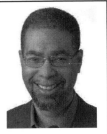

Dexter Shurney, MD, MBA, MPH *is the Chief Medical Director / Executive Director for Global Benefits, Health and Wellness for Cummins, Inc. Dr. Shurney was the Chief Medical Director of the Employee Health Plan for Vanderbilt University and Medical Center. During his tenure at Vanderbilt he also held joint faculty appointments as Assistant Clinical Professor, Division of Internal Medicine and Public Health, and Adjunct Faculty, Owens Graduate School of Management. Dr. Shurney sits on the editorial boards for the peer-reviewed journals Population Health Management and The American Journal of Lifestyle Medicine. Dr. Shurney is co-author of the book Integrating Wellness into Your Disease Management Programs. He was also the most recent Chair of the Business Strategies Committee for Centers for Disease Control and Prevention (CDC)/National Diabetes Education Program (NDEP). Dr. Shurney is board-certified in general preventive medicine and public health.*

The Pain Elimination Solution

David Bullock, DO

Before I became a vegan, I had a severe car accident in 1991 that nearly killed me. For 10 years afterwards, I continued to suffer such immense and frequent migraine and tension headaches and acute neck and back pain that I started every morning taking narcotic pain medications. Although I tried multiple treatment options, including acupuncture, chiropractic, and multiple physical modalities, it was not until my Osteopathic residency that I discovered diet's role in pain management.

During residency, I adopted Dr. Joel Fuhrman's "Nutritarian" lifestyle, a plant-based, vegan diet with an emphasis on "superfoods." Superfoods have the highest micronutrient density. Micronutrients have been shown to help repair DNA damage, or 'evict' toxins from cells (keeping them healthier), and support normal function far better than processed foods or animal products (or even simple starchy plant foods). For example, a recent study on prostate cancer and walnuts found that eating the equivalent of two ounces of walnuts a day both slowed growth and incidence of prostate cancer. The more micronutrients, the greater the ability to cope with illness, prevent disease, and reverse chronic conditions such as diabetes, coronary artery disease, and various auto-immune conditions as well as prevent strokes and dementia. Leafy greens (such as kale, red chard, and baby spinach) are one type of of superfoods that are strongly correlated with longer life in multiple studies. Research done by the National Institute on Drug Abuse and the Department of Neurosurgery showed that blueberries, spinach or spirulina reduced ischemic injury and cerebral infarction (stroke) damage significantly and improved recovery of muscle function after the stroke.[2]

Meat and dairy products are low in micronutrients and antioxidants and promote inflammation, which continues the cycle of swelling and damage to muscles and nerves that inevitably promotes and prolongs pain. Although most people point to the added antibiotics and hormones in meat as dangerous, rather it is the natural components in meat and dairy which contribute to increased pain, inflammation, and disease.

six

A HEARTY PROBLEM

Cardiovascular disease is the leading illness in the world today and is completely preventable. This disease should not even exist. The cause of heart disease is plaque or fatty deposit build up in the 60,000 miles of veins and arteries throughout our body, not just our heart. The culprits are saturated fat and cholesterol from animal-based products.

What would happen if we cut back on animal protein? Would it really "solve" heart disease? In the 1970s Finland's mortality rate from heart disease was the highest in the world. In an effort to reduce heart disease, Finland's government decided to cut back on meat, eggs, and dairy products. Finland implemented nationwide programs that reduced intake of saturated fat from cheese, chicken, cakes, and pork. They even switched dairy farmers to berry farmers. The result? There was an 80% drop in heart disease deaths and the cardiovascular and cancer mortality was cut in half.[1] Remarkable? We think so.

The most amazing news, as the following leading cardiologists and experts in this chapter indicate, is we can reverse and prevent heart disease by eliminating these foods from our diet. In contrast to animal based foods, plant-based foods contain nutrients that improve the overall health of our arteries by minimizing fat and cholesterol. Instead of looking at the history of heart disease in the family, we need to look at our family's breakfast, lunch, and dinner plates.

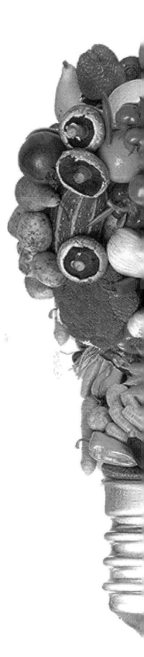

Your Heart on Plants

Robert J. Ostfeld, MD, MSc.

Today cardiac health should be on everyone's mind. On average, 2 heart attacks happen every minute in the United States.[1, 2] If you have a 30 minute commute to work, 60 heart attacks occurred during your trip.

Ten years ago, I would not have picked up this book or any other that offered a plant-based diet as a panacea for heart disease. Throughout my training with physicians and scientists at Yale and Harvard, the impact of a whole food plant-based diet was not featured. I was trained in the world of pills, procedures, and modest lifestyle changes.

After my cardiology fellowship, I began working at Montefiore Medical Center in New York City. Initially, I did all of the things I was trained to do. I followed medical guidelines and prescribed evidence based medications, gave advice regarding exercise, and reviewed a Mediterranean style diet. I even asked my patients to sign onto a plan where they would agree to both exercise more and lose weight.[3, 4] And this worked. A little. We slowed the progression of their heart disease but it did not stop. We were losing the battle. What could we do better?

After reading *The China Study,*[5] and meeting with Dr. Caldwell Esselstyn, the author of *Prevent and Reverse Heart Disease,*[6] I more fully appreciated the importance of diet in preventing and treating heart disease. In his groundbreaking work following 24 patients with severe coronary artery disease for 12 years, among the 18 patients who embraced the whole food plant-based diet, only 1 had a coronary event, and that patient had strayed from the diet. More importantly, those who remained on the diet were alive and doing well.

The biological rationale and research behind a whole food plant-based diet in preventing heart disease is strong.[5,6] Studies show that parts of the world where people eat largely a plant-based diet, such as in rural China or Central Africa, heart disease is extremely uncommon.[7,8] In contrast, in the United States, approximately two out of every three *12 year olds* have early signs of cholesterol disease in the blood vessels that nourish their hearts.[9] Cholesterol disease leads to heart attacks and strokes and is the *number one* killer of adult men and women in the United States.[10]

Based on this research, we started a Cardiac Wellness Program at Montefiore where we encourage patients to eat a whole food plant-based diet with the goal of preventing and reversing disease. We have had the joy of observing the dramatic improvements patients experience in both their health and quality of life. It has been an incredible journey that I have learned is never too early to begin and never too late to start. Before we discuss the science behind why a plant-based diet works, here are three inspiring patient examples:

1. Maria* is in her 60s and could barely walk one block before having to stop. This prevented her from seeing family and friends. She was overweight and had been experiencing uncontrolled diabetes, hypertension, and high cholesterol for years. Although initially resistant to lifestyle changes, after just a few weeks, Maria lost about 10 pounds, her high blood pressure and diabetes medications were decreased, her low-density lipoprotein (LDL) cholesterol (otherwise known as the "bad" cholesterol) fell 40 points, and she was walking 3 to 4 blocks. She literally cried from joy when describing her excitement for the future.

2. Mark, also in his 60s, is married with kids and is a vibrant member of his community. All of that nearly came to an end when he developed crushing chest pain. Major cholesterol blockages in his heart were the cause. Mark did not want an invasive procedure like a coronary stent and despite being placed on all of the appropriate medications his symptoms persisted. He had been eating what he thought was a "healthy" version of the western diet, low in fat with lean meats and some vegetables. After 5 months of embracing a whole food plant-based diet, he lost about 25 pounds, his LDL cholesterol fell 70 points and he was walking more than a mile without chest pain. Now, 2 years later he says he feels better than he did in his 30s!

3. Jay did not fit the picture of a heart patient. In his 40s, he is athletic, exercised regularly, and played in a band. He did not have any known risk factors. One night after a show, he felt intense chest pressure. He was having a heart attack. It was the kind that doctors darkly label the widow maker, because it usually ends in fatality. Fortunately, Jay received immediate care and shortly thereafter made the decision to embrace a whole food plant-based diet. More than a year and a half since his heart attack he has lost weight, his cholesterol is down, he is more active, and he has had no further signs of heart disease.

Traditionally, taking care of patients like Maria, Mark and Jay would have meant dispensing the standard pills, procedures and vague general advice to be healthier. Although pills and procedures can be very important and often do a lot of good, they frequently do not address the "heart" of the problem.

What Is The Whole Food Plant-Based Diet?

Basically, the "diet" consists of nutrient dense foods including all vegetables, fruits, 100% whole grains, beans, spices, lentils, seeds, walnuts, avocado, salads, almond milk, and soymilk. It excludes red meat, chicken, fish, dairy (such as milk, yogurt and cheese), eggs, processed foods, and simple sugars. It's pretty simple: stay away from something with a face or made from something with a face. There is no need for calorie counting.

So why is it good to eat a whole food plant-based diet? Honestly, given what we already know, it amazes me that we are having this debate. Why are we still assuming that the standard American diet, which is associated with multiple health problems including high cholesterol, heart disease and cancer, is the appropriate way to eat?[5,8] Think of it this way: do we really need to prove that parachutes are important when jumping out of planes?[11] That is common sense to us. The Western dietary link to heart disease should no longer be in question.

Preventing Heart Disease with Diet

In my decade of practice, outside of interventions following an extreme medical emergency, like someone having a large heart attack and receiving a stent, I have never seen anything come close to the breadth and depth of benefit that a whole food plant-based diet provides.

Let's look in more detail at a few of the benefits, starting first with cholesterol. Cholesterol has many important functions but in excess is harmful. It is a waxy substance that is used to produce certain hormones, Vitamin D and bile acids that are essential for digestion. Reassuringly, our brilliant bodies make all of the cholesterol we need. We do not need to eat any. Not a drop.[12]

When we are born, our LDL cholesterol is wonderfully low- at about 30-70 mg/dl, and[13] over the years we may munch our way up to much higher levels. The "average" "normal" adult in the United States has an LDL level of about 120 mg/dl.[14] Yet, half of all heart attacks occur in adults with "normal" cholesterol levels.[15] Hence, to me, normal is not normal.

Lower Cholesterol with a Plant-Based Diet

How can cholesterol levels fall with a plant-based diet?

Although this explanation is an oversimplification of a complicated process, cholesterol levels fall because we absorb less and excrete more. If there is no cholesterol in your diet you won't absorb it from your diet. Animal-based foods have cholesterol, and plant-based foods essentially do not.[46,47] Hence, when we eat a plant-based diet, there is for all practical purposes no cholesterol to absorb. Furthermore, the fiber found in a whole food plant-based diet binds to some of the bile acids leading to their excretion, further reducing our cholesterol levels.

When LDL is in excess, a condition that frequently arises from eating animal products, it makes its home in the body's arteries, creating deposits called plaque. LDL burrows into the walls of your arteries-kind of like sliding under wallpaper. In the arteries, LDL is very irritating, like a splinter, causing inflammation and the production of toxic free radicals. White blood cells are directed into the wall of the artery to try and gobble up the intruding cholesterol, but they only wind up making the problem worse. The cholesterol plaque slowly grows, gradually clogging the artery, making it harder for blood to flow. This process may go on for years, further damaging the artery until one day, its inner lining, the "wallpaper", cracks, exposing the blood directly to the growing gob of toxic junk living inside the vessel wall. When that happens, the blood flowing in the center of the artery clots nearly instantly. If the clot is big enough, all blood flow in that artery stops, killing the tissue it feeds. This causes a heart attack. Even if the "wallpaper" doesn't ever crack, the whole cascade is damaging to the health of your blood vessels and hence, to you.[16]

> **Fun Fact:** All the endothelial cells in your body would cover about 7 tennis courts.[48] That's a lot of cells that we can either keep healthy, or not.

Science tells us that blockages take years to develop[16] and they may take years to reverse.[8] So how can symptoms from cholesterol blockages like chest pressure or shortness of breath get better in just a few weeks with a plant-based diet? Our endothelial cells come to the rescue.

Cardiologists often say that you are as young as your endothelium. Endothelial cells, or the endothelium, line the innermost wall of your arteries. On a whole food plant-based diet, endothelial cells more readily make a substance called nitric oxide.[17, 18] Nitric oxide, among its many beneficial effects, helps arteries dilate so that it is easier for blood to get to where it needs to go, like turning a one-lane street into a three-lane highway.[19] For example, if you go for a walk, your leg muscles will need more blood. The healthy endothelial cells lining the blood vessels in your legs will then make nitric oxide, directing more blood to your leg muscles and giving them the oxygen and nutrients they need. The same goes for your heart, your brain, your skin and every other organ in your body. When those organs need more blood, healthy endothelial cells make nitric oxide, directing blood to the organs that need it. It's like a beautiful symphony. Treat your endothelial cells well and they will treat you well. Treat them poorly and they will treat you poorly. How do we keep them healthy? The answer, of course, lies on the end of our fork. Even one unhealthy meal can transiently damage those endothelial cells.[20]

We have only scratched the surface of what healthy endothelial cells can do. Its product, nitric oxide, not only helps blood vessels dilate; it helps blood flow more smoothly and makes blood less sticky. It quiets the inflammation and free radicals brewing within

Animal- Based Foods Produce Toxins that Damage Blood Vessels

Fascinating new work further highlights the toxic effects of animal based foods. In recent studies, when omnivores were fed steak or eggs they made a substance called trimethyl amine oxide (TMAO). TMAO adversely impacts cholesterol transport in a way that is toxic to endothelial cells, promoting diseased blood vessels. However, when people who ate a plant-based diet for at least one year were fed the same steak or eggs, they made virtually no TMAO. The reason has to do with the bacteria in our gut. We all have tons of bacteria in our gut and many of those bacteria are our friends and they help us digest and absorb nutrients we need. Omnivores and vegans have different compositions of bacteria living in their guts and omnivores have more of the specific bacteria that make TMAO.[49, 50]

the cholesterol plaques in our arterial walls, potentially slowing and even reversing the process while simultaneously making our blood vessels healthier. [21, 22]

Healthy endothelial cells can even help with high blood pressure, which is called the silent killer, because even though you don't feel it, it can kill you.[23,24] If you are 55 years old and living in the US, your lifetime risk of developing high blood pressure is about 90%.[25] High blood pressure also causes strokes, heart attacks and kidney damage.[24] Although an oversimplification, blood pressure falls on a whole food plant-based diet because healthy endothelial cells help arteries relax, leading to less pressure on their walls with each heartbeat.

In the office, I frequently get asked 2 questions about this dietary change. First, "where will I get my protein?" With a varied whole food plant-based diet your protein needs will easily be met.[5,26,27] In fact, broccoli is approximately 35% protein![28] And, many other vegetables are superb sources of protein as are nuts, seeds, hemp and beans. We should also note that animal based protein has detrimental effects. For example, it creates a toxic acidic environment in our bodies, which, among other things, leeches calcium from bones, promoting osteoporosis.[29-32] Furthermore, protein in cow's milk is associated with promoting cancer, autoimmune diseases and even kidney stones.[33-42] I have never seen one of my follow-up patients walk in with a protein deficiency. I have, however, seen them walk out much healthier.

The second question is whether eating a plant-based diet improves erectile function. The short answer – yes! To put this problem into perspective, up to 40% of men aged 40 and older and up to 70% of men 70 years and older have some degree of erectile dysfunction.[43] Achieving an erection is a complex process that involves psychology, the nervous system and our blood vessels.[44] The same kinds of factors that damage the blood vessels to our heart, brain and body also damage the blood vessels to our penis. The process is so similar, in fact, that erectile dysfunction is often called the canary in the coal mine for heart disease. Why the canary? Because the blood vessels that feed the penis are smaller than those that feed the heart so blood flow to the penis may become compromised sooner than blood flow to the heart. Accordingly, a healthier lifestyle improves erectile function.[45] And, on a whole food plant-based diet, many of our patients report improved erectile function.

Listen to Your Heart

If you are reading this you may already be plant-based or interested in exploring the wonders of a plant-based diet. Wherever you are in this spectrum, I can say this – as a practicing physician of over 10 years, I am confident that it will change your life. And as someone who is plant-based, I can vouch for the fact that it changed mine, both personally and professionally.

My patients have been able to reduce or completely discontinue medications for high blood pressure, diabetes and high cholesterol. They have lost weight, report fewer colds, have clearer skin, feel more energetic and describe clearer thinking. I have never seen anything so remarkable. And a great part is that the patient is in control. They know that what they put on their fork helps determine their health.

The hard truth is that none of us are immune from the modern day plagues caused by the western diet. Far too many otherwise healthy looking adults come into the hospital with heart attacks and strokes. Being thin, athletic and young does not make you immune.

In general, when we are born, our bodies are like turbo engines. Years of burgers and chips later, we turn those turbo engines into clunkers. Let's turn back the clock, because we can.

Robert Ostfeld, MD, MSc., *a cardiologist, earned his BA from the University of Pennsylvania; his MD from Yale University School of Medicine; his Masters of Science in Epidemiology from Harvard School of Public Health and completed his residency at the Massachusetts General Hospital, and his cardiology fellowship and research fellowship in Preventive Medicine at Brigham and Women's Hospital, Harvard teaching hospitals. He is the founder and director of the Cardiac Wellness Program at Montefiore, an Associate Professor of Clinical Medicine at the Albert Einstein College of Medicine and the Associate Director of the Cardiology Fellowship at Montefiore-Einstein. Dr. Ostfeld was elected to the Leo M. Davidoff Society at Einstein for outstanding achievement in the teaching of medical students.*

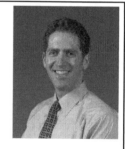

Patient names and identifiers have been changed.

Ending the Coronary Heart Disease Epidemic[1]

Caldwell B. Esselstyn, Jr., MD

The cause of coronary artery heart disease is no longer a mystery. We know that cultures whether by heritage or tradition consume plant based nutrition have virtually no cardiovascular disease. Individuals with established coronary artery disease who completely transition to plant based foods can halt and reverse their disease.

Just suppose all Americans took it upon themselves to help this nation eliminate its crushing debt from the skyrocketing expenses of Medicare and Medicaid. The PDAY (Pathobiologic Determinants of Atherosclerosis in the Young) study of 1999 determined that disease of the coronary arteries was ubiquitous in the autopsy finding of young Americans between the ages of 17 and 34 years who had died from accidents, homicides, or suicides. Chicago Economists, Topel and Murphy reporting back in 1999 in the Chicago University Press calculated a $40 trillion dollar savings for the nation if we just eliminate heart disease – a tall order yet possible. However, since 1999, the incidence of heart disease has dramatically increased and so have the healthcare costs.

At the time you graduate from high school in this country you receive a diploma and the early formation of coronary artery disease. Western world foods cause vascular endothelial injury and compromise the capacity of the endothelial lining to manufacture the gas NO (nitric oxide) which is the guardian and life jacket of our blood vessels.

The injurious foods are oil, dairy, meat, fish, fowl, eggs, coffee with caffeine, and sugar (fructose). Recent Cleveland Clinic research discovered an additional way these foods injure arteries as omnivores possess intestinal bacteria which convert animal foods into TMAO (trimethylamine oxide) which is a molecule that promotes vascular injury but not in those consuming plant based foods which do not possess intestinal bacteria capable of making TMAO. This research and our knowledge of nitric oxide production destruction by oil and animal based food is powerful validation of why whole food plant-based nutrition is successful.

Experts in coronary artery disease concur that injury to the endothelial lining of blood vessels is the inception of heart disease. The typical western diet of milkshakes, cheeseburgers and pizza lead to intracellular adhesion molecules (stickiness) of intravascular cellular elements. This phenomenon results in LDL cholesterol migrating beneath the endothelial lining into the sub-endothelial space where LDL cholesterol is oxidized by free radicals to small, hard, dense LDL cholesterol. White blood cells within the tissue as macrophages ingest the oxidized LDL molecules creating a storm of oxidative inflammation. As these reactive oxygen species accumulate, the size of the plaque increases. The macrophage once filled with oxidized LDL particles is now renamed a foam cell. The foam cell manufactures powerful enzymes which erode the cap over the plaque on the wall of the artery. The weakened cap may eventually rupture spilling plaque content into the flowing blood. The spilled plaque content activates platelets to initiate clotting which may rapidly clot the entire artery. The fully clotted artery now deprives the heart muscle downstream from the clot of all oxygen and nutrients and it dies. This is a heart attack and how 90% of them occur.

This disastrous flow of events need never happen. It is not caused by your genes. The good news is that without pills and drugs, or entering a cardiac cathedral for stents or bypass surgery, you can be empowered to prevent, halt, and reverse this lethal cascade of coronary artery heart disease through following the lessons of cultures without heart disease that thrive on whole food plant- based nutrition.

In 1985 I initiated a study utilizing whole food plant based nutrition in a small group of severely ill patients with coronary artery disease. My eureka moment came a year later with a patient in his 50s that had significant vascular disease of his heart and right leg. He initially reported he had to stop 5 times with right calf pain while crossing the skyway to my office. A pulse volume study revealed a markedly diminished ankle pulse. Nine months into treatment he reported he no longer had to stop crossing the skyway as all calf pain was gone. A repeat pulse volume was now doubled in comparison to his earlier baseline study. Since statin drugs were not in use at this time, this was confirmation and proof of concept that whole food plant based nutrition alone could halt and reverse cardiovascular illness.

Twelve years later we reviewed the cardiovascular events of our 18 patients. We found during the 8 years prior to entering our study, while in the hand of expert cardiologists, they had experienced 49 cardiac events reflecting disease progression, whereas, during the 12 years in our study 17 of the 18 experienced no further events. One initially adherent but subsequently after 6 years non-adherent participant developed angina and the need for bypass surgery. This illustrates the need for compliance.

Twelve of our early group had follow up catheterization angiograms. Four (33%) confirmed significant disease reversal. We now had evidence that consuming whole food plant based nutrition could not only eliminate future cardiac events but could also achieve selective angiographic disease reversal. Even those without angiographic reversal benefit from a powerful more subtle reversal. The health of their endothelial cells and their capacity to produce more nitric oxide is restored. The robust antioxidant nutrition of whole grains, legumes, red, yellow, and especially green leafy vegetables and fruit enables them to diminish the oxidative inflammation of plaques and foam cells thus strengthening the cap over these plaques. A strengthened cap cannot rupture and adherent participants have now made themselves heart attack proof without expense, risk, ineffective drugs, stents, and bypass surgery.

A frequent comment by skeptics of my original study is that it was too small and a larger group might not comply. I recently submitted, with colleagues, an updated study of 200 participants with significant cardiovascular disease followed almost 4 years. This manuscript is presently in press with a peer reviewed journal to be published by early 2014. The adherence rate was close to 90%. We, the authors and the editors, anticipate it may be a significant contribution capable of swaying physicians to the benefits of whole food plant nutrition.

Our approach succeeds because the patients have been instructed as to causation of their disease. This renews the covenant of trust between the caregiver and patient recognized since the days of Hippocrates: whenever possible treat the cause of the illness. While this approach is not used in cardiovascular medicine today, the high-risk expensive therapy this specialty employs accounts for 45% of Medicare expenses. Many cardiovascular specialists are caring and compassionate but are simply not aware of the studies on the success of plant based nutrition or if aware they have no idea how to achieve it as they never receive nutrition study in their training. Numerous physicians admit to being uncomfortable discussing lifestyle transition with their patients. Even those who believe are unable or unwilling to find the time in their schedules to achieve successful behavioral modification. Physicians deserve compensation for their time and effort in this activity yet the insurance system is sadly lacking in creative support. The financial conflict created with this simple effective whole foods plant-based approach qualifies as an enormous threat to medicine's biggest cash cow of drugs, stents, bypasses and hospital income.

Nevertheless, the environment today is quite different than 30 years ago. Physicians attend and apprentice with our 5 hour intensive counseling seminar and employ it in their practice with equal effect. Patients are more inquisitive about plant-based alternatives and are challenging the usual interventional techniques.

Present cardiovascular therapy does not cure patients, it does not end the cardiovascular disease epidemic, and it is financially unsustainable. However, it is perhaps unfair to ask cardiovascular medicine to shoulder all the burden of this lifestyle transition. They have busy schedules, lack training in this approach, and may lack motivation. Those with a passion and knowledge of lifestyle medicine will welcome the opportunity to work synergistically in the spirit of cooperative endeavor with cardiovascular colleagues to enable those participants in need of this lifestyle transition to become empowered to eliminate their disease.

In my opinion, it is unconscionable for physicians not to inform patients of this powerful option. A seismic revolution in health is possible for the United States. This revolution will not come about from the invention of another drug, another procedure, or another operation. It will come about when those of us in the healing profession have the will and determination to share with the public the lifestyle which empowers them to be the locus of control to eliminate common chronic killing diseases.

Caldwell B. Esselstyn Jr., MD *received his B.A. from Yale University and his M.D. from Western Reserve University. Dr. Esselstyn presently directs the cardiovascular prevention and reversal program at The Cleveland Clinic Wellness Institute.He is the best-selling author of Prevent and Reverse Heart Disease, featured on CNN and has authored over 150 publications. Dr. Esselystn trained as a surgeon at the Cleveland Clinic and at St. George's Hospital in London. Since 1968 he has been associated with the Cleveland Clinic, serving as President of the Staff and as a member of the Board of Governors. In 1991, Dr. Esselstyn served as President of the American Association of Endocrine Surgeons, That same year he organized the first National Conference on the Elimination of Coronary Artery Disease. In 1968, he was awarded the Bronze Star as an Army surgeon in Vietnam. He was a member of the victorious United States Gold Medal rowing* 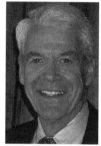 *team in the 1956 Olympics. Dr. Esselstyn and his wife, Ann Crile Esselstyn, have followed a plant-based diet for more than 26 years. The Esselstyns have four children and eight grandchildren.*

Eat to Cure Heart Disease

Carl Turissini, M.D., FACC

As an Interventional Cardiologist, by the time patients are referred to me and I place a stent in one of their greasy coronary plaques or, worse, send them to bypass surgery, they are already manifesting an end stage coronary disease process. When I started practicing two decades ago I did not see a significant association between diet and heart disease. I was trained in high tech, cutting edge cardiology where diet seldom was considered. Sure, we realized the American diet was unhealthy, but whatever role diet played we thought could be overcome by medicines and medical procedures.

Over the last 10 years, I have seen a dramatic change in the profile of my patients. They are younger, more obese, and lacking many of the traditional cardiac risk factors such as smoking or family history. It is more and more common for me to place metal stents in patients in their 30s and 40s and have the vast majority of my patients present with elevated blood sugars (either glucose intolerance or Type 2 diabetes). Two decades ago, the only patients I treated in this age group were either heavy smokers or cocaine users. While we expounded the virtues of lean meats and less fat, the dismal result has been younger, fatter, and sicker patients. The American Heart Association predicts that heart disease will cost our country $818 billion dollars per year by 2030. To an observant cardiologist, the link between diet and coronary disease is clear. My understanding of this relationship between diet and heart disease led me to a career change I never expected: a plant-based Interventional Cardiologist.

The statistics are alarming. In just 30 years, Americans have packed on so much weight that now nearly two thirds of all Americans are overweight and one third are obese. Diabetes has increased fourfold since 1980. While most diabetic patients tell me that their problem is genetic, it is actually impossible for this rapid increase to be genetic. There is no way the human genome can mutate that fast to cause this diabetic epidemic. Our diet and lifestyle are the only plausible explanations.

So what happened? I think the answer lies in understanding how our diet has changed over the past several hundred years with the advent of modern agriculture and more recently with food processing. Our closest relatives, the chimpanzees, are probably the best living example of what our diet looked like before modern agriculture. Chimpanzees eat plants and fruit all day, but eat meat only about 9 days per year.[1] In the past 100,000 years, humans evolved with a diet that was primarily the same—low- fat and plant-based. We seldom ate meat.[2] Our bodies were not designed to capture prey, and our tools for hunting and fishing were primitive. Even more recently and closer to home,

Americans 200 years ago seldom ate meat. In the early 1800s, meat was too expensive and too impractical for most Americans. Only the rich ate meat on a regular basis, which is why gout, caused by the breakdown of protein, was called the "rich man's disease." Most Americans would only eat meat on special occasions such as Easter and weddings.

However, by 1910 advances in farming and transportation increased consumption to 100 pounds of meat per capita, and by 2007, to an astounding 220 pounds of meat per person. During the same 200 years, our per capita sugar consumption rose from 15 pounds per year to 160 pounds per year. Since this change in diet occurred over the course of many generations it went largely unnoticed, and established dietary habits learned early in life were never questioned.

For example, drinking milk is still a rather recent event in the human evolutionary time span. Milk is generally accepted as a healthy food source even though it is essentially liquid flesh and comprised of fat, protein, and cholesterol found in meat. We are the only species to drink milk after weaning and the only species to drink the milk from another species. The mere fact that two thirds of all adults are lactose intolerant shows a lack of evolution towards milk as a food source.

More recently, processed food has become the norm. Processed food by design is laden with fat, sugar, and salt to increase market share. The result is a near addiction to all three. We find it acceptable to continue to eat unhealthy cholesterol laden foods and, at the same time, take cholesterol medicines with potential side effects to lower our cholesterol. Yet, despite all of these advances in technology and pharmaceuticals, the incidence of heart disease-- as well as obesity, diabetes, hypertension, coronary disease, and cancer-- continues to rise. All of these can be both prevented and, in some cases, reversed by adopting a whole food, low fat, and plant-based diet.

Evidence of the benefits of a plant-based diet is observed even today in some cultures where cardiovascular disease is virtually nonexistent. The Tarahumara native Mexicans, Papua New Guinea Highlanders, and residents of rural China and rural Africa are all very culturally diverse but they share two common characteristics: all lack heart disease, and all follow a plant- based diet.[3]

Although low fat, plant-based diets dramatically reduce cholesterol and weight, the marked benefits of a low fat, plant-based diet are much greater than these. The improvement in nitric oxide may account for this remarkable reduction in risk. Nitric oxide is so important that it was called the "molecule of the year" by Science magazine in 1992.[6] Nitric oxide is a molecule produced by the endothelium, or the lining of our

Type 2 Diabetes, Heart Disease & a Plant-Based Diet

Even mild elevations of blood sugar (greater than 100 mg/dl) can greatly increase the risk of coronary disease. Insulin resistance, due to the American diet, is the main culprit in type II diabetes. Insulin resistance is reduced and hyperglycemia is improved by a whole food plant-based diet.[4] In fact, type II diabetes can be completely reversed with a whole food plant-based diet.[5]

blood vessels. Nitric oxide has many roles: it is a potent vasodilator, it regulates artery health, and more importantly protects against the development of coronary plaques. Nitric oxide is suppressed by diabetes, high cholesterol, and cigarette smoking. It can even become suppressed by just one fatty meal. Dr. Robert Vogel showed that just one meal of sausage and hash brown potatoes compared to oatmeal can markedly suppress nitric oxide function for up to 4 hours, despite no changes in serum lipids.[7] Since Americans eat fatty meals 2 to 3 times a day, nitric oxide is being continually suppressed. Over time, this can significantly contribute to the development of atherosclerosis or plaque buildup in the arteries.

Plant-based diets improve intestinal bacteria, which studies show plays a role in many diseases. The human gut is filled with bacteria that are greatly influenced by diet and especially meat intake. L-carnitine is an amino acid found abundantly in red meat. L-carnitine is metabolized by intestinal bacteria to trimethylamine (TMA), which is converted to trimethylamine-N-oxide (TMAO) by the liver. It is well known that both L-carnitine and TMAO cause cholesterol deposition in arteries. A study in which vegans, vegetarians, and meat eaters were all given a high carnitine meal found that meat eaters had a much higher level of TMAO after carnitine ingestion than did vegetarians or vegans. When these researchers fed L-carnitine to mice, they found double the incidence of arterial plaques. When the mice were treated with bacteria-suppressing antibiotics the plaque forming effect of L-carnitine was blocked, proving the causative role played by intestinal bacteria. This helps explain why vegans and vegetarians have lower heart disease incidents and why red meat consumption is associated with more cardiovascular disease than other meats or fish.[8]

As a cardiologist, I tell my patients that there is no need for heart disease to exist at all. Of the many plant- based health benefits, the prevention and reversal of coronary disease probably has the most scientific support. Dr. Nathan Pritikin was one of the first to show that a low-fat primarily plant-based diet markedly reduced cholesterol and obesity. In the 1980s, Dr. Dean Ornish showed that a vegetarian diet combined with lifestyle changes such as exercise and smoking cessation can actually slow regression of coronary plaques.[10] The Framingham study evidenced that persons with total cholesterol less than 150 mg/dl are virtually protected from coronary disease.[9] Caldwell Esselstyn Jr., MD demonstrated a plant-based diet's role in both prevention and reversal of coronary disease in his patients. His 12 year longitudinal study, evaluated 40 patients all of whom had coronary disease. Eighteen patients (originally 24 but 6 were noncompliant) whom collectively had 49 cardiac events (defined as heart attacks, strokes, need for revascularization, and death) in the 8 years prior to the study, agreed to follow a low-fat, plant-based diet. During the 12 years on the diet none experienced cardiac events. By comparison, the 20 patients still following the standard American diet had 45 cardiac events collectively in the 12 years follow-up. Of the patients on the plant-based diet, coronary angiograms showed that all the patients had arrested the progression of coronary disease and 73% actually showed reversal of the coronary disease.[11] These dramatic results, zero cardiac events and regression of disease, are far superior to any achieved with any other diet, statin drug, aspirin or Plavix, cardiac stents, or bypass surgery.

In contrast, the Lyon Diet Heart Study placed patients with known coronary disease on a Mediterranean diet consisting of olive oil, bread, fruit and vegetables, fish, and a moderate amount of dairy (mostly cheese) and wine. In just 4 years, 25% of the Mediterranean diet patients went on to have a cardiac event.[12] In the Courage Trial, patients were treated with optimal medical therapy including intensive cholesterol medication, Aspirin or Plavix, diet, exercise, and blood sugar control. Even with these aggressive medical interventions, 23% had cardiac events in the subsequent 4.5 years.[13]

A plant-based diet is as delicious as it is healthy. It does take time for the body and taste buds to adjust to this way of eating, and it can take up to a year for the sugar addiction to subside. Many will have to learn an entire new ways of shopping, cooking, and eating that are unfamiliar to them. However, with substantial education and support, we cannot only achieve a lifetime free of heart disease and diabetes, but a better quality of life. When faced with the alternative of coronary stents, bypass surgery, and multiple medications, a low fat plant-based diet is the only appropriate course of action.

Dedicated to Caldwell Esselstyn Jr., MD
It takes courage and perseverance to shift the paradigm.

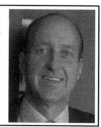

Carl J. Turissini, MD, FACC, *is the Director of Interventional Cardiology at Hallmark Health System, and Staff Physician, Department of Cardiology, Massachusetts General Hospital, and Clinical Associate at Harvard Medical School. Dr. Turrisini has practiced Cardiology for over 20 years and is board certified in Internal Medicine, Cardiology, and Interventional Cardiology. Dr. Turrisini routinely lectures on plant based benefits and has appeared as a guest on "About Health with Jeanne Blake." For more information, please visit: www.eat2cure.org*

The Statin Concept—Medication vs. Prevention

Richard A. Oppenlander, D.D.S.

The most widely prescribed medications in the world belong to the statin family—Crestor, Lipitor, Pravachol, Lescol, and Zocor—garnering over 6% of all medication purchases. Annual sales of statins globally have reached $26 billion. Only 1 out of 100,000 people have genetically transmitted or familial hypercholesterolemia (a condition where the body is producing hundreds of milligrams of cholesterol daily); these individuals need cholesterol medication. Rather than relegating oneself to taking a statin pill every day and being confronted with the possibility of stents, quadruple bypass surgery, and other procedures for cardiac and circulatory vessel collapse, it should be an easy choice to simply not eat animal products.

My Darling Cholesterol, Treat Me Right

Joaquin Carral, MD

Why is cholesterol so bad if we need it to live? Cholesterol is a lipid (fat) molecule that is synthesized by the liver and other organs of our body and is transported to all the cells in our body so that they can use it.[1] We can produce all the cholesterol that we need in our liver and other cells.[2, 3] Cholesterol is essential for all animal life and vital for normal body function. But dietary intake of cholesterol from meat and dairy sources increases cholesterol levels, which subsequently contributes to today's leading chronic conditions such as atherosclerosis and heart disease.

Cholesterol has three main functions in our body:

1. It helps the cells keep their membranes flexible, so it's in the lining or membrane of every cell in our body.

2. It is the precursor of many vital hormones like estrogen or testosterone.

3. It helps us absorb fat in our digestion. The liver creates the bile components from cholesterol, and when they are secreted to the gut, they help coat the digested fats so that we can absorb them.

All the cholesterol that we need is made by our own cells and it is transported to the whole body so that it can be used where it's needed. After the liver has produced the cholesterol, it is packed into transporter molecules and sent to the blood. These molecules are known as *lipoproteins*. They are classified based on their density, and referred to as high density lipoprotein (HDL), intermediate density lipoprotein (IDL), low density lipoprotein (LDL), very low density lipoprotein (VLDL), and chylomicrons. These transporter molecules are like buses that take cholesterol and other fats from the liver to the organs or back from the organs to the liver.[4]

When you hear the terms *good cholesterol* and *bad cholesterol*, doctors are talking about these cholesterol transporters. After the cholesterol is synthesized in the liver, it is packaged into a very low density lipoprotein (VLDL) or a low density lipoprotein (LDL) and sent to the blood. Most of the cholesterol that goes from the liver into the organs or arteries (blood vessels) is transported in the form of low density lipoprotein cholesterol (LDL-C). This is the bad cholesterol because it takes the cholesterol to the arteries.

The route that goes the other way—from the organs or arteries to the liver,—gets transported in the high density lipoprotein cholesterol (HDL-C). This is the good cholesterol because it takes the cholesterol from the arteries and helps them get healthy, and sends it back to the liver where it is not harmful. This is why our doctors want our LDL-cholesterol to be lower and our HDL-cholesterol to be higher.

Cholesterol in the blood can be abnormally elevated when we eat dietary cholesterol and saturated fat from animal products like dairy, eggs, chicken, meat, and fish.[5] Although certain genetic diseases can elevate cholesterol, they only affect 0.3 to 0.2 percent of the population,[6] so in most cases the cause of elevated cholesterol is from food sources. Since we produce all the cholesterol that we need, we don't need extra cholesterol from external sources. But in the standard American diet (SAD) we get so much cholesterol and saturated fat that our cholesterol is dramatically elevated.

Having elevated cholesterol is very dangerous. It is one of the major causes of the number-one killer in the Western world—heart disease. Because it is so dangerous to have elevated cholesterol, many of the top selling drugs in the world treat elevated cholesterol. The most used ones are statins like atorvastatin (Lipitor) or rosuvastatin (Crestor).[7]

When we have too much cholesterol it is reflected in the amount of LDL-C in the blood, this transporter travels to the arteries and drops off its passenger, cholesterol, into the wall of the blood vessel. When the cholesterol is in between the cells of the vessel, it chemically reacts and becomes even more dangerous. The body tries to fight this invader and sends cells, some of which will try to eat up the cholesterol, but they end up malfunctioning from the cholesterol inside and become big goblets of cholesterol sitting in the artery. This process creates more and more inflammation. After some time a bump (like a pimple) appears in the wall of the blood vessel. This bump is called *plaque*. The plaque can do two bad things. One is grow into a "stable plaque" and restrict the flow of blood into the organs. The other more dangerous effect is that it can rupture ("unstable plaque") and create a clot that will block the flow of blood completely. This is when heart attacks or strokes happen.[8]

How Does Cholesterol Affect Me?

Around the heart there is a system of arteries that supply the blood to the pumping muscle. When there is stable plaque in those arteries called *coronaries,* we can develop chest pain, also called *angina,* and we may have shortness of breath because of the lack of flow into the coronaries. This is like someone squeezing the water hose, so we can't get the blood flow that we need. This type of plaque usually does not rupture, and doctors put in stents to restore the blood flow.

Almost all heart attacks happen where there is unstable plaque. This unstable plaque is a thin buildup of cholesterol that has so much inflammation that it can burst open at any point. When that happens, our blood will try to heal it quickly by creating a blood clot. But this blood clot will block all the blood flow and create a heart attack. Since this unstable plaque is small, we can't see it so easily, and therefore we can't put stents in it. But as Dr. Ornish's study showed we can eat healthier to regress this plaque. [9]

Strokes are the equivalent of a heart attack that happens in the brain. There are two types of strokes. One is a blockage of blood flow as in a heart attack, and the other is bleeding inside the brain. The most common one is a blockage of blood flow into the brain. This can happen in two ways. A blood clot can travel all the way to the brain, usually from the heart or the neck and brain blood vessels. When this clot reaches the point where it can't travel any further, it sits there blocking all the blood flow to that area of the brain, and this brain tissue starts to die, creating a stroke. When these events happen again and again, they can damage little parts of the brain over time. This process can cause the second most common cause of dementia after Alzheimer's, called vascular dementia. [10, 11, 12]

Even our legs can be affected from excess cholesterol, called peripheral artery disease. When blood flow is reduced due to cholesterol plaque buildup, the legs can't get the blood they need to move. Usually people with this problem have tired or painful legs while walking a few blocks. This pain usually goes away after resting for a couple of minutes. In the extreme case of lack of blood flow, there can be gangrene, where all the parts of the leg die because they are not getting any blood.

Excess cholesterol affects all of our organs causing erectile dysfunction,[13] stroke, and peripheral artery disease among other problems. The good news is that there is a way to prevent this buildup from getting worse, or even reverse it completely by eating a whole food plant-based diet. [14, 15, 16, 17]

Joaquin Carral, MD, *grew up in Mexico and attended Anahuac University in Mexico City. He completed his residency in Internal Medicine at St. Luke's Roosevelt Hospital center in New York, where he served as the Chief Resident. Dr. Carral has worked with Dr. Neal Barnard in the Physician's Committee for Responsible Medicine and with Dr. John McDougall in his ten day program in Santa Rosa California. Currently, he is a Fellow in Preventive Cardiology in New York University to continue to help patients to live a healthier life.*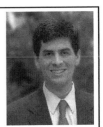

Don't Have a Stroke- Eat Plant-Based!

John Pippin, MD, Cardiologist

The elevated risk for coronary heart disease and heart attacks from diets high in red meats, processed meats, and other dietary sources of animal fats is widely known and incorporated into dietary recommendations for heart disease risk factors. Less often considered, however, is the similarly elevated risk for stroke associated with these dietary components and the typical Western diet characterized by beef, poultry, seafood, egg, and dairy consumption. This dietary link to stroke risk has been demonstrated in prospective studies and meta-analyses for both men and women in the U.S. and other countries. Comparative studies have also shown the protective effects of plant-based diets for heart disease and stroke. Similar dietary risks are confirmed for peripheral vascular disease as well, so it is prudent to conclude that diets high in meat, eggs, and dairy products – sources of animal fats – confer serious risk for morbidity and mortality throughout the cardiovascular system.

Atherosclerosis: A Preventable Pandemic?

Rick Koch, MD, FACC

Atherosclerosis, or coronary artery disease, is far and away the number one killer of both men and women in the United States. Atherosclerosis is a hardening or buildup of plaque in the arteries, particularly in the coronary arteries. By age 53, 50% of white males have measurable coronary disease and by age 66, 50% of white females have measurable coronary disease.[1]

We are facing a pandemic problem and are already on the verge of breaking the American medical system. There were 600,000 deaths from heart disease in this country last year and 365,000 deaths from heart attacks alone.[2,3] The obesity and diabetes trends we are seeing with children are worrisome. We are now seeing the first pathogenesis of atherosclerosis, and cholesterol streaking of the arteries in children as young as age 11.[4] With the advent of obesity and early onset of type 2 diabetes in children, this age range could be even younger. The lifestyle modification needs to be implemented as early as possible.

Our current medical system is more concerned with cleaning up problems, rather than focusing on prevention. **Eighty percent of adverse cardiovascular events are deemed preventable.**[5] through a combination of lifestyle modifications, meaning diet, exercise and healthy lifestyle choices, such as not smoking and preventing high blood pressure, diabetes, and high cholesterol.

The Relationship between Cholesterol, Triglycerides, and Heart Attacks

A heart attack is a rupture of plaques that build-up in the arteries. Current misinformation about the contributing factors to heart attacks and coronary blockage is that cholesterol plays little role and sugar- driven triglycerides play a larger role. Yet cardiology research says the exact opposite.

Cholesterol comes from 2 important sources. The first is we produce our own cholesterol without any dietary intake in the liver. The second source comes from food sources. To be clear, dietary intake of cholesterol only comes from animal products. When we lower LDL, low-density lipids, portion of cholesterol, we can reverse cholesterol deposits that have built up over decades in our arteries. We find when the LDL cholesterol is lowered to less than 70 it reduced existing cholesterol deposits by 13% 6 months later.[6] Additionally studies have shown that blood flow to the heart muscle improved in those with significant blockages when they were placed on vegan diets.

A study in Britain which compared those who consume meat to vegetarians and vegans, found that vegetarians have a 24% reduction in adverse cardiovascular events (heart attacks, stroke and deaths) and lifelong vegans had 57% decrease.[7] As the only difference in the vegetarian and a vegan cohort is dairy and eggs, there is just as much benefit from cutting out dairy as meat. LDL cholesterol, associated with heart attack risk, is more affected by meat and dairy products. This same study found that when they put people on a vegan diet, they saw a 33% reduction in LDL cholesterol in 2 weeks, whereas normally it can take up to 6 to 12 weeks to see changes on medications.[7] This challenges some of the information disseminated in society that dairy and meat don't have a significant impact on heart attack risk as research data directly and definitively goes against these implications.

If heart attacks and arterial blockage was primarily associated with triglycerides, then fish oil, which is very effective at lowering triglycerides and contain omega 3 fatty acids, would lower heart attack rates. However, this has not been evidenced. There is a sugar component to heart attack risk as it relates to weight gain. However, current scientific evidence refutes the notion that heart attacks are primarily sugar-driven.

Reversing Heart Disease

It is estimated that 50% of people find out they have heart disease with their first heart attack. One of the unfortunate dirty little secrets in cardiology is the fact that 68% of heart attacks occur in coronary arteries that have less than 50% blockage.[8] Even stress tests do not accurately tell if you have heart disease or if you are a vulnerable patient. Sixty-eight percent of the people who have heart attacks presumably would have had a normal stress test. This causes a false security blanket. Sudden death from a preventable disease is unacceptable, especially since heart disease IS reversible.

Heart disease does have a genetic component. If you have a family member who has had a significant coronary disease at a younger age that means you are 2 to 4 times more likely to have significant heart disease yourself.[9] That's the power of genetics. If you are someone at risk, you can lower your risk through the following: maintaining a lean body mass, stop smoking, exercise regularly (at least 30 minutes 6 times a week) and ensuring you get screened for diabetes. While you can't change your genetic predisposition, you do have the power to lower and treat you cholesterol levels and diet is an incredibly potent way to do that.

Currently, statin medications are commonly used to lower cholesterol. Statins predominantly lower LDL cholesterol but also affect triglycerides, which can play a role in heart attacks by modifying how your liver produces cholesterol. While statins, have had an impact on lowering the rates of heart attacks on a per capita basis, diet can also drastically lower and maintain healthy cholesterol levels.

The only way to completely eliminate dietary cholesterol is to remove animal products from your diet, and eat a whole food, plant-based diet. Even if you are genetically pre-disposed, by eliminating dietary cholesterol from animal products you can bring your levels to your natural cholesterol production. If you lower your blood concentration of your LDL cholesterol significantly enough – (LDL 40-60)- it could be enough to both halt the development of atherosclerosis and reverse atherosclerosis that's already there. It took decades for the cholesterol to build up so it will similarly take decades for it to reverse that process. It's never too late to start making those changes.

We underestimate the impact of eliminating animal protein. Inflammation from both animal protein and sugar make the plaques vulnerable to rupture. Our body tries to stabilize inflammation and over time the soft cholesterol plaques turn into calcium. When they calcify, this is referred to as the "hardening of the arteries."

The coronary calcium screening is a painless, low radiation CT scan that can measure the calcified coronary deposits. A score of zero indicates that there are no measurable calcified deposits but it doesn't mean atherosclerosis doesn't exist as it takes time for the plaque to calcify. This test is not only inexpensive but the single best non-invasive screening testing for asymptomatic individuals. The testing can be a motivating factor for patients as it can show how much heart disease you have and your risk factor. This test is best in individuals at intermediate risk for having heart disease (women > 55 years old and men > 45 years old with at least one risk factor).[10]

By using biomarkers- such as cholesterol (particularly LDL), weight, and blood pressure, we can track these parameters and changes in patients to see the impact of diet. Biomarkers show the patient where they are today and by tracking changes we can visually associate success with decrease in weight, cholesterol, and ability to reduce medications.

With knowledge comes power and knowing what you can do breeds empowerment. The science and evidence we have seen now tells us that we need to expand our minds and stop underestimating the impact of diet and lifestyle. This healthy lifestyle can have significant effects on all of us. The economic burden for heart attacks this year alone is an estimated $109 billion dollars.[11] Heart disease and strokes combined cost an estimated $312 billion dollars through a combination of the direct costs for critical care, medications, and loss of productivity.[11] This number is expected to increase to $818 billion dollars by 2030 unless we interrupt this cascade.[11]

As a physician, I am here to partner with my patients. It is my responsibility to explain what the potential benefit is and strongly recommend following a well balanced whole food, plant-based diet, especially, if you do not want to be on drugs indefinitely.

I encourage my patients to find a local support network either within their local community or virtually. It is important and powerful to have support as meal times provide an opportunity for support or difficulty, especially in homes where not everyone is committed. Remember, changing habits is not easy but you have the power to prevent a cardiovascular tragedy.

Rick Koch MD, *attended University of Chicago's Pritzker medical school as well as completing his Internal Medicine Residency and Cardiology Fellowship at University of Chicago Hospitals where he remained active in academic research publishing many papers. Dr. Koch is board certified in Cardiovascular Diseases, Internal Medicine, Echocardiography, Nuclear Cardiology and Cardiovascular CT. Initially, an engineer, he received his BS in Electrical Engineering from Rensselaer Polytechnic Institute and worked as a software engineer for Hewlett-Packard. He currently practices as a non-invasive cardiologist at Bend Memorial Clinic in Bend, Oregon where he serves as the Director of Advanced Non-Invasive Cardiovascular Imaging.*

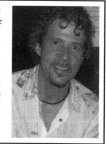

Diet and Atherosclerotic Disease

Kristofer M Charlton-Ouw, MD, FACS & Scott J Aronin, MS, CSCS, CES

What do heart attacks, strokes, and amputations have in common? These conditions are all caused by a gradual clogging of our arteries known as atherosclerosis. Although our genetic make-up might influence our susceptibility to atherosclerosis, our biggest modifiable risk factors for preventing this condition and its consequences are in our control.

Atherosclerosis is a systemic inflammatory process that causes plaques to build up in different arteries around the body. The plaques consist of inflammatory cells and fatty acids such as cholesterol and triglycerides. These plaques can grow and eventually completely block the artery. When this happens, the organ supplied by that artery, such as the heart, may not get enough blood flow and is deemed *ischemic*. Even relatively small atherosclerotic plaques that do not significantly limit blood flow can cause trouble when the plaques rupture. The ruptured plaque causes platelets and clot to form around the plaque. These clots then break off and block other arteries.

Although atherosclerosis can affect arteries all over the body, the specific location of the plaque determines the patient's symptoms. For example, atherosclerotic plaque in the carotid artery that supplies the main blood flow to the brain is a major cause of *stroke*. Plaques that block the heart arteries can limit blood flow and cause *angina* or chest pain when exercising. When these plaques rupture and suddenly block the smaller downstream arteries, it causes a *myocardial infarction* or heart attack. Plaque that builds up in the arteries supplying the leg causes pain with exercise or *claudication*. Many patients are surprised at the bulk of their plaque, which can be seen and felt without magnification. When enough arteries are blocked, ulcers and gangrene occur in the toes and feet and is the leading cause of leg amputation. Complications of atherosclerotic peripheral arterial disease are the most common reasons for the estimated 65,000 leg amputations performed in the U.S. each year.[1]

Interventional cardiologists and vascular surgeons can crush plaques by causing controlled plaque rupture in arteries using a balloon inside the artery. Severe atherosclerotic disease can also be surgically treated. Most of us have heard of bypass surgery where surgeons create new channels around arteries blocked by plaque. Despite advances in medical and surgical care along with new drugs to lower cholesterol and antiplatelet agents, there is no question that prevention of atherosclerosis would save many people from heart attacks, strokes, and amputations. Diabetes, family history, obesity, tobacco smoking, exercise, and diet play a role in causing atherosclerosis. We have little control over our family history and the genes we inherit that make us more susceptible to atherosclerosis. However, our biggest modifiable risk factors for atherosclerosis prevention are smoking, exercise, and diet. This chapter focuses on the role of diet and atherosclerotic disease

The Relationship Between Diet and Atherosclerosis

Based on the process by which atherosclerotic plaque forms, it seems clear that there are dietary connections to the development of clogged arteries. The United States dietary patterns are connected to a higher incidence of atherosclerosis. When examined, this same association is not true for other populations around the world that have dramatically lower rates of atherosclerotic disease.[2,3]

The body of medical literature on diet and atherosclerotic disease is large. Studies have evidenced that a plant-based diet[4,5]; diets that contain more fruits and vegetables by quantity and proportion[6,7]; that contain less sugar[8,9,10]; more fiber[11]; lower quantities of refined carbohydrates of all types; and lower trans-fat, cholesterol and saturated fat diets are all associated with lower rates of atherosclerotic disease.[12] It also seems possible that diets with more whole grains as opposed to refined grains,[13] and with less refined Omega-6-heavy vegetable oil[14] are also protective against atherosclerosis and other diseases, like diabetes, cancer and arthritis.[15,16]

Further, some related studies show an actual reversal of arterial blockage in subjects who adhered to dietary regimens such as low fat (10% of diet), vegetarian or similar diet, and who quit smoking (in some cases), engaged in stress reduction training and activities and, in other cases, undertook regular aerobic activity.[17,18] It should be noted that a "plant-based" diet evaluated in studies contained no animal products.

Let us look more closely at these studies to see why the above dietary factors are connected to lower atherosclerosis disease rates.

A Note on Dietary Studies

There are some limiting factors to finding clear effects of one specific dietary factor on health outcomes, including atherosclerotic disease. For example, obesity and overweight are independent risk factors on their own through mechanisms of hyperleptinemia or too much of the appetite control hormone, leptin, in the blood. Other shortcomings include: differentiating between types of fat and protein, relying on people to give accurate accounts of their own diets, and lifestyle factors that can accompany a certain type of eating. In a number of important studies that showed the actual reversal of plaque buildup in arteries, study subjects were also engaging in stress-reduction training and the effects of these interventions were not independently known.

Dietary risk factors for atherosclerotic disease include body weight and obesity, low density lipoprotein cholesterol (LDL), total cholesterol, triglycerides, hemoglobin A1C (a measure of sugars bound to hemoglobin which indicates average plasma glucose concentrations over the previous weeks to months), blood sugar/diabetes, hypertension, C-reactive protein (CRP) and other markers of inflammation[19] as well as homocysteine. Diets associated with these risk factors are higher in fat, protein and cholesterol. For instance, diets high in fat and cholesterol yield high blood cholesterol and triglycerides. They are also directly linked to atherosclerotic lesions and insulin resistance. Dietary cholesterol has been shown to increase plaque formation, serum triglycerides and insulin resistance. Diets higher in protein (usually also higher in fat and cholesterol) are linked to increased atherosclerosis in a dose-dependent manner.[20] These components are associated with higher consumption of meat and dairy products.

On the other hand, plant-based diets demonstrate lower serum cholesterol and triglyceride levels, decreased incidence of cardiovascular events, and even reversal of arterial atherosclerosis. In general, vegetarians have lower incidence of atherosclerosis, cardiac events, and all-cause mortality. Large studies indicate the best effects were associated with diets that were completely plant-based and not just vegetarian. In a trial of Seventh Day Adventists, vegetarians had much lower than average rates of death from heart attack and other causes.[21]

Can Exercise Reduce Your Risk?

Interestingly, although obesity rates were much lower in the Cornell China study population, calorie intake was actually higher by 30% This was explained to be a likely result of the higher rate of physical activity in rural China- even office workers tended to bicycle to work. Exercise itself reduces risk and incidence of atherosclerotic disease. However, a case cannot be made that the increased exercise can explain all of the differences in cardiovascular deaths between this study population and the overall American population.

Across-cultural large trial, The Cornell China Study, showed how rural Chinese had a fraction of the death rate from heart disease compared to Americans. American men had almost 17 times the death rate from atherosclerotic heart disease and American women had 5.5 times higher mortality from the same cause. The average Chinese dietary fat intake was less than half as a proportion of diet, fiber intake was 3 times as high and animal protein intake was comparatively very low at less than 10% of that in the US diet, and vegetable intake was much higher. The rates of atherosclerotic disease were positively associated with meat intake and sodium intake but decreased in relation to consumption of green vegetables and plasma levels of mono-unsaturated fatty acids. Although the project did not set out to study vegans or plant-based diets, the conclusion was that a plant-based diet is the most preferable way to avoid atherosclerosis.[22]

Plant-based diets also minimize the risk of sugar and excess protein intake, which are risk factors for atherosclerosis.[23] Added sugar intake is associated with both higher incidences of atherosclerotic disease and also rises in related risk factors like blood cholesterol. In addition, protein intake is also positively correlated to cardiovascular disease. In large population studies it is unclear if the detrimental health effect is a result of the protein intake itself or the fact that higher protein diets were also higher in animal foods and the fats (many saturated) and cholesterol that they contain.[24] Either way, plant-based diets tended to mitigate this risk.

The body of literature on diet and atherosclerosis suggests that plant-based diets confer lower risk of cardiovascular events. Plant-based diets are associated with lower serum cholesterol and triglycerides, less obesity, decreased systemic inflammatory markers, and lower blood glucose and homocysteine levels. Vegetarians and vegans certainly have lower rates of this disease than the American population as a whole. It seems that beyond just reducing animal food intake, increasing vegetable and overall fiber intake, reducing consumption of added sugar and increasing the ratio of Omega-3 to Omega-6 fatty acids in the diet all reduce the risk of atherosclerotic disease, as well as the other primary disease killers in western populations.

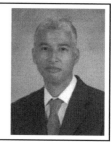

Kristofer M Charlton-Ouw, MD, FACS *is Board Certified as both a Vascular and General Surgeon. He works in the Department of Cardiothoracic and Vascular Surgery at the University of Texas Medical School in Houston, Texas.*

Scott J Aronin, MS, CSCS, CES *heads the Professional Fitness and Wellness Consulting, Lords Valley, PA.*

Lower Blood Pressure and Reverse Atherosclerosis

Jennifer Rooke MD, MPH

High blood pressure (BP) is the most common chronic medical condition in the world. One in every three adults in the world has high BP and over the age of 60 the rate jumps to 1 in every 2 people, or every other person.[1] If you are over 55 years old and live in the US, you have a 90% chance of developing a high BP at some point in your lifetime, [2] but that risk varies around the world. Rural India, for example, has the lowest rates (3.4% in men and 6.8% in women) and Poland has the highest rates (68.9% in men and 72.5% in women).

What is Blood Pressure?

The blood vessels in your body are divided into 2 main categories: those going from your heart to the rest of the body, called arteries, and those going from the body to the heart, called veins. The arteries carry blood with oxygen and nutrients to nourish the cells in all parts of body while the veins carry "empty" blood back to the heart and lungs for a refill. The heart is a pump that is continuously contracting and relaxing to push blood into the arteries. In between contractions the heart fills up with blood from the veins that it will push back out into the arteries when it contracts again. When the heart contracts and pushes blood out into the arteries, the force of blood flowing in the arteries under pressure is the systolic pressure (top number). When the heart is relaxed and filling, the pressure in the arteries is the diastolic pressure (bottom number).

$$\frac{130}{85}$$

What does this mean?

The medical community has generally agreed that the upper limit of the "normal" BP range is 140/90 mmHg, if your BP is consistently above 140/90 on three separate occasions your health care provider will diagnose hypertension, but an ideal BP is actually around 115/75 mmHg. This is where the BP-related risk of death from heart attacks and strokes is near zero. Every 20 mmHg increase in systolic pressure or 10 mmHg increase in diastolic pressure doubles the risk of death from a heart attack or a stroke.[3] You can see that at 140/90 your BP may be in the "normal" range, but you actually have double the risk of death from a heart attack or a stroke as someone with a BP of 120/80.

A high BP is a warning sign that blood is not flowing smoothly through your arteries. The most common reason for decreased blood flow through arteries is atherosclerosis, an inflammatory disease of the artery walls characterized by fatty pus filled abscesses called plaque that narrow the space where blood flows. More force is required to push blood through narrowed arteries and this increases the pressure in the arteries.

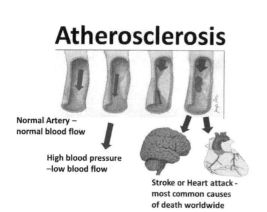

Atherosclerosis

Normal Artery –
normal blood flow

High blood pressure
–low blood flow

Stroke or Heart attack -
most common causes
of death worldwide

When an atherosclerotic abscess ruptures the debris and blood that spills into the artery can form a clot and completely block blood flow. If the blocked artery supplies the heart the person will have a heart attack. If the blocked artery supplies the brain, the person will have a stroke. In some cases the pressure to push blood through clogged arteries in the brain can rise so high that a blood vessel will break and bleed into the brain, this is a hemorrhagic stroke. ***Although we think of heart attacks and strokes as separate diseases they are both outcomes of the same underlying disease - atherosclerosis.***

Heart attacks and strokes are dramatic life-threatening events, but atherosclerosis decreases blood flow to all parts of the body and, over time, the results can be equally devastating. Decreased blood flow to the brain may result in shrinkage which leads to vascular dementia and possibly Alzheimer's disease. Decreased blood flow to the kidneys causes sodium retention which further increases BP and can lead to renal failure and require dialysis for survival. Decreased blood flow is the most common cause of erectile dysfunction. While it may not be a life-threatening problem, it can decrease quality of life. High BP can be controlled and all of these conditions can be reversed by reversing atherosclerosis.

The only way to reverse atherosclerosis is with a cholesterol-free plant-based diet. Atherosclerosis is not a new disease; CT scans of Egyptian mummies and the remains of ancient hunter-gathers from different parts of the world show that they too had atherosclerosis.[4] Doctors reported seeing it on autopsies for centuries, but it was thought to be a normal part of aging. In the early 1900s pathologists showed that this was not the case when they produced atherosclerotic lesions in rabbits by feeding them cholesterol containing foods; food without cholesterol did not produce atherosclerosis.[5] Since then there has been much debate in the scientific community about how cholesterol causes atherosclerosis but the fact remains that dietary cholesterol does cause it. Reversal of atherosclerosis occurs when cholesterol containing foods are removed from the diet.

In 1990 Dr. Dean Ornish showed that atherosclerosis could be reversed by feeding humans a mostly plant based diet with stress management and exercise.[6] In 2001 Dr. Caldwell Esselstyn demonstrated that eliminating cholesterol containing foods would completely reverse atherosclerotic plaques.[7] There are no medications that can reverse atherosclerosis, and the severity does not seem to be related to the serum cholesterol level. In a 2008 study, over half of the patients who were hospitalized with heart attacks had normal serum cholesterol levels.[8] Lowering cho-

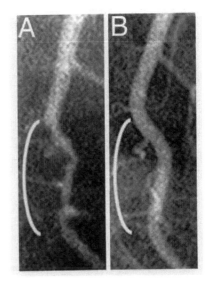

lesterol levels with medications such as statins may not be protective and the American Food and Drug Administration warns that statin may increase the risk of type 2 diabetes, muscular pain, memory loss and mental confusion.[9]

The only way to unclog arteries without costly cardiac catheterization and stents- which re-clog without dietary changes - is to eat a cholesterol-free diet. The only foods that contain cholesterol are animal products: cheese, eggs, fish, milk, chicken and every kind of meat, including grass-fed and organic meat. Cholesterol cannot be cut away from lean meat as it is in every single cell of the animal's body.

A - Coronary angiogram of clogged arteries before study.

B- Coronary angiogram after 32 weeks on a cholesterol-free plant based/vegetarian diet.

The scientific-evidence is very clear. From *Prevent and Reverse Heart Disease* by Caldwell Esselstyn, MD

The only standard medical advice on diet and blood pressure is to limit salt. Sodium raises blood pressure by increasing blood volume and causing vasoconstriction, but the effect of salt is worse if arteries are already clogged and narrowed by atherosclerosis. Potassium has the opposite effect to sodium (salt) as it is a mild diuretic and mild vasodilator-- it decreases blood volume and opens arteries. Increasing sodium intake by 100 mmol (about 1 teaspoon salt) increased systolic blood pressure by an average or 3mmHg while the equivalent amount of potassium decreased systolic blood pressure by 6.1 mm Hg.[10] You can see that the balance of potassium to sodium is more important than just limiting salt. All unprocessed fruits, vegetables, nuts and seeds have relatively high potassium to sodium (K: Na) ratios. These foods also contain the amino acids necessary to make all the proteins needed for optimal human function. In kidneys that are already damaged by low blood flow, high blood pressure, or other renal disease diets high in animal protein can increase the rate of functional decline.

Stress is also a factor in high blood pressure because stress can cause vasoconstriction which further narrows already clogged narrowed arteries. Reversing atherosclerosis by eating a cholesterol-free and high potassium to sodium ratio diet will not eliminate life stresses, but it will decrease the impact that stress has on increasing blood pressure.

If your blood pressure is consistently above 130/80, with or without medications consider this a warning that it is time to eliminate animal products from your diet, eat more foods with a high potassium: sodium ratio, learn how to counter your stress response with relaxation, and get regular physical activity. "But," you say, "There is nothing I can do because high blood pressure runs in my family." Stop thinking that now. Your blood pressure is more a reflection of your lifestyle habits than your genes. If you have a family history of hypertension it is even more important for you to make lifestyle changes now that will protect your children by example in the future.

Jennifer Rooke, MD, MPH, *is the Medical Director of Advanced Lifestyle Medicine and author of "Lifestyle Interventions to Prevent and Reverse Hypertension." Dr. Rooke is board certified in both Public Health/Preventive Medicine and Occupational Medicine. She is a fellow of American College of Occupational and Environmental Medicine, and the American College of Preventive Medicine and serves as an Adjunct Clinical Assistant Professor in the Department of Community Health and Preventive Medicine at Morehouse School of Medicine and in the Department of Family and Preventive Medicine at Emory University. www.advancedlifestylemedicine.com*

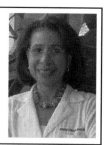

Hypertension: A Silent Dietary Disease

James Craner, MD, MPH, FACOEM, FACP

Hypertension, or high blood pressure, is one of the most prevalent chronic diseases in the United States and other westernized nations. It occurs in adults of all ages and disproportionately affects certain minority populations and individuals above age 60.

High blood pressure is an insidious, *asymptomatic* condition. If left uncontrolled over many years, hypertension significantly increases the risk for fatal or debilitating cardiovascular outcomes, including: myocardial infarction (heart attack), stroke (cerebrovascular accident), congestive heart failure, dialysis-dependent kidney failure, peripheral vascular disease (PVD) including major artery obstruction, aortic aneurysm, carotid stenosis, ischemic bowel disease, and erectile dysfunction in men. [1-4] These diseases account for 50% of all deaths in adult Americans, hence hypertension's reputation as the "silent killer." Direct complications of advanced hypertension include hypertensive crisis (nosebleeds, severe headaches, encephalopathy, myocardial ischemia), acute and chronic heart failure, cerebral (brain) hemorrhage and infarct (a form of stroke), and retinopathy leading to loss of vision.

Much of the economic and emotional burden of hypertension—and nearly all its related vascular diseases—can be prevented or substantively reduced by changes toward a low-fat, plant-based diet.

What Causes Hypertension?

Approximately 95% of hypertension is categorized as having an 'unknown' cause, and is euphemistically referred to as "essential hypertension." Only a very small proportion (<5%) of hypertension is caused by specific diseases of the kidney, endocrine organs, collagen vascular diseases, medications or occupational toxins, or other uncommon, treatable conditions.

However, a plethora of epidemiological and clinical studies published over the past 50 years collectively demonstrate that diet plays the most critically important role, and genetics a lesser role. [5]

Numerous population studies confirm a direct, strong relationship between obesity and risk for hypertension. [4, 6-9] As many as 60% of hypertensives are overweight or obese. [10, 11] In a large prospective study of US nurses, obesity and overweight were directly associated with increased risk for hypertension, while weight loss was associated with reduced risk.[6] The combination of a "family history" of hypertension and obesity is associated with a 3 to 4- fold risk of developing hypertension.[12] Not all individuals who consume an unhealthy diet are overweight, but being overweight or obese is a strong marker for such dietary choices.

The Standard of Care Treatment: Ineffective Diet, Medication for Life

Most of the approximately 50 million Americans diagnosed with hypertension—and the many more who have the disease but have not been diagnosed—are treated with one or more of medications.[19] Total annual costs for medication, complications, and treatment of complications in the US exceed $15 billion (in 1996 dollars).[20] Research has shown that among those with moderate to severe hypertension, the risk of heart attack and stroke is lowered with blood pressure reduction, but no research evidence exists that any medication actually *reverses* the disease.

The incidence of adverse side effects from anti-hypertensive medications is significant. The billions of dollars from treatment of side effects often exceed the costs of the drugs themselves—an important windfall for the "health care" industry.[21, 22]

Vegetarian Diet to Prevent and Treat Hypertension

Cross-sectional studies of populations throughout the world that adhere to vegetarian diets, and interventional studies in people with elevated blood pressure, have demonstrated that vegetarians and plant-based diets significantly reduced risk for hypertension and cardiovascular diseases.[5, 23-27]

Although direct scientific "evidence" to justify treatment or prevention of hypertension with a vegan (i.e. completely plant-based) diet is lacking, dietary studies have provided substantive "evidence" of how a plant-centered diet impacts development or progression of hypertension and related diseases. A number of small research studies demonstrate how dietary changes positively reduce blood pressure in people with hypertension as well as people with normal/high blood pressure over about 6 weeks time.[28-30] In a study of 29 individuals, all of whom had been taking medications for hypertension for at least 8 years, nearly all had significant reductions in blood pressure even after stopping their medications after one year of a vegan diet.[31]

The most aggressive and successful vegan intervention program was conducted by John McDougall, MD in Santa Rosa, CA.[32] The study followed 500 self-referred hypercholesterolemic subjects with a variety of health problems who attended a 12-day residential lifestyle modification program. They consumed a very low fat (5% of calories from fat), **vegan** (i.e., no animal products) diet with no restrictions on portion size. They also exercised and practiced stress management techniques. In most cases, all blood pressure medications were stopped shortly after beginning the program. Within 11 days, subjects experienced an average drop of -9/-4 in blood pressure, while those with higher blood pressures on admission had the most dramatic declines (-17/-13 average). Lipid profiles and weight similarly improved, and participants typically left the program free of medication not only for hypertension but also for other chronic vascular diseases. This investigation demonstrated the rapid, significant physiological effects on blood pressure with an idealized vegan diet that only restricts the type but not amount of food ingested.

The Ornish *et al* study demonstrated that a 1-year regimen of very low fat, lacto-vegetarian diet combined with regular exercise and meditation in individuals with advanced coronary artery disease (CAD) and risk factors, including hypertension, reduced the extent of CAD and blood pressure.[33] However, changes in blood pressure may have been due to the ongoing use of medication in both groups, since CAD lesions, and not risk factors *per se*, were the targeted endpoint for measurement.

Among the many studies of vegetarians and vegetarian diets, no single nutrient source has yet been identified as a principal blood pressure-lowering factor.[34]

Implications

Most of the burden of hypertension and its related conditions is practically preventable or reversible through primarily dietary means. The available scientific evidence accumulated in the past 30 years collectively indicates that the widespread adoption of low-fat, plant-based diet accomplish this goal and thus represents the safest, most cost-effective means of primary and secondary prevention (i.e. treatment of early disease).[35]

Even dieticians, the bastion of the *status quo*, have come to accept and even advocate plant-based diets based on the available research evidence of their beneficial effects on disease prevention and reversal.

To accomplish population-wide change in dietary practices and reduce the massive burden of this and related diseases, the perverse economic priorities that propagate the *status quo* must be effectively challenged and overturned. Physicians[37], the health care industry, pharmaceutical companies, the food industry, and ultimately the public—the "stakeholders"-- must have real incentives to change their behaviors.

This chapter is excerpted from his chapter, *Hypertension*, in Carlson P (Ed.), The Complete Vegetarian: The Essential Guide to Good Health published by University of Illinois Press, Urbana, IL, 2009.

James Craner, MD, MPH, FACOEM, FACP *is a graduate of Princeton University and Harvard Medical School. He completed residencies in Internal Medicine (Rhode Island Hospital/ Brown University School of Medicine) and Occupational & Environmental Medicine (Rutgers Medical School), as well as a Master of Public Health from Rutgers University. Dr. Craner is board certified in Occupational Medicine and Internal Medicine (1991-2012). He also serves as an assistant clinical professor in Occupational Medicine at the University of California, San Francisco (UCSF) School of Medicine. Dr. Craner has practiced Occupational & Environmental Medicine and Internal Medicine for 20 years based in Reno, Nevada USA. He is the developer of webOSCARä, a web-based system that companies use to better protect their employees' health. As a long-time vegan, Dr. Craner actively promotes sustainable approaches to human and environmental health.*

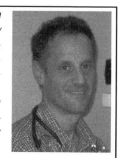

The Most Effective Tools for Preventing and Treating Heart Disease

Heather Shenkman, MD, FACC

Medications, stents, and CT scans have become synonymous with treating heart disease. But what role does diet play and how effective are these technological tools in actually saving lives?

What is Coronary Artery Disease and How is it Detected?

Coronary artery disease consists of plaque buildup in the arteries of the heart. This can lead to angina, which is pain or shortness of breath due to lack of blood flow to portions of the heart, a heart attack, or even sudden death. Although risk factors for coronary artery disease like age and genetics are out of our control, there are several risk factors associated with increased incidence, such as blood pressure, cholesterol, diabetes, smoking, and stress that can be addressed through lifestyle changes. Medications, along with a plant-based diet and regular exercise, can treat and even reverse coronary disease.

How Can Stress Tests and CT Scans Help?

I see many patients who come in for a consultation with me worried about whether they have coronary disease. Some patients, based on their risk factors and symptoms, are certainly justified in seeking cardiology evaluation. However, only if I feel their symptoms are suggestive of coronary artery disease, will I proceed with a stress test. As nuclear stress tests transmit quite a bit of radiation, (one single test can emit more radiation than a person would otherwise be subjected to over the course of one year), it is imprudent to do an unnecessary stress test because of the possible harm, such as increasing risk of several forms of cancer.

Stress tests don't necessarily predict heart attacks, either. In fact, news anchor Tim Russert had a "normal" stress test one month before he died of a massive heart attack. Stress tests are designed to look for areas of the heart that may not be getting enough blood flow. Typically, these would be areas of the heart with major coronary artery blockages of 70% or greater. However, these severe blockages are not where heart attacks originate. Heart attacks generally occur when moderate plaque, typically a 40-50% blockage, ruptures and travels downstream and suddenly blocks blood flow.

It is important to weigh the possible harm versus any benefit that can come from a test. For example, in the event that a low-risk, asymptomatic patient undergoes a stress test, and the stress test results are abnormal, odds are that the test results are a "false positive" rather than a truly abnormal test. This abnormal test can then lead to more invasive and more risky testing. In the case of an abnormal stress test, the next step is usually a coronary angiogram, also called a "cath." This invasive test involves feeding catheters through the major arteries of the body to the heart, injecting dye, and taking x-ray pictures. While the test is considered "low risk", there is a 1 in 1000 chance of major complications, including stroke, heart attack, need for emergent heart bypass or vascular surgery, bleeding, infection, or damage to the kidneys from the dye used. In the case that a significant blockage is found, and the patient receives an angioplasty- a procedure to open up a severe narrowing of an artery (often with a stent), the risk of complications rises to 1 in 100.

What about coronary CT scans? These tests are not appropriate for patients at low or high-risk. However, for a patient who is considered to be at intermediate risk, a coronary CT scan can be beneficial to reclassify a patient as either low-risk or high-risk. This may help a physician and patient decide on a future course of care. It is also important to know that coronary CT scans do not specifically convey how much disease is in the coronary arteries; rather they illustrate how much calcium is present. Further, they are not functional tests, as they do not assess whether various areas of the heart are compromised by lack of blood flow during stress.

Setting the Record Straight on Stents

I hear many patients talk about the stent that "saved their life." The truth, though, is that unless an angioplasty is performed in the setting of a heart attack, stents do not save lives but rather simply open arteries and improve blood flow which can decrease symptoms such as chest pain or shortness of breath.

The COURAGE study shook the cardiology community upon its publication in 2007. Researchers looked at patients with chronic stable angina- chest pain and symptoms attributed to coronary artery disease. Patients were randomly assigned to 1 of 2 treatment groups. One group received invasive treatment with either an angioplasty or bypass surgery to improve blood flow. The other group was assigned to medical therapy alone. Medical therapy, in this circumstance, consisted of appropriate doses of medication to lower blood pressure, aspirin, and statin medication to lower cholesterol to appropriate levels and collectively improve blood flow through narrow arteries. Researchers concluded that in patients with chronic stable angina that invasive treatments such as stents and bypass surgery don't prolong life beyond what proper medications alone can do.

Cholesterol Medicines Don't Save Lives

In my experience as a physician, when I struggle to get a patient's cholesterol low enough with medications, their lifestyle tends to be far from ideal. The patient is generally not exercising enough or not practicing healthy eating habits. The "standard American diet" containing large amounts of animal products and processed foods and minimal amounts of fruits and vegetables, along with lack of physical activity, predisposes the masses to abnormal cholesterol numbers.

Statins are cholesterol-lowering medication for lower low-density lipoprotein levels, also called LDL. LDL particles deposit cholesterol in the arteries. In patients with coronary artery disease, statins can stabilize and even reverse the amount of plaque build-up in the coronary arteries, and reduce the risk of a heart attack or stroke.

However, there is minimal literature on statins' effectiveness in patients who have not had a cardiac event, which is when the majority of statins are prescribed. Studies have demonstrated that statin medication can reduce risk of a heart attack or stroke in this population, but the yield is very low. In those studies demonstrating benefit, a physician would need to treat 100-200 patients with daily statin medication over the course of 5 years to prevent a single cardiac event. There is no data demonstrating that giving statins to this patient population reduces the risk of dying.

Studies do show, though, that there is a significant risk of side effects related to statin use. About 10% of patients treated with statins will develop muscle aches. The risk of diabetes is also increased as evidenced in the meta-analysis from The Lancet, showing a 9% increase in diabetes in patients taking a statin compared those who are not.[1] In fact, more potent statins such as rosuvastatin, atorvastatin, and simvastatin, are associated with an even greater risk of developing diabetes than the less powerful statins such as pravastatin and fluvastatin.[2]

Statin medications are not completely benign drugs and should be only used in appropriate patients. If your cholesterol is high and you have never had a heart attack or stroke, you will get a much greater benefit from improving your lifestyle through eating a whole-food, plant-based diet, exercising, and maintaining a healthy weight than from taking a statin medication. These healthy habits are known to not only lower cholesterol, but also reduce risk of heart attack and stroke and ultimately prolong your life.

Reduce Blood pressure and Stress through Lifestyle Choices

Stress can in fact cause a heart attack. A Takotsubo cardiomyopathy, sometimes referred to as "broken heart syndrome," can occur in people without any plaque in their arteries. This type of heart attack is actually far more common in women than in men. Regardless of whether stress ultimately induces a heart attack, it is not good for the heart.

Emotional stress often keeps us from making the right choices, such as eating foods that negatively impact our body's performance, smoking, or not exercising. Managing your stress is important to reducing your risk of heart disease.

Blood pressure, however, is not just lowered by medication. Exercise and weight loss are quite potent in lowering blood pressure. Because blood pressure is tied to body weight and diet, lifestyle choices can severely affect the direction of your health. Even if you are placed on blood pressure medications, it is possible to come off of them once you make changes to your lifestyle.

How Do I Keep My Heart Healthy?

Being heart healthy isn't complicated. The key is in your daily life choices. Studies by Drs. Caldwell Esselstyn and Dean Ornish demonstrated reversal of plaque buildup in the arteries with a whole food, plant-based diet consisting of plenty of fruits and vegetables, unprocessed foods, whole grains and avoiding meat, dairy, oil, and added sugars. Making good choices, such as exercising, not smoking, and eating healthy, can help keep you out of my office and out of the hospital.

Heather Shenkman, MD, FACC, *is an interventional cardiologist practicing in the Los Angeles area. She earned her BS and MD together at Rensselaer Polytechnic Institute and Albany Medical College. She completed her residency in Internal Medicine at Henry Ford Hospital in Detroit, MI, her cardiology fellowship at the University of Rochester in Rochester, NY, and her interventional cardiology fellowship at Tufts Medical Center in Boston, MA. Dr. Shenkman has followed a plant-based diet for nearly 9 years and is an accomplished runner and triathlete. She has completed in several triathlons of all distances including Ironman Lake Placid in 2010. She has competed internationally at the Maccabiah Games in Israel in the summer of 2013 earning a bronze medal.*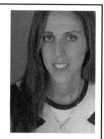

Food Prescription for Better Health

Baxter Montgomery, MD

I have discovered a simple but amazing fact—*when it comes to disease reversal and prevention, nutritional excellence is everything*. As a cardiologist, I know that moderation is inadequate at best, and potentially deadly at worst. The vast majority of illnesses we suffer from are merely side effects of the bad food we eat. The body is designed to perform its own rebuilding and repairing when properly nourished. Once we eliminate foods that are harmful to our body, we allow it to start rebuilding itself in a way that restores its ability to carry out physiological functions in an optimal manner. *How* we nourish our bodies is important and goes beyond keeping track of calories, protein, fats, carbohydrates, and portion sizes. Simply stated, the best form of medicine is optimal nutrition.

During the years I have spent practicing internal medicine, cardiology, and cardiac electrophysiology, I have witnessed substantial advances in medical science. And yet today, I am seeing more young people than ever before plagued by chronic illnesses. I noticed over time that my LDL cholesterol had risen to 138 by the age of 38. It should have been less than 100 mg/dL. As a cardiologist with a genetic predisposition to diabetes and heart disease, I knew this was a significant problem and researched alternative ways to achieve optimal health and wellness.

Healthcare professionals are trained to offer drugs and surgery. Collectively, we think of medications as near cure-alls. This is simply not true. Often, what is really going on with such treatments is just the masking of symptoms. Studies have shown that chronic illnesses are the direct result of our poor lifestyle choices, the most damaging of which is our food choices. We eat too many unnatural, processed foods that are toxic to our bodies,

Heart Disease in America[9]

- 1.26 million Americans are estimated to suffer an initial or recurrent heart attack each year.

- About 452 million people die each year from CHD.

- Over 10 million people suffer from angina pectoris—symptoms caused by poor blood circulation to the heart.

- It is estimated that 500,000 new cases of stable angina occur each year.

- 17.6 million people today have a history of heart attack, angina pectoris, or both.

- Approximately 7.9 million Americans, age 20 and older have experienced a prior heart attack.

in place of foods that are natural and supply our bodies with what they need. We need a paradigm shift in our approach to healthcare. Our efforts need to start with removing unnatural foods from our diet, and replacing those foods with ones that are "natural," as a way of reversing illness and facilitating health.

Reversing and Controlling Disease

Most chronic diseases are progressive in nature, meaning they continue to get worse over time. The irony of chronic diseases is that they are the most common and most costly of all health problems and the most preventable.

Cardiovascular diseases (mainly heart disease and stroke) are the leading causes of death in the U.S. Much of what happens to our arteries can be traced back to the foods that we eat. There are two major, mechanisms through which animal protein contributes to atherosclerosis that are well understood. First, increased intake of fat and cholesterol from animal foods contributes to build-up of fatty substances within the walls of the arteries. The fat and cholesterol molecules are "packaged" in special protein substances known as lipoproteins. These lipoproteins travel throughout the blood stream and their levels can be increased in part due to the amount of cholesterol and fat that is eaten. Special cells that are part of our immune system engulf or "swallow" these lipoprotein molecules and carry them to our cell walls. Excess buildup of lipoproteins in our blood vessel walls can contribute to abnormal blood vessel function.

When someone consumes meat, poultry, and fish they are introducing a foreign substance into their body, which triggers a chronic process of inflammation. Inflammation frequently occurs as a result of injury or foreign invasion within the body and is primarily mediated by the body's immune system. In the early phases of coronary artery disease, arteries within the heart become damaged due to the buildup of fatty molecules and associated low levels of inflammation within the arterial walls. Essentially the consumption of fish, chicken, pork, and beef contributes to coronary heart disease by increasing the amount of fatty molecules in the blood and the blood vessel walls; and, more importantly, through the development of a chronic process of inflammation that can have acute flare ups which are the underlying causes of heart attacks.

A heart attack occurs when the plaque becomes acutely swollen or unstable and bursts, resulting in a series of chemical reactions in the blood that causes the blood to form a clot. The blood clot blocks the artery and results in the sudden loss of blood and oxygen delivery to the part of the heart muscle that is "fed" by that artery. This causes sudden death of that part of the heart muscle, triggering a heart attack. We can think of the flare up and rupture of a plaque as similar to the flare up and rupture of an acne pimple, which is also caused by chronic inflammation.

Individuals often live with heart disease until it progresses to advanced stages, which is why for about forty percent the first symptom of coronary heart disease is cardiac arrest.

Why Diet is Important

The World Health Organization projects that by the year 2015, 2.5 billion adults globally will be overweight, and another 700 million will be obese.[1] As of March 2013, the WHO reports that at least 2.8 million adults die each year as a result of being overweight or obese. In 2011, more than 40 million children under the age of 5 were overweight.[1]

Nearly 100% of my patients and wellness clients agree in theory that following a diet based on good nutrition has a significant influence over their health and well-being. Unfortunately, too many do not recognize what a nutritionally sound diet consists of and have bought into the perception that anything consumed in moderation is okay.

The Nutritional Sufficiency of a Plant-Based Diet

The best way to classify food is by its origin—plant-based or animal-based. Plants provide humans with an abundance of vitamins, minerals, carbohydrates, fats, protein, phytonutrients, and water for nourishment. In fact, when consumed in adequate amounts, plants can theoretically provide humans with all of their nutritional needs other than sunlight and B12, which can be effectively addressed in a supplement.

Although the majority of Americans position animal products at the center of their diet, there is significant scientific evidence that shows plant-based foods to be superior to animal-based foods for human health.[4] The American Dietetic Association (ADA) came out with the following proclamation in 2009: "…well-planned vegetarian diets are appropriate for individuals during all stages of the life cycle, including pregnancy, lactation, infancy, childhood, adolescence, and for athletes."[5] This is likely because vegetarians tend to consume fewer foods containing saturated fats and cholesterol while favoring fruits, vegetables, whole grains, nuts, soy products, fiber, and phytochemicals.

Are Unprocessed Plant Foods Better than Processed Plant Foods?

Studies confirm that, through the cooking process, vegetables lose some of their nutritional value.[6] We can have the freshest, most nutrient-dense, organically grown vegetables available, but after boiling them, we end up pouring what our body needs for good health right down the drain. Research also shows that there is a correlation between the length of time food is exposed to heat and the amount of toxins that develop in food as a result of increased temperatures. Grilling, baking, frying and microwaving at high temperatures have adverse effects on foods. When vegetables are additionally deep-fried or battered they constitute a higher fat content and, as a result, become associated with adverse health conditions.

Some forms of processing, specifically raw juicing, may actually be beneficial.[7] Peer reviewed scientific journals and books report on the numerous health benefits of raw fruit and vegetable juices for various medical conditions.[8] I have personally observed clinical benefits of juicing through my patients with conditions such as coronary artery disease, congestive heart failure, arthritis, diabetes, hypertension, and many other chronic diseases.

True Health

If we were to closely evaluate our current national health condition we would find that our lives are progressively becoming unraveled by our poor health. We regularly suffer from headaches, allergies, mood disorders, insomnia, impotence, loss of libido, fatigue, attention deficit disorder, aches and pain from arthritis, and a generalized decrease in mobility. These common health conditions are often associated with many advanced disease states such as heart disease, cancer, diabetes, and more. Unfortunately, many of these diseases begin *before* the prime of our lives. Our current solutions to these problems consist of over-the-counter and prescription drugs, artificial vitamins and herbs, invasive medical procedures and surgeries.

There is a need for revolutionary change in how we address chronic illnesses in this country and around the world. If we continue in our current approach of trying to find the next "magic bullet" pill, manipulate the next lethal gene, or design the next high tech surgical procedure while ignoring the obvious underlying cause of why we are ill, the problem will only persist. In this setting, we will pass on a legacy of sickness and disease to future generations.

Our new paradigm will be one in which we address chronic illnesses from the perspective of our lifestyle behavior, with optimal nutrition being the central theme. It is recognized that congenital abnormalities, physical injuries, and the like will continue to contribute to our overall health condition, and in many cases will require the best that medications and surgery have to offer. However, the major burden of chronic illnesses on our collective health could be heavily reduced or nearly eliminated, by shifting focus to our new health care model.

True health should be a process of optimal living with continual improvement in our actions over time. We should always strive to eat better, think more positively, exercise longer and more effectively: this mindful process can begin at and continue through any age or clinical condition. With a better understanding of human physiology and nutrition, we can create a healthy, disease-free society just by changing the way we eat.

Baxter Montgomery, MD, *is a cardiologist in Houston, TX and founder of Montgomery Heart and Wellness program. He is a Clinical Assistant Professor of Medicine in the Division of Cardiology at the University of Texas and a Fellow of the American College of Cardiology. Dr. Montgomery is the author of Food Prescription for Better Health and a member of the Physicians Committee for Responsible Medicine.* http://www.drbaxtermontgomery.com/

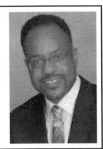

seven

FOR MEN ONLY

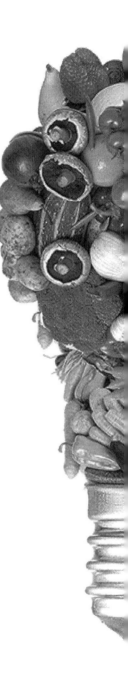

Guys, if you are having problems standing erect, the culprits are most likely high intake of saturated fat and cholesterol from dairy and meat. Two of the most common issues today- erectile dysfunction and prostate cancer- are largely associated with the "manly" meat and dairy diet.

Although a sensitive issue- erectile dysfunction- is actually one of the first signs of heart disease. While we tend to focus on the plaque build-up in our coronary arteries, the problem is if you have clogged arteries anywhere, you have clogged arteries everywhere! Our arteries are smaller as we travel south making the penal arteries the first to be affected. Companies have built billion dollar businesses around pills for erectile dysfunction however the solution to your sexual woes is on your plate, not in the form of pills.

Prostate cancer is also affecting more men at younger ages. Prostate cancer is slow growing and many men live with it for many years before detection. There is a stunning difference in prostate cancer risks around the world, despite ethnicity, which signifies that this cancer is more diet related than age or genetic related. For instance, a recent 2011 study found that men who ate 2 or more servings of red meat a week were twice as likely to be diagnosed with aggressive prostate cancer. This is the equivalent of having a roast beef sandwich for lunch and steak for dinner, a typical American man's diet. However, cruciferous vegetables such as cauliflower, broccoli, brussels sprouts and cabbage are some of the strongest antioxidants as they contain phytochemicals that activate enzymes in the body which weaken cancer causing agents.[1]

These doctors discuss why a plant-powered prostate is the best way to prevent prostate cancer, keep your arteries clear, and enjoy your love life.

Pills or Plants? The Hard Facts on Nutrition and Sexual Health

Joel Kahn, MD

The last I checked, the heart is about 3 feet above the genitals so what is a cardiologist doing counseling patients on sexual performance? In the nearly 30 years I have been caring for heart patients, I have seen over and over that erectile dysfunction (ED) can be an important warning sign to silent heart disease. Although harder to quantify, the same is probably true for some women with sexual dysfunction. The failure to perform adequately during sexual activities is often a clue to an ailing endothelium. The endothelium is the single layer of cells lining all the arteries of the body. When healthy, the endothelial lining of arteries makes a miraculous gas called nitric oxide that causes arteries to expand or dilate and also helps them resist clotting and atherosclerosis (hardening of the arteries). The endothelium can be injured throughout the body by poor lifestyle habits such as smoking and consumption of animal based and processed foods. Poor sexual performance may result from endothelial damage and may be recognized years before the same disease process causes a heart attack.

Picture this: Draw one circle about the diameter of a Number 2 pencil and another circle that is smaller and about the diameter of a stirrer in a drink side by side. The larger circle is the approximate diameter of a good sized coronary artery. The smaller circle is approximately the diameter of the pudendal artery, the major blood supply to the penis. It is easy to see right away that the choice of one more burger, one more sausage or one more plate of ribs is much more likely to clog the pudendal artery and impair your sexual performance before your heart gives out, even if both are getting clogged from poor lifestyle choices.

So what does great sex have to do with nutrition? It takes healthy arteries, a healthy endothelium, and a heart capable of pumping out increased blood flow to our pelvis to make it all happen. For both men and women the sexual response requires a surge of blood flow through arteries to enlarge specialized tissues (the clinical term for sexual organs) to prepare for sexual play and climax. No increase in blood flow, no sexual performance. And you thought it was all about flowers and champagne!

For example, in one study researchers selected 53 men with erectile dysfunction (ED) and had them drink pomegranate juice or a placebo for 4 weeks.[1] Pomegranate juice has been shown to reverse endothelial dysfunction (the other ED) and cause artery plaques to reverse in humans. When a global improvement score for achieving erection was measured after 4 weeks, the drinking of real pomegranate juice was more likely to deliver the goods and lead to erections. In another study, 555 diabetic men were surveyed as to their adherence to a Mediterranean diet rich in vegetables and fruits and their ability to achieve erections.[2] The presence of erectile difficulties and particularly severe erectile difficulties was much lower in the plant strong eaters. How about nuts? A group of scientists studied 17 men with erectile dysfunction and had them eat 100 grams of pistachio nuts a day.[3] At the end of 3 weeks, cholesterol values were lower, blood flow measured in the penis was higher, and measures of the ability to have erections were improved.

Why bother with eating healthy, why not just eat the burger with blue cheese and take the blue pill? The blue pill, or Viagra, and the 2 other available prescription drugs for erectile dysfunction does not work in everyone. The medications also require a healthy endothelium and healthy arteries capable of providing increased blood flow to work. If the sex organ arteries the size of a Twizzler stick are severely diseased, there will be no "badda boom badda bing" an hour after taking them. These medications only work by enhancing the natural effects of a healthy endothelium. Here's how it works: when the lining of the arteries is healthy and a lot of nitric oxide is made, this miracle gas diffuses into the artery and causes a chemical called cyclic GMP to increase.[4] Cyclic GMP or cGMP results in the blood vessel relaxing and dilating but it is a very short lived chemical. The drugs for erectile dysfunction prevent cGMP from being broken down as fast as normal. The longer cGMP hangs around, the more blood flow will increase (no that is not where the expression well hung comes from). But if the endothelium is sick from fatty, toxic blood full of recently ingested animal products and fatty foods, the nitric oxide will not be released as expected and the result will be less than satisfactory. The biochemistry of the male sexual response is understood better than the female response but even Viagra has shown a therapeutic benefit in the sexual response of diabetic women so the basics are universal.

So why do vegans have an easier time with peak sexual performance? At present, there is no known dietary agent that mimics the blue pill and directly boosts cGMP by blocking the same enzyme that Viagra does. However, vegans front load the beginning of this pathway by increasing the production of nitric oxide, the miracle gas. Nitric oxide is generated in the blood vessels by the amino acids L-arginine and L-citrulline cycling back and forth. This system is particularly active when you are less than 40 years of age. If you want to boost your levels of nitric oxide for better overall artery health and superior sexual responsiveness, why not eat healthy foods high in these amino acids? Foods that are particularly high in L-arginine include pine nuts, peanuts, walnuts, almonds, pistachios, and Brazil nuts. Grains, including oats and wheat germ, also have significant amounts of L-arginine. And what about L-citrulline? Watermelon has the highest concentration in nature (particularly the white rind), followed by onions and garlic. Just one standard serving of yellow watermelon provides enough L-citrulline to boost sexual performance. My advice is that you might want to stick to watermelon and not onions and garlic to boost your nitric oxide production before going on a date!

There is another way to generate nitric oxide and its blood flow-enhancing effects. Chemicals called nitrates and nitrites, found in many foods and generated in our saliva, are directly converted to nitric oxide. You may be thinking *I thought nitrates and nitrites are bad for you?* In fatty meats this may be true as they get converted to nitrosamines but in the healthiest foods, particularly vegetables, they are a load of fun. What foods are packed with nitrates, nitrates, and the antioxidants that make them rush to convert to nitric oxide? Which of these can make you master of your domain? Arugula, rhubarb, kale swiss chard, spinach, bok choy, and beets are the top of the list. Finish your diet off with grapes, pomegranates, apples and green teas and you have a dynamite erotic potion that will supercharge your endothelium both in your groin and your heart.

Nutrition is of course just one part- albeit the biggest part- of an overall heart healthy lifestyle. Not smoking, exercising regularly, avoiding diabetes and obesity, and achieving adequate sleep are proven ways to maintain endothelial health and sexual performance. A low fat vegan diet along with exercise, stress reduction, no smoking, and social support led many participants on the Esselstyn diet with advanced heart disease to enjoy improved sexual performance.

Over 400 years ago, Thomas Sydenham said, «A man is as old as his arteries.» Four centuries later, we know just how right he was. Eat plants to protect your brain, eat plants to protect your heart, but also eat plants to power your sexual life even if it seems hard at times. What may seem hard will keep you hard.

Joel Kahn MD, *is a Clinical Professor of Medicine at Wayne State University School of Medicine and Director of Cardiac Wellness, Michigan Healthcare Professionals PC. He practices at William Beaumont Hospital, Royal Oak, and Troy. He is a Summa Cum Laude graduate of the University of Michigan School of Medicine. He lectures widely on the cardiac benefits of vegan nutrition and writes for Readers Digest Magazine as the Holistic Heart Doc. Dr. Kahn's first book, The Holistic Heart Bible, will be published by Readers Digest in January, 2014.*
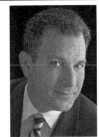

Prevent Prostate Problems with Diet

Ira Michaelson, MD

Benign prostatic hypertrophy (BPH) is a condition affecting millions of older American men. As we age, the prostate gland enlarges, causing problems. The prostate sits below the urinary bladder. It encircles the urethra, where voiding occurs. As the prostate enlarges symptoms develop, including frequent urination often disrupting sleep, dribbling after urination, blood in the urine, and bladder infections. Typical treatments include drugs called alpha blockers, which relax the bladder muscles and make it easier to urinate. Surgery is also a common treatment that involves removing a portion of the gland. Sexual dysfunction may result from this procedure, among other side effects.

Fortunately, we now know that diet has a great influence on the prostate. Studies have shown that lycopene found in plants decreased the prostate-specific antigen levels (a marker of prostate disease levels) and inhibited prostate growth.[1] Studies have also found that a diet low in fat and rich in vegetables may reduce the risk of prostate cancer, which often follows BPH.[2-5] The phytoestrogens or plant estrogens are helpful because they inhibit prostate growth, and enzymes such as tyrosine kinase used in cellular proliferation, a major factor in development of BPH. For instance, capsaicin, found in hot peppers, has been found to promote apotosis (cell death) in prostate cancer cells in mice.[6] While a plant-based diet is not a cure-all for BPH, there is evidence that it is significantly helpful in preventing development of prostate cancer.

Erectile Dysfunction and the End of Health

Lawrence J. Derbes Jr.,MD, FACC

Just as puberty marks the end of childhood, Erectile Dysfunction or ED marks the end of good health. Erectile dysfunction (ED) is usually defined as the recurrent or persistent inability to attain or maintain an erection in order for mutually satisfactory sexual performance. It's very common; Americans make up only 8% of the world population, but have 30% of the world's erectile dysfunction. In fact, 40-50% of men in the USA over the age of 40 are impotent.[1]

Erectile Dysfunction is known as the canary in the coal mine of health that heralds a future of heart attacks, strokes, pain, procedures, and surgeries. One would expect that the advent of sexual dysfunction in mid-life to be a cause for great concern, leading to physician visits and a tenacious inquiry into its causes and cures. The problem is many men rarely volunteer the presence of ED to their physicians, as most men still aren't comfortable talking about impotence. It remains taboo unless asking for the magical blue pill. However, the implications of erectile dysfunction are far worse than the problems of "getting it up."

This is because coronary artery disease and erectile dysfunction are different manifestations of the same disease - atherosclerosis. Atherosclerosis is a disorder that destroys all our arteries with inflammation, calcification and thrombosis. How does atherosclerosis happen? Plaque from fatty foods such as meat, dairy and processed products gradually accumulates inside all of our arteries impeding blood flow. This is why the advent of ED is associated with a 50-fold increase in heart attack risk in men aged 40 - 49 years. Treating erectile dysfunction, therefore, is more than just achieving an erection, as the diagnosis is an opportunity to reduce cardiovascular risk.

WOMEN – diet also affects your sex life more than you know. 40% percent of US women age 20 - 65 report sexual problems. And the most distress occurs in the prime of life. High lipid levels is associated with significantly lower arousal, less orgasms and lubrication, and much lower satisfaction scores, compared to 21% of women with normal lipid studies. So, listen up - everything about ED below also pertains to you.

Why does erectile dysfunction usually manifest before coronary artery disease? The leading hypothesis involves the size of the arteries. Because penile arteries are only half the size of coronary arteries, the same amount of plaque will narrow them more significantly. This makes sense as one would expect the smaller arteries to be impaired first as plaque gradually accumulates over the years. The organs connected to the smaller arteries manifest the symptoms first. Even prior to the development of ED symptoms, decreased penile artery blood flow accurately predicts the onset of coronary artery disease.

From the onset of symptoms of erectile dysfunction to the first manifestation of coronary artery disease (heart attack, acute heart failure, serious arrhythmia, or sudden cardiac arrest) there is, on average, only 2-5 years.[2] That is, 67% of men suffering a heart attack became impotent about 3 years before. An exception to this rule is unstable plaque syndrome. When unstable plaques rupture it leads to heart attacks. This is important because it means not all men have ED as a warning, some have a heart attack first. The lucky ones are the guys who develop ED first; they have a warning. Guys, the clock is ticking.

The good news is we can listen to the warning signs and reverse the process that underlies both atherosclerosis and erectile dysfunction. Medical treatment focuses on the immediate problem - lack of erections. The common drugs Viagra, Cialis, and Levitra block PDE5, allowing the buildup of cGMP. With more cGMP, erections are easier to achieve and sustain as nitric oxide levels are higher. The drugs work well to help maintain erections - and so the immediate manifestation is erased. However, these medications come with side effects. But the real reason not to rely on these drugs is that they only mitigate symptoms; they do nothing for the underlying cause. At best, they are a temporary fix. At worst, they mask the underlying problem with the continued decline in health. This removes the stimulus to change the behaviors that promote the underlying disease and can lead to fatal heart attacks.

The Science Behind an Erection

Humans rely on fluid hydraulics to enlarge and stiffen the penis as we do not have a baculum, or penile bone. For the process to work, good blood flow through the arteries is needed. With sexual stimulation, nitric oxide (NO) is released from nerve endings and endothelial cells in the corpus cavernosum, or the spongy erectile tissue of the penis. This activates the enzyme guanylate cyclase, which then increases cyclic guanosine monophosphate (cGMP) levels. cGMP causes the smooth muscle to relax, which increases blood flow that then leads to an erection. cGMP is then hydrolysed back to the inactive GMP by phosphodiesterase type 5 (PDE5). When the penile arteries are blocked, calcified, and stiff the nitric oxide produced is not sufficient to make the arteries open enough to cause an erection.

What Changes have Proven Outcomes and are Cost-Effective?

A systematic review and meta-analysis of the literature on the effect of lifestyle modification and cardiovascular risk factor reduction on erectile dysfunction was published in

2011.[3] The effect of statins, weight loss, physical activity, and dietary changes were studied. The results indicate that dietary changes produce the most substantial effects to mitigate and reverse erectile dysfunction. For example, a recent study of 173 men with ED using the highest dose of the statin simvastatin for 6 months, showed zero difference in improvement compared to the placebo group.[4] In comparison, a study of dietary intervention only, using the Mediterranean diet for 2 years, in 65 men with the metabolic syndrome, 13 men in the diet group had IIEF scores of 22 or higher compared to just 2 in the control group. Thirty-seven percent of the men on the Mediterranean diet regained normal sexual function. The changes in IIEF score were related to the intake of fruits, vegetables, legumes, nuts, and the ratio of polyunsaturated to saturated lipids.

Stimulating plant-based foods shown to improve erectile dysfunction and decrease blood pressure and cholesterol are watermelon, papaya, and pistachio nuts. All produce arginine, the precursor to NO.[1] Why risk drug side effects when a plant based diet can fix the underlying problem, and the side effects of a plant-based diet are all good?

In addition to improving erectile dysfunction, the vegan diet has been shown in many studies to prevent and even reverse coronary artery disease. Drs. Ornish and Esselstyn have proven this beyond a shadow of a doubt. Indeed, "A substantial body of knowledge demonstrates that the abundant consumption of food of plant origin, including vegetables, fruit, and whole grain, and the dietary patterns rich in these foods, convey a markedly lower risk of coronary disease."[5]

But why wait for the heart attack? The first one just might be the end of you.

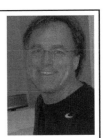

Lawrence Derbes Jr., MD, *is a long time vegan and a board certified cardiologist. Dr. Derbes was the Assistant Professor of Clinical Medicine at Tulane University Health Sciences Center. He currently lives and works on the Big Island of Hawaii with his family and enjoys training for triathlons.*

Take Charge of Prostate Cancer

Ron Allison, MD

ancer is not as genetically driven as we assume. Diet is at the forefront- both in the creation and control of cancer. In the Western world we have access to an excess amount of calories and food products, particularly meats, which are relatively unhealthy, when compared to other diets around the world.

For instance, let's take someone eating an Eastern Diet (mainly vegetarian) from Asia, and move them to Hawaii, with a Western Diet (mainly meat and dairy). Even though they are from Asia, where the incidence of prostate cancer and other cancers are low, when they change their diet, we are seeing the same high rates of cancer within a single generation. Once individuals consume a Western diet, cancer and heart disease rates jump up. Critically, the reverse is also true. If we were to take men from the United States, which has a tremendous prevalence of prostate cancer, and switch their diets to a more plant-based diet, these men would certainly not experience the same high rates of prostate cancer and other health problems. Further, they could avoid the serious complications and financial expense affiliated with prostate treatment.

Types of Prostate Cancer

Today we consider 2 main types of prostate cancer, the more common hormone sensitive prostate cancer and hormone insensitive prostate cancer. Hormone sensitive prostate cancer has the best possibility of being treated. However, when hormone sensitive cancers continue to grow they tend to become hormone insensitive, which have fewer treatment options available.

High Fat, High Protein Diets Cause Cancer

Fat is key to cancer development as not only does it feed cancer growth, but it also functions as a storage component in our body. The problem is fat stores the nasty toxins, pesticides, and antibiotics that accumulate in the animals we consume. Each time we take a bite of a greasy burger, fried or grilled chicken, processed foods or eat cheese, we are getting a mouthful of carcinogens and cancer promoting agents that are stored in the fat in our body.

Dairy and meat products are filled with both natural and artificial growth hormones that feed cancer. "Hormone Free," declared milk is a misnomer as dairy contains natural hormones by virtue of its purpose for baby calves. Additionally most animals today receive artificial growth hormone injections. For example, cheese, composed of mainly fat, is a highly processed and concentrated source of these toxins.

Dairy, like meat, also contains more protein than our body can process. Despite advertisements, our bodies cannot process such high levels of protein. This inability injures our kidneys and liver. More worrying, proteins that are not broken down completely become carcinogens.

Essentially, we get the worst of everything in meat and dairy: excess fat which causes cancer to grow, toxins concentrated in the fat from animal-feed, and excess protein that become carcinogens if not digested completely. Further, meat and dairy are completely devoid of fiber, which is an extremely protective agent against many cancers.

Processed Foods: The Most Fantastic Mechanisms for Causing Cancer

Another contributor to cancer is processed foods. Think about this: it is possible to go to any fast food chain, in any place in the entire world, at any time, 7-days-a-week and the food will taste exactly the same as it would 10,000 miles away. Chemists have created something that looks like a beef patty or a chicken patty but in reality it is just a chemical conglomeration.

Processing involves literally thousands of different chemicals that our body has absolutely no history of eating because they are man-made. If they were made of a natural substance, the body would have thousands of years to create defense mechanisms against it. Since processing has only been developed in the last 100-years or less, your body has not had a chance to develop any mechanisms to fight against the negative effects of these weird chemicals that are put into your body. Processed foods might just be one of the more fantastic mechanisms of causing cancer and particularly prostate cancer.

The Best Approach to Cancer is Prevention

The best way to deal with cancer is to prevent it. By replacing, or eliminating animal-based food products, with plant-based products we can decrease chance of developing the most common cancers, colorectal, breast, and prostate, between 50 to even 90%. This is a tremendous difference.

Let's look at the Seventh Day Adventists in the United States as an example. As a largely vegetarian and vegan population living in similar environments who do not smoke or drink alcohol, they provide an ideal population to study the effects of diet on cancer. Adventists who eat a plant-based diet live 10 to 12 years longer than those in the same group who eat meat, smoke, and/or drink.

The foods that protect against cancer are plant-based. One of the main protectors found in plant-based diets is fiber. Fiber assists in pulling out the fat from our bodies, which decreases the risk of breast, prostate, and other cancers, as well as pulls out the carcinogens from our colon and rectum, decreasing the rate and risk of colorectal cancer.

Tofu and soy products, a good source of protein, have also been shown to help prevent as well as heal cancer. Both contain components that bind to and attack cancer cells as well as chemicals that can cause cancer growth. Tofu and soy products can be very potent tools in terms of treatment and health. For example, of the breast cancer patients who have been diagnosed, and treated, those who ate more tofu have less recurrence, and live longer than those who do not eat tofu. Since breast and prostate cancer are very similar, the same could apply to prostate cancer patients. (Note: this does not apply to processed soy beans but the natural form of soy.)

The Marriage Curse

Most men do not think about their prostate in terms of health until they have a problem. However, many older men begin to experience prostate growth or benign prostatic hypertrophy (BPH). Since there is little room for an enlarged prostate to grow, it can squash the urethra, making it very difficult to empty your bladder. The prostate can also grow large enough to press on your rectum, which also causes bathroom problems.

There is connection between what is stimulating the prostate to grow and stimulating cancer cells to grow. It appears that hormones cause the unneeded prostate to grow. These hormones are from fats. Meat-based diets, including low-fat meats, are by definition high in fat. There is no safe way of eating meat, and there is no safe dose of meat in your diet. This meat-based diet feeds the prostate, and it feeds it to grow in a benign fashion, which is BPH.

The treatment for BPH, and prostate cancer, involves agents that block hormones. A plant-based diet blocks these same hormones via phytoestrogens. Phytoestrogens are plant components that are essentially hormone mimickers. They prevent BPH and cancer growths. A plant-based diet also has beneficial vitamins, and minerals, and other chemicals that help prevent growth of cancers and reverse conditions like heart disease.

What Happens If You Do Have Cancer?

I recommend that everybody consider the standard of care treatment, because although it has significant side-effects, it is often quite successful. That being said, if diagnosed with cancer, our diet can help control the cancer, slow the spread of it, and even help reverse growth for most cancers. Prostate cancer is one of the more sensitive cancers to dietary prevention. Altering your diet is a really powerful way of complementing treatment that is inexpensive and has no side effects. **It is surprising that people think dietary change is more radical than surgery, radiation, and chemotherapy.**

I have been treating patients with cancer for 25 years. One of my patients, Nick had a very advanced state of prostate cancer. Conventional treatment did not look like it would be successful. When Nick became a vegetarian, he lost a lot of weight (one of the greatest assets of plant-based diet). Despite having an extremely aggressive form of prostate cancer, he is healthier now than he has been for years. His PSA level, which is often used to measure prostate cancer growth, has been undetectable for years. Although one is never truly in the clear once diagnosed with prostate cancer, Nick is a success story.

There is a misconception amongst men when it comes to their overall health in general. Most men spend more time thinking about what kind of tires to put on their car, than they do about the effects of their diet on cancer and other diseases. Yet, the benefits of a plant- based diet goes way beyond prostate cancer: aiding in the prevention of many other common but preventable chronic health problems.

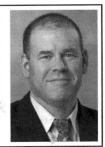

Ron Allison, MD *received his MD from State University of New York (SUNY) Downstate Medical School. He completed his Radiation Oncology residency at SUNY Health Science Center and named chief resident. He joined SUNY-Buffalo and the NCI designated Roswell Park Cancer Institute as attending physician and Associate Professor. In 2000, Dr. Allison joined ECU's Brody School of Medicine as Professor and Chair of Radiation Oncology. He served as director of the Leo W. Jenkins Cancer Center. Since 2010 he has been medical director of 21st Century Oncology. Dr Allison has presented over 300 scientific abstracts and published over 100 peer reviewed publications. He has served as principal investigator for PDT trials.*

Whole Food, Plant-Based Diet in the Prevention and Treatment of Prostate Cancer

Gordon Saxe, MD, PhD

Prostate cancer (PC) is the most commonly occurring cancer among males in Western populations, second only to skin cancer. In the U.S., 1 man in 6 will develop invasive PC in his lifetime.[1] In 2007, there were over 218,000 new cases and over 27,000 deaths from PC.[2] Although most cases progress slowly and may never become clinically apparent, the disease is the second-leading cause of death from cancer in men and the most common cause in male nonsmokers. Further, because of its strong association with age, the number of new cases and deaths from PC is expected to increase dramatically over the next 25 years with the aging of the American population.

More than 80% of cases are asymptomatic and present only with an elevated prostate-specific antigen (PSA) level or palpable nodule on digital rectal examination (DRE). PSA screening is far more sensitive in detecting PC than DRE and can pick it up at an earlier stage. However, a rising serum PSA level in an otherwise healthy man does not necessarily imply that he has "invasive" PC (PC with metastatic potential), only that he has a condition in which there has been an increase in the number or size of prostate cells. A rise in PSA can occur because of invasive PC, but also because of "latent" PC (a histologically cancerous change, commonly observed in the prostates of older men, without metastatic potential) as well as non-cancerous conditions such as benign prostatic hypertrophy (BPH) or prostatitis. It is also a natural concomitant of aging, probably because of the natural tendency of the prostate gland to enlarge with age.

Since the widespread introduction of PSA as a screening test in the mid-1990's, it has become rare for patients to present with overt, radiologically detectable disease outside of the prostate (although undetectable microscopic disease spread beyond the prostate is a more common occurrence than is widely appreciated).[3,4] As a result, the majority of patients elect to receive some form of eradicative primary local treatment in the hope of curing the disease. Most commonly, this takes the form of radical prostatectomy (RP), although a large number opt instead for radiation therapy (RT).

A definitive diagnosis of PC can only be made after a positive biopsy, and not solely on the basis of an elevated or rising PSA level or suspicious DRE. The biopsy can provide clues (such as the grade or "Gleason score") to the potential behavior of the PC, but it cannot perfectly distinguish more aggressive cancers from those with low metastatic potential. While eradicative primary treatment may be life saving in some individuals, often individuals who undergo RP or RT do not have cancer with malignant potential. What this means is that the success rate of these treatments is not only probably over-estimated, but also a significant percentage of patients may be over-treated-- unnecessarily exposing them to potential treatment complications and morbidity. Unfortunately, there is no certain means for differentiating those individuals who will benefit from treatment from those who will not. Additionally lowering the sensitivity threshold of the PSA test has the unavoidable trade-off of increasing detection and over-treatment of PC's with little or no metastatic potential.

In spite of the potential for earlier diagnosis afforded by PSA screening as well as ongoing advances in surgical technique, it has been observed that approximately 35% of patients will experience PSA-detected progression, commonly referred to as "biochemical recurrence" (BR), within 10 years of primary treatment. BR can have a highly variable course and is not an automatic death sentence. Overall, about a third of patients who have experienced BR will develop metastatic disease within the subsequent 5 years, and upon detection of metastases, the average length of survival is under 5 years.[5,6]

Role of Diet and Nutrition in Prostate Cancer

Interest in the role of diet and nutrition in development and progression of PC has grown considerably in recent years. Accompanying this has been increasing focus on use of dietary modification or nutritional supplementation as adjunctive treatments for PC.

The possible impact of diet on PC development and progression is supported by evidence from a variety of epidemiologic, laboratory, and human clinical trials. One of the first suggestions that diet might be implicated in the genesis of PC derives from the observation of dramatic international variations in age-adjusted PC incidence and mortality rates. For example, during the period from 1978-1982, Qidong County, China, had an age-adjusted incidence rate of only 0.5 per 100,000 men, and Osaka, Japan had a rate of 6.7 per 100,000, whereas the rate in the U.S. at the same time was 102.1 per 100,000.[7,8] These differences were observed long before the development of the PSA test and therefore could not have been accounted for by differences in rates of PSA screening in the U.S. compared with China and Japan.

Further, upon migration to the U.S., PC incidence in Japanese men increases 4 to 9 fold within the first generation (i.e. in the migrants, themselves) and mirrors the incidence in the U.S. by the second generation (in the offspring of the migrants).[9-11] While this does not rule out the possibility that genetic inheritance may be part of the causal chain in some cases, it does suggest that environmental or lifestyle exposures-- rather than one's genes-- appear to account for most of the risk.[12] Japan is a densely populated, heavily industrialized country whose population, perhaps even more than that of the U.S., is exposed regularly to many potential carcinogens. This suggests that pollution is not the critical factor in explaining higher PC incidence in the U.S. Numerous studies, therefore, have focused on lifestyle factors (smoking, physical activity, sexual history, occupation, diet) and patterns in search of the explanation for the differences in incidence. With the exception of diet and body weight, however, most lifestyle factors have not been strongly associated with PC incidence or progression.[13-22]

Epidemiologic investigations suggest that diet, particularly meat and dairy intake, may constitute an important set of environmental factors impacting development and progression of PC. As reviewed by Kolonel, 16 of 22 studies (14 case-control and 8 cohort) found a positive association of meat intake with PC risk, with 15 showing odds ratios or relative risks of 1.3 or more.[23] Similarly, in a review by Chan et al, 12 of 23 studies (14 case-control and 9 cohort) found positive associations of dairy foods with PC risk.[24] Consumption of red meat and dairy products, as well as calcium, has also been associated with increased risk of advanced PC.[25] For example, in the Health Professionals Follow-up Study of 51,000 men, those whose calcium intakes (from dairy foods and supplements) were greater than 2,000 mg./day, compared with those whose intakes were less than 500 mg./day, had a relative risk of 4.6 for metastatic and fatal PC.[26] More recent studies have called the dairy and calcium associations into question. For example, a recent meta-analysis by Huncharek et al found no association of either dairy or calcium intake with PC risk.[27]

However, weighing the evidence from over 20 epidemiologic investigations of dairy foods, the World Cancer Research Fund and the American Institute for Cancer Research noted that "most of the studies showed increased risk with increased intake. Meta-analysis of cohort data produced evidence of a clear dose-response relationship between advanced/aggressive cancer risk with milk intake and between all PC risk and milk and dairy products." They went on to add,

"Calcium can be taken to be a marker for dairy intake in high income populations... High calcium intake down regulates the formation of 1,25 dihydroxyvitamin D3 from vitamin D, thereby increasing cell proliferation in the prostate... Diets high in calcium are a probable cause of prostate cancer."[28]

One possible explanation for the adverse effect associated with meat and dairy origin relates to their content of arachidonic acid (AA). AA has been shown to stimulate the growth of both LNCaP (hormone-sensitive) and PC3 (hormone-insensitive) PC cell lines and is as effective as testosterone in stimulating growth of hormone-sensitive LNCaP cells.[29] An explanation for the increased PC risk observed in association with dairy foods is that high calcium intake due to increased consumption of these foods may lower concentrations of 1,25-dihydroxy vitamin D, a hormone thought to promote cellular differentiation and protect against PC.[30,31]

Cancer Protective Properties of Plant-Based Foods

In contrast with foods of animal origin, plant-based foods – rich in an array of potentially beneficial phytonutrients – appear to be protective. Plant-based foods, including whole cereal grains, vegetables, legumes, and fruit have been examined in cohort and case-control studies with respect to their potential for protecting against prostate carcinogenesis. A review summarizing 8 of 16 studies (13 case-control and 3 cohort) reported inverse associations of specific or total vegetable intake with PC risk, whereas 8 reported no association. However, none reported increased risk. The strongest protective effects were seen for legumes, pulses and nuts, carrots, leafy greens, cruciferous (cabbage family) vegetables, and tomatoes.[32]

In particular, cruciferous vegetables have been found in 2 population-based studies to be associated with a reduction in PC incidence.[33,34] This may be due in part to indole-3-carbinol (I3C), a compound found in cruciferous vegetables. I3C inhibits the growth of PC-3 human PC cells by inducing G1 cell cycle arrest (thereby leading to apoptosis) and also regulates the expression of apoptosis-related genes.[35]

Carotenoids, found primarily in vegetables and fruits, may also impact PC risk. Carotenoids promote differentiation of epithelial tissues, perhaps in part through the provitamin A properties of certain members of this class (such as b-carotene). Carotenoids may also exert anti-cancer effects independently of provitamin A effects through anti-oxidant protection against free radical damage to DNA, carotenoid-regulated production of gap junction proteins, or other mechanisms.[36] Recently much interest has focused on lycopene as a result of in vitro studies suggesting an inhibitory effect on PC.[37] However, epidemiologic support for a protective effect has been mixed, with only one of eight cohort and case-control studies, but 2 of 3 plasma studies, showing inverse associations.[38]

Growing evidence suggests that nutritional factors may influence not only PC incidence but also risk of recurrence and progression. Consumption of red meat and dairy products has been associated with increased risk of metastatic PC.[39] Vitamin E supplementation has been associated with a decreased risk of advanced and fatal PC's among smokers[40-42] and may delay disease progression.[43] Adoption of plant-based diets has been associated with prolonged survival and instances of remission of bone metastases in men with advanced disease in uncontrolled studies and case studies.[44] Refined carbohydrates, because of their associations with total energy intake, may also be directly associated with body weight.[45] Body weight, perhaps through its effect on circulating sex steroid hormones, may be an important mediator of a possible dietary effect on prostate tumor progression. Obesity has been associated with lower serum levels of sex hormone-binding globulin[46] and therefore could lead to higher circulating levels of dihydrotestosterone, a putative prostate tumor promoter. Obesity has also been linked to insulin resistance and increased levels of insulin growth factor-1 (IGF-1). IGF-1 stimulates the growth of both normal and PC cells in the prostate gland.[47] While body weight has not been strongly linked to PC incidence, several studies[48,49] have found associations between body weight at diagnosis and risk of recurrence.[50,51,52]

Dietary Strategies for Primary and Recurrent Prostate Cancer

There appears to be a growing consensus regarding some of the broad brushstrokes of what might constitute an ideal dietary strategy for both preventing and slowing or stopping progression of PC:[53] a largely whole food, plant-based diet emphasizing whole kernel grains, vegetables, beans and legumes, fruit, seeds and nuts;[54] limitation or avoidance of most foods of animal origin, particularly red meat and dairy and others high in pro-inflammatory AA,[55] added emphasis on foods with suspected anti-PC properties such as brassica and allium vegetables, sea vegetables, soy (particularly fermented soy foods), turmeric, and green tea;[56] emphasis on rectification of the prevalent imbalance in the omega-6:omega-3 fat ratio within the context of an overall reduction of omega-6 fats; and[57] portion control and reduction of refined carbohydrates that may contribute to excessive calorie intake and obesity.

This dietary pattern is consistent with the recommendations of various dietary traditions that have been employed as alternative medical practices by numerous cancer patients. Perhaps not surprisingly, there have been a significant number of anecdotal claims, including several medically documented cases, of remission of distant metastases, particularly bone metastases, in men with metastatic PC.[58] To date, there have been 3 reports of clinical intervention trials that have employed a similar dietary strategy in combination with stress management training.[59-61] All 3 studies combined stress management along with plant-based diets and all found a reduction in the rate of PSA increase, as well as improvements in body weight, serum lipids, and other health parameters.

It should be noted that the 2 studies (2 by Saxe et al) that found the largest reduction in the rate of PSA increase were focused on patients who had already undergone BR, a subset that: (a) may select for more aggressive – and potentially more diet-linked PC's, and (b) had to overcome less background "noise" in the PSA tests they employed because they focused on men who had already undergone RP and therefore had no contribution to their PSA from non-PC sources. In contrast, the third study (Ornish et al) examined men who had lower-grade PC's, were undergoing "watchful waiting" (and therefore still retained their prostates), and therefore had more non-PC factors impacting their PSA (and possibly partially concealing the "signal" of the true impact of the intervention). A fourth dietary intervention study, which promoted a low-fat, soy-supplemented diet in patients with BR, detected a more modest improvement in PSA. Unlike the first three trials, the latter study did not utilize a whole food, plant-based dietary approach and also did not employ stress management training.[62]

The magnitude of the societal impact of PC has been growing along with its prevalence. Diet and nutrition appear to play an important role in PC development and progression and evidence is growing that dietary and lifestyle modification may offer a safe and effective option – that actually addresses and corrects underlying causes of the progression of this cancer, especially for patients with recurrent disease. There is still much to learn about the optimal dietary approach and more rigorous studies are needed. It is important to remember that although latent PC is common in older men, diet and environmental factors may "water the lawn" and increase the risk that latent or lower grade PC's develop into more aggressive and invasive forms of this disease. Finally, cancer risk is not confined to the patient. A whole food, plant-based diet may reduce the risks of cancer and other chronic diseases for the entire family.

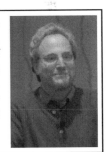

Gordon Saxe, MD, PhD *received his MD from Michigan State University, his PhD in Epidemiology from the University of Michigan, his MPH in Nutrition from Tulane University, and his BA from Brandeis University. He completed residency training at the University of Massachusetts and is board certified in General Preventive Medicine and Public Health. Dr. Saxe is a founding member of the UCSD Center for Integrative Medicine and its Director of Research. He is also the Medical Director of the UCSD Natural Healing & Cooking Program. He is most well-known for his pioneering work in the combined use of a plant-based diet and mind-body stress reduction to control the progression of advanced prostate cancer.*

eight

DIABETES, YOU DECEIVE ME

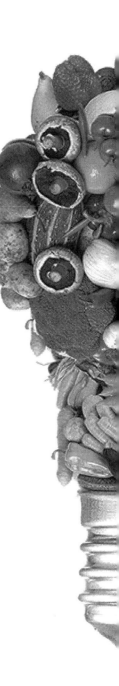

Diabetes mellitus has been around as far back as 1500 BC in ancient Egypt, but its cause remained a mystery for thousands of years. In ancient times physicians diagnosed diabetes by tasting the urine of patients to evaluate its sweetness. Even though physicians Sushruta and Charaka recognized over 2000 years ago that it was better to prevent this disease than treat it, today's escalating rates of Type 2 diabetes indicate we have done little to follow this ancient warning.

We commonly view diabetes as strictly a "sugar" problem, which is why all too often dietary advice focuses on calorie and carbohydrate restriction. However, diabetes occurs when fat blocks our insulin receptors leading to a buildup of sugar in the blood. As the following diabetes experts will demonstrate, Type 1 and especially Type 2 diabetes are closely associated with our high in fat meat and dairy based diets. Recent findings from the EPIC study in Europe that followed women over a 14 year period found that those who ate a diet high in meat and dairy had a 56% chance of developing diabetes, compared to those who ate a diet high in fruits, vegetables, and legumes.[1] In fact, cross-cultural studies show a diabetes map of the world that is directly associated with dietary patterns.

By removing meat and dairy and switching to plant-based diet, we can lower our blood sugar better than medication! For example, Amla or Indian gooseberry, not only has one of the highest antioxidant contents of any food, but also recent studies show it can lower blood sugar better than glyburide, a modern pharmaceutical used to treat type 2 diabetes.[2] As these doctors will demonstrate, we have the prescription to not only better manage diabetes but also in many causes reverse it with a nutritious diet plan.

The Not So Sweet Story About Diabetes

Eddie Ramirez, MD

I still remember as if it were yesterday. The topic of the medical school class was type 1 diabetes, and the professor informed us that we currently do not have any idea what causes this type of diabetes. Surprised by the comment, I raised my hand and said, "There is evidence that cow's milk may be a culprit." The whole class started to laugh. I happened to carry the book that every medical student is required to read in their pathology class and quoted from it: "Children who ingest cow's milk products early in life have 1.5-fold increased risk for type I diabetes."[1] There was an immediate silence in the room, as I had just "won" the argument.

Type 1 diabetes is one of the fastest growing diseases in the world.[2] There are many possible etiologies for type 1 diabetes that we are still learning about, but there is significant evidence that milk may be one of the most important causes.[3] One possible explanation is that cow's milk has a protein that is similar to a protein in the pancreas.[4] In certain people, the cow's protein is identified as a foreign substance in the body, and the immune system tries to get rid of it. It is eliminated from the blood, but since there is a similar protein in the pancreas, there is destruction of the insulin-producing cells of the pancreas. The American Pediatric Association recognizes that "early exposure of infants to cow's milk protein may be an important factor in the initiation of the beta cell destructive process in some individuals," and "the avoidance of cow's milk protein for the first several months of life may reduce the later development of IDDM or delay its onset in susceptible people."[5]

Understanding the Most Common Type of Diabetes: Type 2

In the Marshall Islands, diabetes was virtually unknown before the 1950's. In March 1, 1954, the US tested a nuclear head that was 1,000 times larger than the bomb dropped in Hiroshima. As a result of the radiation, many islanders were affected and sued the US government, winning the suit and getting a big settlement. What did they do with that money? They changed their whole lifestyle from simple plant-based foods to Spam™, frozen turkey tails, and fast food full of fat, salt, and sugar.[6] Today the Marshall Islands have one of the highest rates of diabetes in the world.

In the US, the lifetime risk of diabetes for Hispanics is 53% for females and 45% for males and for Caucasians 39% for women and 33% for males.[7] The main problem with diabetes is the associated complications including kidney failure,[8] amputations,[9] nerve and ligament problems,[10] and cognitive decline.[11] Three out four diabetics will have high blood pressure[12] and 80% of diabetics will die of stroke[13] or heart disease.[14] Diabetes is also the number one cause of blindness in the US.[15]

These complications are the result of abnormally high levels of glucose. Insulin glucose will "stick" to everything in the body, causing problems. The good news is that most of these complications can be avoided all together[16] if we are willing to change our habits permanently.

What are the Symptoms of Diabetes?

Some classic symptoms of diabetes are a manifestation of how the body is trying to compensate for the abnormal levels of glucose and insulin in the body. Classic symptoms[17] include extreme hunger (due to the body not able to use the already high levels of glucose); extreme thirst (since water will dilute the sugar levels and therefore lower them); frequent urination (secondary to taking so much fluids); and weight loss (since the body is not able to use the sugar, the body enters a catabolic state in which it "destroys" tissue in order to survive). In addition to these classic symptoms,[18] one can also experience low energy, fatigue, blurred vision, irritability, tingling or numbness in hands or feet, frequent infections, cuts or bruises that are slow to heal, nausea or vomiting, dehydration, and even reduced conscious level. I usually check blood sugar in people that have gained or lost weight recently, have a depressed mood, or have a strong diabetic gene in the family.

The Link Between Animal Product Consumption and Type 2 Diabetes

Recently I visited one of the best archeological museums in Mexico City where they recreated a pre-Columbian market scene-- you could see corn, beans, squashes, and avocados, but no meat, chicken, or dairy products, since Spaniards brought them to the Americas.[19] Similarly, in the rural areas in Africa people have access to simple plant-based foods. As they emigrate to the big cities or affluent countries, they tend to exchange their traditional diet for a richer diet in animal products. Subsequently, diseases like diabetes,[20] heart disease,[21] and cancers[22] (among others) dramatically increase.[23] One of the common denominators in this transition is the inclusion or increase in animal product intake.[24] This is a phenomenon we are now experiencing on a world scale; you can literally see geographical diabetes maps[25] of disease directly related to income and animal product intake. Animal products are naturally pro-inflammatory, which is one of the triggers of diabetes. One study showed that high levels of inflammation were created in just half an hour by a typical breakfast of sausage and eggs.[26] Regular consumption of these types of foods creates havoc in the human body. We need to return to a simple plant-based diet to prevent or reverse these problems.[27]

Help Heal Yourself in Days

My personal experience is that the majority of diabetics can either stop the progression or completely reverse their disease if they are willing to make permanent changes in their lifestyle. In regards to diet, the focus should be to adopt a wholesome, low-fat, non-inflammatory diet that has a low glycemic load[28] (i.e. food is digested slowly) that can help to lose weight, specifically lose visceral fat.[29] The best diet is based on legumes (beans, lentils, garbanzos, etc.), whole cereals, and vegetables that grown from the ground.[30] Note: if you are going to eat roots, like potatoes, make sure you eat them with high fiber foods (such as legumes) to reduce the glycemic load. Whole northern fruits (fruits that grow in the north like pears and apples) tend to have less sugar and higher levels of water. Small daily portions of nuts and seeds should also be added to the diet.[31] The diet should be free from animal products, animal fats and hydrogenated vegetable oils. It is best to eat most of the calories early in the day (before 3 PM) and have a very light supper, such as of fruits as well as complement this regime with an hour of exercise six times per week.

Current dietary guidelines from the American Diabetic Association push a "westernized" diet. They clearly ignore the health needs while encouraging a "sanitized version" of the Standard American Diet and the fast-food culture with animal proteins, sugars, and too much fat. It is like trying to use gasoline to extinguish a fire. This advice does not reflect the scientific knowledge we have accumulated so far. For example, the use of chicken and dairy products will not increase the glucose levels of patients on the short term, but rather the excess protein will put an extra burden on the kidneys and will increase insulin,[32] cholesterol,[33] and inflammation levels.[34]

I have never seen, in my 18 years of experience, a single patient that has reversed their diabetes by strictly following the American Diabetic guidelines. It is common to hear some of my patients say, "I just can't understand what is happening. I am following the guidelines, eating mostly chicken and turkey, but my cholesterol still has not come down that much!" Animal protein alone will increase cholesterol. A landmark study in 2006 shows the clear advantages of a vegan diet against the current ADA diabetic guidelines.[35] The vegan group was able to control glucose much better and improve other health markers such as cholesterol and weight.

Although sometimes diabetes cannot be completely reversed, we can control our diabetes with diet. For example, a recent patient had gained a lot of weight and was battling depression. Nobody had checked her glucose recently; her 10 hour fasting glucose was 138 (7.6 mmol/l), and further testing confirmed her diabetic state. I put her on a temporarily raw vegetable diet for 7 days. This has amazing results for their blood sugar as the patient will not feel the need to snack between meals, and the patient will quickly lose some weight. This plan works so well that it is imperative to monitor their glucose and medications so they don't fall into hypoglycemia (reading of less than 70 mg/dl (4 mmol/l)[36] in their fasting glucose). By the end of the week her fasting blood sugar was 106 (5.8 mmol/l), she had moved from a diabetic state to a barely pre- diabetic state. After following a plant-based diet, in a few more days her sugar was in normal levels and her depression was on its way out. A diabetic state will create changes in the pancreas. The ability of the pancreas to continue to secrete sufficient insulin is a strong predictor of reversibility.[37] Even if the diabetes cannot be completely reversed, a change to a full plant- based diet will help to keep sugar under better control and, in many cases, will lead to less diabetic medication.[38]

Eddie Ramirez, MD, *graduated at the top of his medical class from CEUX in Baja. Dr. Ramirez is the founder of a successful bilingual diabetes club and has worked as a clinician, speaker and researcher on 3 continents. Follow him on Twitter @EddieRDMD*

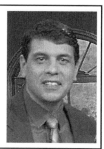

Diabetes Can Be Defeated

Veronika Powell, MSc

Diabetes has reached epidemic proportions around the world and numbers are rising. Type 2 diabetes usually develops in people over the age of 40 however; it is rapidly becoming more common in young people of all ethnicities. This is predominantly ascribed to the increase in childhood obesity. The best available medication and current dietary recommendations are unable to limit the growth of this disease, never mind reverse it. Problematically, diabetics are likely to develop various health complications, reducing their quality of life and potentially leaving them with damaged eyes and kidneys, prone to heart attacks and amputations, and in constant pain due to neuropathies – which can eventually lead to depression and premature death. Lifestyle and diet changes are recognized as necessary for diabetes management, but none of the mainstream recommended dietary changes are truly effective.

The only diet that has proved to be effective in reversing diabetes, bringing blood glucose levels under control, inducing weight-loss, and significantly improving the health of diabetics is a vegan, low-fat, low GI (Glycemic Index) diet. This approach works on basic biological principles and strikes at the very core of the condition. Although genes can play an important role in the development of diabetes, lifestyle, and environmental factors determine whether the disease actually develops in the first place.

What is Type 2 Diabetes?

Diabetes mellitus is a condition characterised by high levels of glucose (sugar) in the blood which the body cannot properly use and which is eventually excreted in the urine, along with a good deal of water. As glucose passes through the kidneys, it attracts water which results in frequent trips to the toilet to urinate and a feeling of thirst caused by fluid loss. In type 2 diabetes, commonly called adult onset, the pancreas does not produce enough of the hormone insulin or the body stops responding to insulin, as cells develop insulin resistance which is the most common scenario.

Insulin is a hormone produced by the pancreas and acts as a key allowing glucose into the body's cells. Glucose is a vital source of energy for cells and is the main fuel for the body's processes. It comes from digesting carbohydrates, but is also partially produced by the liver. When glucose is prevented from entering the body's cells, they are denied their basic and most important fuel. This can result in tiredness, one of the symptoms of diabetes. Other symptoms are irritability, nausea, hunger, thirst, weight loss, blurred vision, tingling sensations in the hands and feet, and dry, itchy skin.

Most mainstream diets for diabetics recommend limited carbohydrates. This approach fails to work because when the body cannot obtain enough energy from carbohydrates, it uses fat instead, but this inevitably disturbs the biochemical balance of the body. This energy fuel substitution affects metabolism to a large extent, causing increases in blood lipids, including cholesterol. It might seem desirable that the body is burning fats, but human metabolism is not adapted to fat being the main source of energy. Unless the diet is really low in fat, the condition cannot improve significantly.

Link Between Animal Products and Type 2 Diabetes

The conventional diet recommended for diabetics does not limit animal products - the main sources of saturated fat in the diet. Eating just one serving of meat per week significantly increases the risk of diabetes,[1] and the more meat we eat the more likely we are to develop type 2 diabetes.[2]

What is it that makes animal products so detrimental to health? The main enemy is fat. Diets high in animal protein force both liver and kidneys to work harder in order to filter nitrogen byproducts (of protein metabolism) out of the bloodstream in the process of producing urine. Kidneys dilate their blood vessels to filter out protein waste-- and animal protein causes greater dilation than plant protein. Plant-derived proteins are lower in sulphur and demand less from the kidneys' filtration system.

A series of studies[3,4,5,6,7] discovered that people with various degrees of insulin resistance had microscopic drops of fat inside their muscle and liver cells, and this fat interfered with the cells' ability to correctly react to insulin. Muscle cells normally store small quantities of fat as energy reserve, but in insulin-resistant people fat had built up to levels 80% higher than in healthy people. For example, when young healthy men (average age 23 years) were put on a high-fat diet (50% of calories came from fat), after just 3 days the amount of fat in their cells had increased considerably which showed how fast the accumulation of fat inside cells is.[8] This type of fat is not necessarily reflected in physical body shape as slim people can also have this fat accumulation in their cells causing insulin resistance.

Further tests revealed that fatty foods have a profound effect on the genes and proper functioning of mitochondria (cell's metabolic units). In fact, fatty foods turned off those genes that normally help mitochondria to burn fat. A high-fat diet therefore caused the body to accumulate more fat in muscle cells while at the same time slowing down the body's ability to burn this fat; this can be explained by our evolutionary history when fat storing was a necessary mechanism for times when food would be scarce.[9] This significantly inhibits the ability of the cells to respond to insulin.[10]

The Principles to Defeating Diabetes with Diet

It is possible to decrease and control blood sugar levels, limit medication, cut the risk of complications, and even reverse type 2 diabetes with a low-fat, low GI diet.[12,13,14,15,16,17,18] In 2010, the American Diabetes Association endorsed whole foods, plant-based diets stating that they had been shown to improve metabolic control in persons with diabetes.[19]

1st Principle: Eliminate Animal Products

By eliminating all animal products (meat, fish, dairy, eggs) diabetics avoid eating substantial amounts of fat, and cholesterol. Even lean, white meat and fish contain surprisingly high amounts of fat. For example, 38% of calories from roast chicken and 40% of calories from salmon come from fat-- and most of it is saturated.

Protecting the kidneys is another key issue for diabetics. Animal protein from meat, fish, dairy, or eggs places an additional strain on the kidneys and can damage them.[20,21] Plant proteins do not appear to cause the same problem. Animal products contain no fiber or healthy carbohydrates, while plant foods contain all the essential nutrients we need.

2nd Principle: Low-Fat

In order to reverse or improve the diabetic condition, it is essential to eliminate fat stores within cells.[22] A review of studies on bariatric surgery revealed that type 2 diabetes can be reversed within days of the surgery, even before any significant weight loss is achieved.[23] The main mechanism for this dramatic change is the sudden decrease of triglycerides and free fatty acids in the blood and rapid reduction of fats in liver and muscle cells.

The amount of fat per serving should not exceed 3 grams (or 10% of calories from fat). Diabetics should also limit their consumption of nuts, seeds and vegetable oils. To ensure sufficient intake of essential omega-3 fats, natural sources should be made part of a daily diet - flaxseed (linseed), hempseed, walnuts and their oils (used cold, not cooked) and rapeseed (canola) oil (for cooking and baking).

3rd Principle: Low Glycemic Index (GI)

Glycemic index, or GI, is a measure of the effects of carbohydrates in food on blood sugar levels. Carbohydrates that break down quickly during digestion and rapidly release glucose into the blood have a high GI. Carbohydrates that break down more slowly, releasing glucose gradually into the bloodstream, have a low GI. Low GI foods will not cause a sharp rise in blood glucose levels, which is exactly what diabetics require. It allows better control over blood sugar and reduces the likelihood of complications caused by hyperglycemia.

Glycemic Index of Selected Foods (from Glycemic Index Database and the GI Diet Guide)	
Classification	Examples
Low GI	Most fruits and vegetables, pulses (beans, soya, peas, lentils, chickpeas), barley, buckwheat, hummus, pasta, nuts and seeds, sweet potatoes, dried apricots and prunes, rolled oats, all-bran cereals, wholegrain pumpernickel bread, soya yoghurt, and products low in carbohydrates
Medium GI	Whole wheat bread, rye bread, crisp bread, brown rice, basmati rice, corn, porridge oats, shredded wheat, pineapple, cantaloupe melon, figs, raisins, beans in tomato sauce
High GI	Potatoes, watermelon, pumpkin, white bread, French baguette, white rice, rice cakes, corn flakes, processed breakfast cereals, dates, sugary foods

Whole grains are rich in complex carbohydrates, high in protein and fiber, and have a low GI. Virtually all vegetables have a low GI and contain many essential vitamins and minerals, as well as cancer fighting antioxidants. It is a common misconception that fruits should be avoided by diabetics. In fact, nearly all fruits have a low GI, the only exceptions being watermelon and pineapple.

A whole foods, plant-based diet constructed on these principles is the healthiest possible for diabetics. Vitamin B12 supplementation is needed and requirements may be higher in diabetics as the commonly taken drug, Metformin, can reduce absorption of this vitamin.

Diabetes does not have to be a fatal diagnosis. Scientific research and clinical studies show that lifestyle is the single most important factor in the development of diabetes and it is therefore never too late to try a new – and effective – approach.

Veronika Powell, MSc, *is a biologist, researcher, and qualified teacher. She is currently at health campaigner at Viva! Health.* www.viva.org.uk/health/diabetes *and* www.veganrecipeclub.org.uk

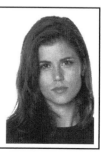

Insulin Resistance as a Source of Chronic Diseases

Eric Slywitch, MD

Vegetarian and especially vegan diets are effective in improving the levels of glucose in the blood and insulin. This metabolic adjustment is very important to understanding how other diseases can be prevented through plant-based diets.

When we have a meal, we eat fats and glucose as a source of energy. Protein can be used as energy also, but only when we do not have enough glucose. Our brain needs glucose to function properly. In an emergency state, the brain can use ketone bodies, produced at the same time as we are burning fat. However, glucose is the main and preferred source of fuel for the brain.

Insulin is a hormone that orders the muscle cells to "open up" and accept the glucose. Think of insulin as a type of key, and the muscle has a type of lock (insulin receptor). In normal production of insulin, the key joins the lock (insulin links with the receptor), and the muscle cells open for the glucose to enter.

In many situations, the receptor (the lock) does not answer the insulin, and the glucose level remains high in the blood. High levels of glucose stimulate insulin production. The more blood glucose, the more insulin is produced. The problem is that, we have high levels of insulin trying to maintain normal levels of glucose. This is insulin resistance, and the consequences affect our entire body.

Let´s address some of the problems associated with insulin resistance in turn:

Fatigue: Our body requires energy for every function from contracting our muscles to thinking. Inside the muscle cells, we have an energy factory: the mitochondria. Glucose is the raw material used to produce energy, or ATP (adenosine triphosphate). If glucose is outside the cells and is not being received into the muscle, it is impossible to produce energy. Every person who has high levels of glucose in the blood is showing us that they have low amounts of glucose inside the muscle cells, and the production of energy is low. This is fatigue.

In this condition, taking vitamins and energetic teas or drinks do not solve the problem. Furthermore, when insulin is high, we cannot burn the adipose tissue. We then gain weight easily and the fat accumulated produces inflammation, the genesis of disease.

Fatty Liver: The liver is an important organ that protects us from glucose, as glucose outside the muscles can hurt our cells. Glucose is a potential cause of immediate tissue damage. Because of this, the liver tries to help the body by removing the glucose that is in excess in the blood. Inside the liver, glucose is converted into triglycerides. Have you ever heard that excess sugar turns into fat? It is exactly this process of converting glucose into triglycerides. In a normal situation, the triglycerides leave the liver and are stored in the adipose tissue or used as a fuel for the muscles. However, when there are high levels of glucose in the blood, we have high levels of insulin also. Insulin does not allow triglycerides to leave the liver completely. We just created a hepatic steatosis, or fatty liver.

This condition affects the functioning of the liver as the excess fat can destroy many of the liver cells in a condition called cirrhosis. This damage is irreversible. To reverse this situation, the insulin must be lowered by not consuming excess calories, avoiding saturated fat and refined grains, and eating rich fibers foods.

High Cholesterol: Fatty liver directly connects to high cholesterol levels and insulin resistance. Insulin stimulates elevated levels of cholesterol by acting on an enzyme called HMG-CoARedutase. This enzyme is the target of the drugs used to lower the cholesterol (statins). Drugs used to lower cholesterol act in the same way the insulin acts on the enzyme HMG, except insulin raises the cholesterol.

Additionally a fatty liver or inflamed liver affects cholesterol production, producing more cholesterol than normal. When the body is inflamed, tissues are damaged and need to be fixed. One of cholesterol's roles in the body is as a raw material to produce new cell membrane. More inflammation thus begets more cholesterol production, leading to high cholesterol levels.

Hypertension: We can think of our blood pressure and blood vessels in terms of pipes and our heart as a water tank or pool. When you inject water directly into the pipes or vessels, excess water will put pressure on the tank, making it overflow. The difference between the pipes and our vessels is the expansion property of our blood vessels. Therefore, when we have water excess inside the veins, they dilate to keep the heart free from pressure, while kidneys remove the water to the urine. This dilation controls our blood pressure and is directly affected by insulin. Insulin does not allow adequate dialysis of sodium by the kidneys. Sodium is difficult to excrete, and water loves sodium. This means that high levels of sodium in the vessels attract water. To accommodate this volume of liquid, the vessels begin to dilate-- the substance responsible for this dilation is called nitric oxide. Insulin, however, does not allow this expansion to occur. Insulin destroys nitric oxide and therefore destroys the possibility of blood pressure control.

Compounding this problem is insulin's ability to activate our sympathetic nervous system-- our system activated by fear or need to fight or escape. When this system is activated, we produce adrenalin. Adrenalin also retains water and sodium and, furthermore, contracts the vessels directly and causes high blood pressure or hypertension.

Cancer: High insulin does not allow the fat to leave the adipose tissue, contributing to weight gain and obesity. Among the various substances produced by the adipose tissue, two enzymes are very important in the context of hormones linked to cancer: aromatase and 5-alphareductase. The first one transforms testosterone into estrogen. The second converts testosterone into dihydrotestosterone. These hormones in high levels can induce breast, prostate, and uterine cancers. When there is insulin resistance the growth hormone is activated by the liver, but when the liver is fatty we have less active hormones. This makes it easier to lose muscle and gain fat—thus adding to cancer risk.

There is also a competition between growth hormone and insulin as both try to act in the same areas in the cells. Therefore, if you have a lot of glucose and consequently high insulin, the growth hormone cannot act properly.

Should We Eat Less Carbs? Simply put: no! Many studies with vegan diets show that a planned diet with low fat and more carbs can be very healthy and helps to control weight and insulin resistance. It is easier to eat more than you need with an animal-based diet. When you choose vegetables and natural sources to eat, you are choosing food with more volume, but fewer calories.

Rules to Lower Insulin and Improve Glucose Control:

1. Eat every 3 hours. When you go more than 3 hours without eating, the levels of glucose in the blood start to lower and our brain needs glucose. Cortisol and glucagon rise and destroy muscle to use its amino acids to produce glucose for the brain. Therefore, we lose muscle. These hormones also destroy the insulin receptor. When you finally do eat, glucose rises in the blood and insulin rises, but the insulin does not find the receptor and more insulin is produced.

2. Maintain a proper weight: Excess fat leads to insulin resistance.

3. Practice physical activity. Cardio exercise helps muscles receive insulin. Exercise for at least 30 minutes every 2 days.

4. Maintain a good level of cortisol, the stress hormone. When cortisol rises, the glucose does not go into the muscle cells. Make sure you are well rested.

5. Improve your fiber intake by avoiding refined and processed food. The large amount of fiber that plant food contains promotes satiety.

6. Avoid saturated fat: the main sources of saturated fats are butter, milk, cheese, eggs and meat. Cheese has about 70% of its kcal as fat. White cheese has 60% of its kcal as fat. Lean cheese doesn´t exist! Saturated fat has two problems in

insulin resistance. The first one is because our cell´s membranes are made of fats and saturated fat is hard. Building your cells with hard fat makes it difficult to transport substances through the membrane, including glucose. The second problem is that liver must remove this fat from the blood, and saturated fat is slower to remove than mono or polyunsaturated fat. The fat that is circulating in the blood reduces the sensitivity of insulin, or worsens the insulin resistance.

Go veg! It is an easy way to improve your health.

Eric Slywitch, MD, *has a Masters in Nutrition and Graduate Degree in Clinical Nutrition. Dr. Slywitch earned his medical degree at the Faculty of Medicine of Jundiai in Brazil. He specializes in nutrology and is the head of the Department of Medicine and Nutrition at the Brazilian Vegetarian Society. Dr. Slywitch is author of Meat free meal (Alimentação sem carne) and I turned vegetarian. And now? (Virei Vegetariano. E agora?). He resides in Sao Paulo, Brazil.*

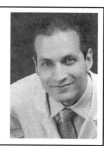

Correlation Between Metabolic Syndrome and Western Diets

Anteneh Roba, MD

Understanding the relationship between diabetes, high blood pressure, dyslipidemia, obesity, and metabolic syndrome is crucial to mitigating the worldwide rise in chronic degenerative diseases. Metabolic syndrome is not as well known or as precisely defined as diabetes or hypertension, so efforts to prevent it are minimal. Most physicians are either unaware or the problem is not addressed until it leads to a disease routinely studied in medical school.

As an attending ER physician, I have seen patients come in that were never properly diagnosed and treated for a constellation of conditions that define metabolic syndrome. Our dietary change from an original, naturally occurring human plant diet to animal-derived foods and processed foods high in simple sugars, is a major factor in the alarming increases in metabolic syndrome as well as diabetes,[1,2] hypertension, cardio-vascular disease, and cancer.[3]

What is Metabolic Syndrome?

Metabolic syndrome, otherwise called metabolic syndrome X, cardio-metabolic syndrome, insulin resistance syndrome, Reaven's syndrome, or CHAOS (in Australia), describes a cluster of conditions that typically include the presence of 3 or more of the following symptoms: elevated blood pressure (hypertension, HTN), elevated waist circumference (central obesity or "belly fat"), elevated fasting glucose (a measure of insulin resistance), elevated triglycerides (hypertriglyceridemia), and reduced levels of "good" HDL cholesterol.

Metabolic syndrome, affecting about one third of the US population, and 20- 30% of people worldwide, is associated with an increased risk of developing more serious chronic illnesses, such as cardiovascular disease and type 2 diabetes.[4]

Obesity as a Precursor to Metabolic Syndrome

As humans have gone from eating mostly plants to significant quantities of highly processed and animal-derived foods, contributing to the rise in obesity, metabolic syndrome has also become widespread in the U.S. As China and other increasingly affluent countries shift toward the Western diet, metabolic syndrome is rapidly becoming a global pandemic, hitting some developing countries before they amass the wealth to support a fundamentally unhealthy populace. By spotting the symptoms early, taking prompt action, and putting the patient on a whole foods, **plants-only** diet, physicians can prevent the dire consequences of metabolic syndrome.

According to the "thrifty genotype" theory, few if any changes in human genes or sequencing of genes have occurred over the past 10,000 years.[5,6] However, environmental changes from consuming processed foods as well as exposure to toxic waste and poor air quality could alter our genetic expression. Consumption of processed and nutrient-poor foods and animal-derived foods and our increasing consumption of highly processed, sugar-filled foods have led to detrimental changes in our physiology. Health-threatening saturated fats are implicated in the clogging of arteries resulting in heart attacks and strokes. Meat takes a particularly long time to transit through the gastrointestinal tract, releasing toxins as it putrefies and decomposes. When these toxins come in contact with the intestinal walls, they become carcinogenic. Adding to impacts on health is exposure to pesticides, herbicides, heavy metals, and other environmental toxins that our bodies cannot eliminate, which cause metabolic disturbances. These lifestyle changes contribute to the genotypic and phenotypic changes we are currently experiencing.

As a physician working in the United States and undertaking humanitarian medical missions in Ethiopia, I have witnessed the consequences of eating animal-derived foods and processed foods high in simple sugars – ubiquitous in America and increasing in affluent communities in Ethiopia. In both locales, the incidence of diabetes mellitus, hypertension, cardiovascular disease, and other chronic degenerative diseases are reaching epidemic proportions. This stands in drastic comparison to the very low incidence of such diseases in most rural African villages where Western "innovative" foods are virtually non-existent.

For example, on one medical mission to northern Ethiopia in 2011, our group of physicians traveled to a mountainous rural community whose diet is more than 95% plants. We saw approximately 800 people with all variety of medical problems and almost all had random blood sugar levels below 70 (most U.S. laboratories consider 70-100 normal) or a BP equal to or lower than 130/75, which is very healthy. When we returned in 2012 and examined nearly 5,000 patients, fewer than 10% of the patients had diabetes mellitus, fewer than 15% had hypertension, and virtually none had symptoms of heart disease. The average random and mostly fasting glucose levels were in the 60s, considered off the charts at the "healthy" end by U.S. standards. Although our first instinct was to administer intravenous glucose, as this level among people is often stereotyped as "deprived" or "developing" in the West, these levels indicated a degree of health superior to counterparts gorging on the western meat and dairy diet in affluent societies.

"An Ounce of Prevention is Worth a Pound of Cure"

Benefits of a plant-based diet for preventing or reducing high glucose levels,[7] elevated blood pressure,[8] high triglycerides, high cholesterol,[9] and increased waist circumference – the quintet that constitutes metabolic syndrome – are well known. Plant foods are rich in nutrients and anti-oxidants which protect against oxidative stress induced by the creation of reactive oxygen species from normal metabolic processes and exposure to environmental toxins- implicated in the aging process, chronic degenerative diseases, and the pathogenesis of cancers.[10,11,12]

The focus of medicine is changing toward prevention, albeit slowly. Too often I see patients for the same chronic problem. The time has come for conventional doctors to educate themselves on how to treat patients holistically by learning how to prevent disease. The only serious way to do that is to include nutrition among other treatment options in the armamentarium used by doctors. A plant- based diet extends beyond the health sphere and has significant social, economic, and environmental consequences. People with severe chronic disease not only experience diminished quality of life, but also serious economic consequences. Thus, a plants-only diet is a factor in a rich and rewarding life.

Anteneh Roba, MD, *is board certified in Emergency Medicine. Dr. Roba is currently doing a fellowship in functional medicine through the Metabolic Nutritional Medicine at University of Southern Florida. Dr. Roba is president and co-founder of international non-profit International Fund for Africa(IFA). He is currently co-editing a book called Africa and her Animals and has lectured throughout North America, Asia, Africa, and Europe. Born in Ethiopia, Dr. Roba currently lives in Houston, Texas with his beloved dogs. www.ifundAfrica.org*

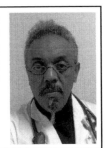

Working Towards a Diabetes- Free India

Nandita Shah, MD

When I became a doctor, about 5% of the adult Indian population was diabetic. Now just 32 years later; the incidence is about 35%. Growing up in Bombay, diabetes, heart disease and hypertension, obesity, and cancer were still uncommon in India. As the consumption of animal products, fried and processed foods increased in India, diseases relating to lifestyle have soared.

Today India is facing a diabetes epidemic as the incidence has spiked ten- fold in just the last 30 years.[1] Lifestyle modifications are all contributing to the increase in type 2 diabetes. The INDIAB research found that 62 million people are diabetic and an additional 77 million are pre-diabetic across the country. With 58% of the population over 50 years old in India diagnosed with diabetes and another 25 % pre-diabetic, India is rapidly becoming the largest diabetic population of any country in the world![2]

Meat and milk products are high in excess protein and fat and contain zero fiber to excrete toxins. Excess fat inside muscle cells is the primary cause of insulin resistance characteristic of type 2 diabetes. When the fat clogs our insulin receptors, it results in a build-up of sugar in the blood stream and an inability for the body to process the sugar and insulin effectively.

Most chronic conditions like type 2 diabetes can be reversible, in many cases. For example, a 21 year old patient with type 2 diabetes was taking 3 insulin injections per day. After switching to a plant-based diet we immediately cut the dose of insulin in half. Within 3 days, he was off insulin altogether. The blood sugar levels were still tested thrice a day to make sure they were ok and they remained normal. Remarkable? I thought so too.

In 2009, Dr. Neal Barnard helped us implement a 21-day diabetes program where 21 participants were put on a whole food plant-based diet, attended daily yoga, meditation, and cooking classes. Complete lab reports were done at the beginning and end of the program, and blood sugar levels were checked daily to closely monitor medications. All 21 participants considerably reduced their need for medications and many eliminated their need for medications altogether in just 3 weeks.

Our body is amazingly self-healing. By implementing a whole food, plant-based diet for just 30 days (with lab reports before and after), most people are able to feel the positive changes in their bodies and see it reflected in their labs. I encourage everyone to learn about our food sources and the environmental implications of our meals. We empower ourselves when we are educated in making healthful choices.

Nandita Shah, MD, *has been practicing homeopathy in India for over 32 years. Dr. Shah founded SHARAN in 2005 and for the past 7 years, she has presented the Peas vs. Pills workshops in India, and around the world, to over 5000 participants inspiring others to make dietary and lifestyle changes. Dr. Shah also conducts health and corporate workshops, cooking classes, and residential programs including a 21-day disease reversal holiday.*

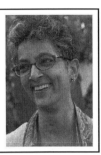

Reverse Type 2 Diabetes Better than Medication

Dana S. Simpler, MD

Lisa* is a 45 year old Caucasian woman who, like many internal medicine patients, had multiple medical problems including hypertension, hypothyroidism, sleep apnea, and migraines.   She developed diabetes, which was very concerning to her, and she agreed to start a whole food plant- based diet. She immediately went completely plant- based and the results were astonishing. Within a few weeks she was calling me with lightheadedness, because her blood pressure medication were now too strong for her and needed to be lowered. In fact, within 1 month she was off of the 2 blood pressure pills she had taken for years. Her weight dropped from 251 to 226 in 2 months, and her hemoglobin (Hbg A-1-C) dropped from the diabetic range to the borderline diabetic range, on NO MEDICATION. Within a year, she had lost a total of 47 pounds and her labs revealed she was no longer borderline diabetic. Her Hbg A1C is now in the normal range and she completely reversed her diabetes on a plant- based diet!

*All patients names have been changed for privacy.

*Please read Dr. Simpler's article, "A Whole Food, Plant-Based Diet: Next Blockbuster Drug of the Year" in What's Missing in Med School chapter

Never Too Late to Cancel Surgery

Dana S. Simpler, MD

Doree* is a 71 year old African American woman, and like many Americans she started with hypertension her chronic medical problems which led to her other chronic medical problems that accumulated over the years. Despite regular office visits and compliance with medications, she developed diabetes, high cholesterol, arthritis, as well as chronic headaches, sinus symptoms, and atherosclerosis that affected her heart and kidneys. Why was she getting sicker when she was taking all the latest modern medications? The problem was we were not treating Doree's underlying cause of all these illnesses, just the symptoms.

Doree had been following the ADA diet (American Diabetes Association), which limits carbohydrates, but still allows considerable amounts of saturated fat, found in animal products. The ADA diet does not treat the underlying problem of insulin resistance. There are small receptors on each cell called insulin receptors, which act like keyholes that need to unlock to allow glucose (sugar) to enter the cells. Insulin functions as the key. But, if there is too much saturated fat in the diet, it 'clogs' the keyholes and the key (insulin) can't connect, causing the glucose (sugar) to buildup in the bloodstream. This condition, called insulin resistance, leads to diabetes.

Doree's arteries were so clogged that her surgeon wanted to do carotid artery surgery. At this time I was just learning the cardiovascular benefits from a plant- based diet. Searching for alternative to surgery, Doree read Dr. Esselstyn's book, **Prevent and Reverse Heart Disease,** and implemented a plant-based diet. Six weeks later Doree told me she felt great! Once Doree stopped eating animal products and saturated fat, her insulin receptors opened up and her insulin resistance and diabetes greatly improved. Also, by cutting off the saturated fat from animal products and losing weight her clogged carotid artery had a chance to open back up as well. Her headaches and sinus trouble were gone, her blood sugar drastically lowered, and we were able to eliminate her need for insulin. Best of all, we cancelled her surgery

*All patient names changed for privacy

*Please read Dr. Simpler's article, "A Whole Food, Plant-Based Diet: Next Blockbuster Drug of the Year" in What's Missing in Med School chapter

The Dietary Connection to Diabetes

Mohamed H. Ismail, MD, MPH

I never took diet as a serious form of treatment until I asked a colleague, a Veteran of the US Armed Forces, how he had achieved some notable health improvements. He gifted me a copy of *The China Study* by T. Colin Campbell, which led to what I consider my "nutritional awakening." Fascinated with Dr. Campbell's work, I followed it by reading Dr. Dean Ornish's *Program for Reversing Heart Disease*, *Dr. Neal Barnard's Program for Reversing Diabetes*, and Dr. Joel Fuhrman's *Eat to Live*. These modern day pioneers of lifestyle medicine came to the conclusion that a 'whole foods, low fat, plant-based diet' could not only assist in weight loss and help prevent illness, but could actually reverse diseases that were otherwise thought to be unrelentingly progressive, such as coronary artery atherosclerosis and type 2 diabetes.

This approach goes against conventional assumptions, as most consider chicken a health food, dairy the only way to get calcium, protein only coming from animals, and plant-based to mean a plate of lettuce. Let's look at type 2 diabetes as an example of how a plant-based diet goes against these assumptions and can protect and reverse this disease.

Type 2 diabetes is a state of glucose intolerance resulting from insulin resistance, whereas type-1 diabetes is caused by a lack of insulin production. Insulin resistance occurs physiologically during growth, healing from injury, and pregnancy; however, it is also linked pathologically to several factors including genes, visceral adiposity, exercise, ethnicity, stress hormones, fatty liver, inflammation, and age.[1-6] A high fat diet (especially saturated & omega-6) and isolated fructose have been shown to induce resistance while omega-3 fats and flaxseed oil may be protective against it.[7-9]

Epidemiological data which show differences in prevalence based on geography indicate the connection between insulin resistance and diabetes, and lifestyle choices such as the amount of meat or sugar consumed. For example, it is clear that the 'American Lifestyle' is associated with an increased incidence of diabetes over the last few decades, though it is hard to pinpoint a definitive single cause since 'lifestyle' includes diverse factors such as processed food and fast food consumption, stress, and lack of physical activity.[10] However, the Adventist health study 2 found that "cases of diabetes developed in 0.54% of vegans, 1.08% of lacto ovo vegetarians, 1.29% of pesco vegetarians, 0.92% of semi-vegetarians, and 2.12% of non-vegetarians."[11,12] This study suggests that eating plant-based is protective and that vegetarians, in general, have a lower risk of diabetes.

The CHIP Pilot Study for Diabetics

I have seen firsthand the benefits and improvements a whole food, plant-based diet can have in treating diabetes through my CHIP study. The complete health improvement program (CHIP), designed by Dr. Hans Diehl, teaches the importance of low-fat whole foods and daily moderate exercise, as well as stress reduction and family bonding. In addition to its 55,000 graduates, it had been proven in multiple peer reviewed works to dramatically improving health and reducing the burden of chronic illness.

After careful scientific planning, my research team and I enrolled 44 diabetic patients into our CHIP pilot program. This program focused on the importance of low-fat, whole foods; daily moderate exercise, as well as stress reduction and family bonding. After 12 weeks, 42 of the original enrollees completed the program (93%). Almost all reported an increase in energy levels. More importantly, their diabetes lab test results improved by over 50% while their diabetes medications were reduced by 50% as well. Cholesterol levels improved and participants lost an average of 1 pound per week. (6 participants lost 20 lbs or more.) Nine participants reached the target of 'controlled' diabetes (HBAIC $\leq$ 7) and 6 participants were able to stop insulin completely. When compared to a control group who had received usual care, the CHIP participants had improved significantly more. A detailed dietary survey of participants showed that by the end of the 12 weeks, they had increased their intake of fruits and vegetables by about 30% and reduced their intake of meats, dairy, fats, and added sugars by close to 75%.

Our pilot group is now several months post-graduation; some continue to do fantastic, while others are working to overcome obstacles that contribute to rising blood sugars. They are dealing with their daily environment-- a reality which is not generally conducive to good health. CHIP's appeal seems to be its promotion of self empowerment and positive supportive environment. As we continue to monitor and support our pilot group, we are well into the planning of an expanded program giving us greater insight into how to sustain this type of lifestyle in a classic care setting. Although using food as medicine is still not yet mainstream, we are confident that we can gradually break through these barriers of resistance.

Mohamed H. Ismail, MD, MPH, *is board certified in Internal Medicine and Preventative Medicine. He received his MPH and trained at Loma Linda University in California.*

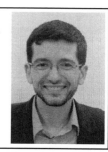

nine

DEAR CANCER

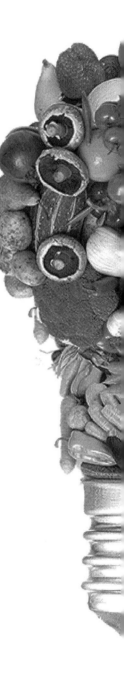

This chapter's leading oncologists will evidence how breast, colon, ovarian, and cervical cancers can be prevented, as well as slowed, and often reversed with a simple dietary change. These doctors attest that we possibly have the cure for 90% of breast cancer cases. Imagine how many mother's and daughter's lives can be saved. As more and more studies implicate processed and red meats in colon cancer, we have the potential to save more men's and women's lives from cancer's grasp. Armed with this knowledge, it's time to eat for the cure.

Did you know we all have cancer cells present in our body throughout our lives? Whether cancer continues to grow or not depends more on our body's environment, largely dictated by our food choices, than our genes. Cancer is a faulty replication of our genes and it can mutate and replicate quickly and unregulated if fertilized by carcinogens. But only about 2 - 3% of all cancers are purely genetic.

It can take 10 years for cancer to grow- meaning our childhood eating habits can set the stage for adult cancer. Some of the largest cancer promoting agents include casein- comprising 87% of milk products, Insulin-like growth factor-1 found in dairy products, processed meats, red meats, cooked meats by producing HCAs, and excess fat.

Simply put, animal protein changes our hormones, cell proliferation, and provides the ideal environment for cancer to grow. Our current diet is cancer-causing. However, switching to a plant-based diet can change about 500 genes, "turning on genes that prevent disease and turning off genes that cause breast cancer, heart disease, prostate cancer, and other illnesses."[1]

*Please note: for more on Prostate Cancer refer to Dr. Gordon Saxe and Dr. Ron Allison in *For Men Only* chapter. On childhood cancer please refer to Dr. Divya-Devi Joshi in *Feeding Kids Right* chapter.

Beat Cancer

Mary R. (Clifton) Wendt, MD

Do you know of someone who has suffered from cancer? Most of us know of someone who has had their lives ruined or shortened by this terrible disease. I have personally worked with over 400 cancer patients in the past 5 years and seen the ravages of the disease far too many times.

Scientists think that all of us have cancer cells in our bodies. Cancer cells are created when normal cells undergo an irregular replication. Instead of this replication resulting in another normal cell, the newly created cell is different. Sometimes the abnormality results in the cell falling out of the normal regulatory mechanisms. Over the next 8 to 10 years those abnormal cells can grow and replicate into a problematic tumor.

Cancer cells that are replicating quickly need direct blood flow to feed their rapid growth. The process of growing new blood vessels for purposes of feeding the cancer is called angiogenesis. Cancer cells attract and develop new blood vessels with a protein called methionine. Methionine is so integral to cancer cell growth that drug companies are spending millions of dollars to identify methionine blockers to slow the progression of cancers. Where does methionine come from? Is there any way to slow the rate of angiogenesis by changing the food we eat?

The highest methionine levels are found in egg whites and fish.[1] That means that the foods with the highest ability to help cancer feed itself by increasing blood flow are eggs and fish. It is both sad and ironic that the "healthiest" animal proteins available are proposed to be fish and egg whites-- fish and egg whites are actually leading contributors to cancer growth in the American diet.

Dairy has also been linked to cancer promotion. One of the main promoters within dairy is Insulin-like Growth Factor – called IGF-1. Studies have found that when IGF-1 is dripped onto cancer cells in the lab, it is like fertilizing a lawn.[2] The cancer cells grow much more rapidly in the setting of IGF-1. IGF-1 is present in all forms of dairy from a glass of milk to a piece of cheese.

It is a fallacy that using organic dairy keeps you from getting any hormones in your milk. Cow's milk is rich in hormones intended to stimulate rapid growth in their baby calves, whether or not it is "organic."

While there is much more definitive information on the connection between milk and cancer growth, there are a number of studies that show that as meat consumption increases, it becomes easier for carcinogens to travel into the cells and stay.[3] Essentially, by ingesting these products, you are making a hospitable environment for cancer to growth.

Antioxidants Fight Cancer

To fight cancer you need a high-level of antioxidants in your blood. There are no antioxidants in meat. Fruits, vegetables, whole grains and beans contain significantly high levels of antioxidants. Increasing antioxidant and fiber intake is associated with the reduction of cancer, heart disease, and all the metabolic problems. Simple changes, like switching from a Diet Coke to a glass of hibiscus tea, can entirely alter your antioxidant level and protect you from cancer every day.

Influencing Prostate Cancer with Diet

One of my patients had a very aggressive reoccurrence of prostate cancer. His PSA level, used to help diagnose prostate cancer, jumped from about a 4 to over a 20 in about 4 months. His cancer was progressing at a rapid pace. He followed my recommended diet for almost 6 months and his cancer remained under control with no changes to his cancer markers. Unfortunately he quit my die. His cancer resurfaced aggressively, with cancer markers doubling in just 1 month. He became strict again with his plant-based diet. It is interesting to see the amazing difference it makes when you take away those dietary stimulatory fertilizers.

Today, especially in Western countries, we eat a diet rich in meat and dairy. When you choose meat, you are choosing to not consume something else with more nutritional value. Not only are you making an unhealthy choice, but you are limiting your intake of healthier choices. Why not let the healthy foods overflow on your plate, instead of trying to moderate your diet with a little good and little bad?

Think about it this way: if you eat 2000 calories per day, and you eat two cookies, that means that 20% of your caloric intake for the day is promoting inflammation, cancer promotion, and heart disease. In the short run it is going to make it harder for you to control your weight but in the long run it will promote much bigger problems.

The study of nutrition and the study of medicine have been separated for far too long. It has become standard for nutritionists exclusively to understand and for doctors to not be familiar with nutrition. Today there is simply too much too data that it is not conjecture. The reality is we have a deeper and clearer understanding of how diet impacts our health.

We can change our behaviors. Doctors are trained that it is a waste of time to talk about nutrition, but I can assure you that it is not a waste of time. The only time I have ever been able to decrease insulin dosages in diabetics or stop blood pressure pills in patients with high blood pressure, it has been because the patient has modified his or her diet. Simple recommendations, such as telling patients to eat more fruits and vegetables, result in increases of patient intake by 1.4 servings per day. 1.4 servings a day increases concentrations of antioxidants in the bloodstream and lowers blood pressure. Talking to your patients about nutrition will change their risk of stroke and heart attack. As doctors, we have power to improve the health of our patients. Now, we must have the courage to do so.

Mary R. (Clifton) Wendt, MD *has been an Internal Medicine doctor for almost 20 years. Dr. Clifton regularly speaks at health and inspirational seminars, medical and health conferences, corporate wellness events, Universities, and for private groups. Dr. Mary is the author of the best-selling book, Waist Away, co-author of the book "Get Waisted: 100 Addictively Delicious Plant-Based Entrees", and CEO of the healthy weight loss program "Get Waisted". Mary most enjoys spending time with her daughters, husband, and reveling in the deliciousness of decadent plant-based food!*

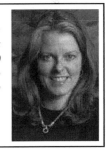

Rethinking Food in the Light of Epigenetics

John Kelly, MD, MPH

Although food is often thought of as a dichotomy of pleasure versus calorie control, the evolving science of epigenetics, the study of the change in gene expression, is revealing that food is much more than calorie-laden pleasure— it is a powerful way to guide the expression of our genes.

Few realize that our genome, the directions inside every cell in our body that largely determine who we are and whether we are healthy or sick, is under the control of the epigenome. The epigenome is a set of 'gene switches' that turn our genes 'on' and 'off' throughout life to make us "us." Food is our most powerful tool for turning the genes we are born with 'on' and 'off'. Exercise and attitude are also very powerful modulators of gene expression, but food has the largest effect on our genes than anything discovered so far. Studies reveal that we can change more than 500 prostate cancer genes in beneficial ways by eating a simple plant- diet.[1] Animal studies reveal that a mother's high-fat food during pregnancy, such as animal foods and fast foods, can alter brain anatomy and function in her adolescent offspring in ways that promote obesity, hyperlipidemia, premature puberty and other untoward effects.[2] Eating DNA-methylating food such as high-folate, leafy-green plant foods during pregnancy, however, can turn 'off' genes causing obesity, diabetes, and heart disease.[3]

The latest cutting-edge genetic science tells us that food is not about calorie-laden pleasure, but about allowing each of us to live healthier, happier lives by muting the unhealthy genes we have inherited and empowering the health-promoting ones. The simplest way to accomplish this is to move away from processed and animal foods to simple, plant foods as grown. Epigenetics is expected by experts to become the epicenter of modern medicine.[4] We must rethink food and see it in its marvelous new light as the remote-control device that can switch genes 'on' and 'off'. Let's learn to use the food-remote wisely.

Plant-Based Diet and Cancer: The Open Secret

Lisa Bazzett-Matabele, MD

I Thought Cancer Was Inherited. What Does Diet Have to Do With It?

People tend to think, "Cancer does not run in my family, so I am not going to get it." Or, "I am going to get cancer because I have family members who have suffered from it." These lines of thinking are common misperceptions about cancer. Only about 5 to 10% of all cancers result directly from gene defects (called *mutations*) inherited from a parent. The rest are acquired throughout our lifetimes based on lifestyle and environmental exposures.[1] In fact, a growing number of cancers are proving to be diet related, and at least one-third of cancer deaths in the United States are due to dietary factors.[2]

Living in New Orleans, we are exposed to typical southern cooking: deep-fried foods, heavy creams and sauces swamping many dishes, and many of the vegetable dishes having animal fats added to 'season' them. Most of the cancer patients I see are overweight, and their list of added medical problems is often extensive. They usually have multiple diseases related to their excess weight, such as diabetes, hypertension, heart disease and joint problems.

As a Gynecologic Oncologist, I treat uterine, ovarian, cervical, vaginal and vulvar cancers. I have never had a patient who chooses a plant-based diet diagnosed with any of these cancers.

How Does Diet Increase Your Risk of Cancer?

There is a developing body of research supporting the fact that obesity increases your risk for cancer, including breast, prostate, uterine, ovarian and colorectal cancers.[3] Looking more specifically at one of the cancers that I treat, uterine cancer, we can see this connection between obesity and this increased risk.

Most uterine cancers result from the body producing excess estrogen. One site of estrogen production in women is in fatty tissue (adipose). In the fatty tissue there is an enzyme, aromatase, which converts testosterone to estradiol, the active form of estrogen. The more adipose we have, the more of this conversion from testosterone to estradiol occurs, creating excess. It is an exponential cycle of production. There are receptors for this estradiol on certain organs in the body, such as the uterus and breast, and when these receptors are over-stimulated by excess circulating estradiol, cancers can develop. Besides overproducing estrogens, increased dietary fat intake hinders our ability to clear these excess estrogens from the body. Our body needs fiber to clear these hormones from our system. Fiber is found only in plants, not in meat and dairy products. Diets high in fat also tend to be very low in fiber, so the hormones are not only overproduced, but without fiber, are also building up in the body. This is why patients who are obese have a much higher risk of developing uterine cancer.

Uterine cancer is the most common cancer of the female reproductive tract. Most of the patients that I see and operate on for uterine cancer are at minimum obese, and often morbidly obese, sometimes in excess of 300 pounds. The diet-related obesity epidemic is leading to an increased number of uterine cancers.

Another type of cancer I treat, **ovarian cancer,** is less studied because it is not as common as a lot of other cancers. However, obesity is now being suggested as one of the contributing factors to its development.[4] Some research also suggests a link between ovarian cancer and a higher intake of dairy products.[5,6] Interestingly, this association has also been made linking dairy products consumption and prostate cancer in men.[7,8,9] Although diet has yet to be extensively studied in relation to ovarian cancer, what we do know is that very few ovarian cancers are genetic, so in most cases, our lifestyle is likely a key contributor.

That being said, I have seen success when one patient with ovarian cancer changed her diet. This patient grew up in New Orleans eating a typical southern American diet and was diagnosed with an ovarian cancer so advanced, involving too many of her vital organs, that it was inoperable. She was treated with the most effective chemotherapy regimen for ovarian cancer, but the tumor continued to grow while on treatment. She was then evaluated at MD Anderson Cancer Center where they suggested an experimental chemotherapy regimen that was questionable whether it would be effective. She was then referred to me to receive her treatment. She decided at that time to switch to a plant-based diet. She is still receiving treatment, and while her cancer is still present, it has not grown in two years, and we are starting to wean her off chemotherapy. She is completely asymptomatic from her cancer and feels great. A result like hers is astonishing!

Cervical Cancer is another cancer I treat as a gynecologic oncologist. Human papilloma virus (HPV) infection is related to over 99% of cervical cancers. It is also the cause of some vaginal, vulvar, anal and throat cancers. A sexually transmitted virus, 80% of women and 75% of men will be exposed to HPV at some point in their lifetimes. Twenty million people in the United States are currently infected with this virus, but not all of these will lead to cancer.[10]

While HPV is necessary in the development of cervical cancer, it alone does not cause the cancer. Co-factors, such as smoking, work in combination with the HPV infection to determine if a person will develop an HPV-related cancer or if they will be able to clear the infection from their system completely and never develop a cancer.[11] We do not know all the co-factors involved, but we do know that smoking and diet are 2 important factors.

Since HPV is a viral infection, any factor that improves our immune system's function and its ability to fight off this infection would therefore decrease our chance that this infection would persist and progress into cancer. Plant-based diets contain an abundance of these antioxidants and natural immune system boosters. It is suggested that folic acid, a B vitamin found in dark leafy vegetables, fruits, peas, and beans may be especially important in preventing HPV-related cervical cancers.[12] While there is a vaccine against some strains of HPV available for young girls and boys, the impact from the vaccine and the decline in the incidence of disease in these young people will not be seen for another couple of decades. In the meantime, and for overall cancer prevention in the general population, we need to continue to consider our diets as our best source of cancer prevention.

Does Soy Cause Cancer?

The relationship between soy, estrogen and cancer is often a topic of confusion. Soy contains very weak plant estrogens called phytoestrogens that are thought to bind to estrogen receptors on cells. When soy binds to these receptors, it inhibits the body's natural estrogen from being able to bind to its receptors, therefore minimizing estrogen's effect. This is an important protective effect in estrogen stimulated cancers, such as some breast cancers. Studies have shown decreased incidence of breast cancer and breast cancer recurrences in women with diets higher in soy.[13,14,15] When you look at cultures that have eaten soy for thousands of years as part of their daily diet, they have significantly less breast cancer rates than we do here in the United States. When women from these populations emigrate and begin eating a Western diet substantially devoid of soy protein and high in animal products, their breast cancer rates increase significantly. It is important to remember that when we talk about soy, we are referring to its most natural form, like tofu, tempeh and soybeans. We are not referring to the isolated soy protein products often used to simulate the taste and texture of 'meat' in processed food products. Isolated soy protein is NOT the same as soy in its more natural form and may act differently in our bodies. People should be wary of including too much of these isolated soy proteins in their diet. It is important to stress that in a plant-based diet, we should always try to consume plant products as close to their natural, whole forms to receive the fullest nutrients and most beneficial effects.

Why Haven't I Heard This Before?

Everyone, both patient and physician, can play an important role in cancer prevention and treatment. While present-day standard treatments for cancer such as surgery, chemotherapy and radiation therapy are necessary and effective in many circumstances, we can do much better. The real *secret* to reducing our susceptibility to cancer is a healthy, plant-based diet. What we choose to put into our bodies every day is of utmost importance. We now have so much good evidence supporting the health benefits of a plant-based diet, it can no longer be ignored; it is no longer a secret.

What people need to understand is that physicians trained in Western medicine traditions are simply not taught in medical school about how nutrition and diet can significantly contribute to disease prevention and overall good health. This absence of knowledge and training follows most of us throughout our careers. Despite all of my training to become a gynecologic oncologist, it was not until years into my practice that I started learning about plant-based nutrition and its effect on our health. Physicians such as John A. McDougall and Caldwell Esselstyn have for years been showing the beneficial effects of plant-based diets on the prevention and treatment of a list of chronic diseases.

Unfortunately, because it is still the minority of physicians who have gained this knowledge, it can then make it difficult for our patients because they may then receive conflicting information from their doctors. For instance, when I tell patients they should avoid meat and dairy, they ask, "Why hasn't my diabetes doctor told me that? Why hasn't my heart doctor told me that? Why hasn't my family doctor who I have seen for 20 years told me that?" Regrettably, our medical culture in this country is preoccupied with treating illnesses and their symptoms, not preventing disease.

Much of what we have been led to believe is healthy for us is often coming from a source that does not necessarily have only our well-being in mind and often seeks to profit from their recommendations. Indeed, the source most of my patients point to when I ask them where they get their information about food is television commercials. It is clever marketing. It is time to get this secret out in the open, talk about it, share it with others, and practice it in our daily lives. A plant-based diet, focused on the most natural ingredients available, is a simple, conscious, daily choice we can make to take control over our bodies to make them and keep them healthy.

Lisa Bazzett-Matabele, MD, *attended the University of Michigan for undergraduate and Wayne State University for medical school.*

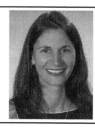

The Role of a Plant-Based Diet in Reducing Cancer Rates

Alberto Peribanez Gonzalez, MD, PhD

Cancer has been the greatest challenge to academic medicine in the last 50 years. The increase in cancer has soared in recent years, particularly in emergent industrialized countries.[1] Despite the rates in the United States being lower than 10 years ago, still 1,600 people a day die from cancer, and each year there are about 215,000 new prostate cancer cases.[2] Worldwide, cancer is spreading in pandemic proportions and now thousands of patients younger than ever before undergo chemotherapy, radiation, and surgery. The next generation may be the first whose life expectancy will be reduced.[3]

A whole food, organic plant-based diet may prevent, relieve, and-- depending on the kind of tumor-- help heal cancer.[4] Today prevention is evidenced in literature, by large population studies relating plant-based diets to a decrease in cancer incidences.[5,6] In addition to conventional treatment when tumors are present, a plant-based diet is a secondary treatment in cancer centers around the world. A plant-based diet is an effective source of anti-cancer phytochemicals that can help prevent secondary tumors and may reduce the progression of all kind of cancers.[7]

Integrating a plant-based diet into conventional treatments can change the prognosis of the disease. The first modern clinical application of a plant-based diet to manage cancer was conducted by Dr. Max Gerson who then authored *A Cancer Therapy: Results of 50 Cases* in which he describes details of healing patients using a fresh and raw vegetable-based juice diet.[8] The Gerson therapy has been mentioned by sectors of academic medicine as "without scientific support" or "with potential hazards," however evidence indicates those who dispute this approach are defendants of only the exclusive conventional treatments).[9]

Epigenetics, a new field that studies gene expression, indicates that even though some people may have genes putting them at a higher risk of cancer, we can influence this predisposition with our diet.[25]

The Good and the Bad Bacteria

Genomic studies indicate that the bacteria in our gut, when sampled together, contain 100 times more DNA than humans. The billions of microbes in our gut play a large role in the proper functioning of our immune system and significantly influence our health.[14]

While good bacteria in our bowel keeps us healthy, our gut also may contain noxious bacterial and fungal colonies. They may produce byproducts (toxins and mycotoxins), which can come from fermentation and environmental toxins, as well as toxins from food products. Food quality has been proven to influence the kind of bacteria which lives in our bowels.[15,16] Eating habits determine if we will have bacteria that stimulate our immunity and produce enzymes and vitamins essential to our cell physiology, or bacteria that produce toxic carcinogenic substances.[18]

Environmental Carcinogens

We currently have unacceptable rates of cancer that can in part be attributed to the toxins environmental toxins from our food products.[34] Brazil is plagued by pesticide use as are many other countries in the world. In Brazil, about 5 to 6 liters of pesticides per capita are annually spread on crops.[35] These pesticides infiltrate our water sources and our food system as the toxins can accumulate in the meat, poultry, and dairy products we eat. Pesticides are carcinogens that were designed to block metabolic routes in insects or microorganisms, and these mechanisms are still present in the food we eat. Since the widespread use of pesticides, there have been an increasing number of cases of cancer, birth defects in babies, and reproductive and hormonal problems.[36] Unfortunately, the response to these problems has so far been limited.

Our gut environment is subject to change depending on the composition of good and harmful bacteria.[19] The physiology of the bowel and liver have a close relationship as the liver receives the blood absorbed from the digestion. When our gut flora changes, these toxins can "leak" into the bowel blood barrier and ultimately reach the liver, compromising the ability of the liver to cleanse our body.[20] When the metabolic clearance rate of the liver is overloaded, these toxic substances can reach greater circulation within the body. Once in the blood, they turn systemic and can induce cells to change their biological characteristics and turn cancer cells on.[21] Our lymphatic vessels drain toxic substances and microorganisms from the tissues, sending them away to the lymph nodes where the immune system may identify it.

However, the overload of sugar and flour in our diet changes our blood and tissue microbiology. These toxins turn into yeast and mold, increasing the mycotoxic load of the tissues and plasma. Most of these mycotoxins are carcinogenic.[22,23]

Our contemporary diet composed of excess sugar and flour, dairy, poultry, and meat (that produces an acidic environment within our body) is essentially carcinogenic or cancer-promoting. PH reduction, or acidity, is related to cell dysfunction and cell death. Our cells and DNA shall best in a neutral pH in order to achieve normal function.[29] All of this acidity accumulates in the tissues, and our kidneys have the task to eliminate it. When renal and respiratory function are not enough to clear acidity, other non-traditional excretory organs like the skin, the lungs, and the stomach are involved, and clinical consequences can include psoriasis, asthma, and gastritis. Acid overload can eventually negatively alter our inner nuclear fluid and DNA.[30]

Cancer cells develop in acidic conditions, and restoring the acid-alkaline equilibrium is instrumental in reducing the growth of neoplastic cells. A plant-based diet high in chlorophyll offers a great amount of alkaline buffers, such as magnesium. Besides magnesium salts, plants offer an infinite number of alkalinizing phytochemicals and enzymes. A well-balanced vegan diet provides alkaline molecules that can easily maintain a normal pH.[31] Additionally when we adopt an organic, high-fiber plant based diet, it induces gut microbes to shift into healthy plant- related bacteria. This probiotic effect of plant-based diet is well described, as its symbiotic bacteria are known as "homeostatic soil organisms."[32]

The impact of a plant-based diet in helping to reducing breast and prostate cancer rates is evident when comparing the incidences of these cancers around the world. Japanese men eat a diet low in meat and dairy and have low rates of prostate cancer compared to men who consume an American diet high in meat and dairy. Additionally the rate of breast cancer in Kenya, which has a vegetable and rice based diet that is low in meat, is only 1 in about every 82 women. These population studies show that diet can play a pivotal role in cancer prevalence.[33]

From acting as probiotics to rid our gut of deleterious bacteria (SBO) ii) to helping maintain the alkaline blood pH (blood-interstitial-intracellular pH) to improving blood sugar balance and influencing gene expression, a whole food, plant-based diet can greatly affect our health (GI).

Alberto Peribanez Gonzalez, MD, PhD *Post graduation in the Institute for Surgical Research/ Ludwig-Maximilian University Munich, coordinator of the Natural Therapy Diabetes Program for Brazil.*

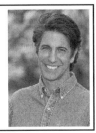

Colon Cancer Prevention

Aurora T. Leon Conde, MD

Colorectal cancer is the second most common cancer diagnosed in both men and women in the United States. The American Cancer Society estimates that there are 102,480 new cases of colon cancer and 40,340 new cases of rectal cancer in the United States in 2013. Although there is about a 5% chance of contracting the disease over the age of 50, even with new treatments and advances in medicine, survival rates are extremely low. Only 40% of those diagnosed with colon cancer are still alive after 5 years.[1,7] Several lifestyle-related factors have been linked to colorectal cancer. In fact, the links between diet, weight, and exercise and colorectal cancer risk are some of the strongest for any type of cancer.

Most colorectal cancers arise from adenomatose polyps. A polyp is a growth in the lining of the colon. Most polyps produce no symptoms and remain clinically undetected.[2] Up to 25% of patients with colorectal cancer have a family history of colon cancer and inflammatory bowel disease. The other 75% have no predisposing characteristics except for their diet.[2,7] Studies investigating different populations diets showed that groups such as Mormons and Seventh Day Adventist (populations in which vegetarian and vegan diets are more common) have lower incidence and mortality rates of colorectal cancer.[2] Similarly, a European prospective investigation found that the incidence of total cancer combined was lower among vegetarians than meat eaters.[9]

Statistics show that mortality is directly correlated with consumption of calories, meat protein, dietary fat, and oil as well as cholesterol. This is one reason why the incidence is higher in Western countries.

A diet that is high in red meats can increase colorectal cancer risk. **Just one 50 gram serving of processed meat (one hot dog) per day increases the risk of colorectal cancer by 21%.** Cutting out meat and animal products reduces your overall risk of cancer as much as 40%.[12] **According to Harvard University studies your risk of colon cancer drops by two-thirds if you stop eating meat and dairy products.**[13,14] Diets in high animal fats are also associated with high cholesterol, which has been linked with the development of colorectal polyps that can lead to cancer development.

Aside from the natural carcinogens in meat, cooking meats at very high temperatures (frying, broiling, or grilling) creates chemicals that might increase cancer risk. This may be in part due to carcinogens called heterocyclic amines (HCAS) that are created by cooking muscle tissue. Additionally fish and eggs contain dioxins that may contribute to colon cancer risk.[3]

Another hypothesis has been linked to insulin resistance and obesity.[10] Insulin resistance is a physiological condition where the cells of our body fail to respond to insulin and our body is unable to process insulin properly. This leads to increased insulin levels and hyperglycemia (increased levels of glucose in the body). All of these factors lead to higher circulating concentrations of insulin-like growth factor type 1 (IGF-1). Studies have found that IGF-1 is a cancer-promoting hormone, involved in every stage of cancer growth, spread, and metastasis. This growth factor appears to stimulate the proliferation of intestinal mucosa that promotes carcinogens. IGF-1 decreases dramatically in people eating plant-based diet.[2,4,5]

Compared to diets high in meat, dairy and cholesterol, diets high in vegetables, fruits, and whole grains have been linked with a decreased risk of colorectal cancer. This is primarily due to high fiber content. This association between dietary fiber intake and colorectal cancer was first proposed by Burkitt in 1971. There are several reasons why fiber has anti-carcinogenic mechanisms. Firstly, the formation of short-chain fatty acids from fermentation by bacteria fights cancer. The second is that fiber tends to reduce the production of bile acids, reducing the chances of cancer producing-bacteria and helps reduce insulin resistance.[11] Fiber also has a major role in regulating normal intestinal function and maintenance of a healthy intestinal tract including the reduction in transit time and increase of stool.[6]If our intestine is healthy we will produce healthy stools, preventing the formation of polyps and adenomas. Fiber supplements do not seem to help, meaning we have to have food rich in fiber and not rely on fiber supplements.[1]

Studies have shown that certain vegetables are better on fighting different types of cancer. In the case of colon cancer they have found that berries, broccoli, black beans, apples and herbal teas are beneficial. Fruits and vegetables are low in fat, high in fiber, and rich in antioxidants, which help to prevent cancer. Among the most potent antioxidants are beta-carotenoids, which can be found in orange vegetables and fruits. Another potent antioxidant is lycopene as found in tomatoes and watermelon.

Antioxidants come in several forms, including the vitamins A, C, and E; plant-derived polyphenols, found in colorful fruits and vegetables, beans, nuts and grains. The antioxidants have the ability to neutralize harmful molecules in our cells. They have the capacity to neutralize free radicals that are highly reactive and can cause damage to our cells and even cause cancer.

Fresh vegetables like cruciferous (broccoli, cauliflower, sprouts) have shown to have the highest anti-proliferative and antioxidant activities toward DNA oxidative damage. If the cell is not able to repair the damaged DNA (our genetic code) this can eventually produce cancer.

A population based study in Western Australia[16] of 1700 people found that the intake of dark yellow (rich in carotenoids) and cruciferous vegetables was significantly associated with decrease of colon cancer risk.

Food sustains our body and is so complex that we still do not fully understand it completely. Yet we do know that a whole foods plant-based diet is beneficial for the prevention and may influence the treatment and even reversal of cancer, so why not start now?

Aurora T. Leon Conde, MD, *was born in Mexico City and raised in northern Mexico. In 2009 she came to the US to continue her career in Medicine. She has always been interested in integrative medicine, a whole-person approach. Dr. Leon is a yoga enthusiast, and she ran NYC marathon on a whole food plant based diet. She participated with PCRM (Physicians Committee for Responsible Medicine) in "Vegeatriano en 21 dias" program*

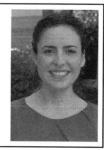

The Intimate Relationship Between Food and Cancer

Jacqueline Maier, MD

I realized the importance of food as medicine in preventing cancer after having completed 11 years of training including specializing in hematology and oncology and 20 years of practice. There was only a small paragraph in my medical school biochemistry book about nutrition. But there was no mention made of how cow's milk contains casein, which studies find promote cancer growth.[1] Casein accounts for about 8.5% of the protein found in cow's milk.[2] I never even learned that the lactaid enzyme is present in large amounts as newborn but as we grow, the production of this enzyme declines rapidly after the weaning stage. This results in lactose intolerance. About 30% of Caucasians are lactose intolerant, and it is almost double that for African Americans and triple that for those of Asian descent.[3]

After graduating from medical school, I robotically treated disease as if there was no possible cure unless it came out of the pharmaceutical industry. It took many years to realize that pushing pills is not the only way. Most of my patients ended up with severe cardiovascular problems, renal failure, diabetes, hypertension, cancer, in other words total body breakdown long before age should have been a big factor. It started to seem like all the different diseases were just different manifestations of the same underlying problem. Just like a car will run for a while on pure alcohol, the motor was not designed to run on pure alcohol. The care might go for a while, but will start to break down sooner than if given gasoline. The same applies to human or any animal body- it will break down much more quickly if not given the right ingredients.

As an oncologist I was drawn to the relationship between food and cancer, especially colon cancer.

Diet's Role in Colon Cancer

Unlike carnivores that can process this amount of meat due to a short intestinal tract and an extremely high level of stomach acid, our bodies are structurally more like herbivores. If we had short intestines like carnivores the transit time of the food would be too quick to be able to do any harm. But we have long intestines with 10 times less stomach acid to digest the meat.[4] The lack of fiber in meat contributes to constipation, which allows carcinogen time to affect the surrounding tissue. Very few vegans develop colon cancer.

To those who say we can't live without animal protein: all proteins are made up of 20 different amino acids and the exact same amino acids make up animal and plant proteins. Although there are different combinations of the 20 amino acids, the only difference between animal and plant proteins is the percentages of the combinations of the 20 different amino acids making up a particular protein that determines plant from animal protein. By eating a varied plant-based diet, one can get all the essential and non- essential amino acids necessary for proper growth, development and maintenance. Therefore even a carnivore could survive on a completely plant based diet if properly administered due to their structural differences. An herbivore however cannot survive on a total animal-based diet. Although amino acids and most proteins are not carcinogenic, food processes such as cooking meat and preservatives can make them carcinogenic.

Preservatives such as nitrates and nitrites are added to meats to preserve color and give a longer shelf life. High consumption of processed meats like cold cuts, sausages, hot dogs, etc are all associated with increased risk of colon cancer in human studies. Nitrites, nitrates and nitrosamines are extremely oxidative to certain tissues, especially the endothelial cells which surround the inner linings of the gut as well as blood vessels. If the linings are destroyed, many other abnormalities develop from there – all kinds of inflammatory changes occur: blood vessels - atheromatous changes; inner gut lining – colitis, leaky gut, and cancer.

The American Cancer Society states that "a high consumption of processed meat over 10 years was associated with a 50% increased risk in cancer of the lower colon and rectum."[5] High consumption was defined as 1 oz per day, 5-6 times a week for men and 1 oz per day, 2-3 days per week for women.

Additionally vegetables and fruits grown in artificially fertilized soil will contain more nitrates and nitrates and according to studies this fact alone may be contributing to the rise in colorectal cancer rates. Ideally, the best diet for everyone would be an organically grown vegan diet.

Jacqueline Maier MD, is a practicing oncologist in New York.

Preventing Colon Cancer is Critical

Ron Allison, MD

Diet has a major influence in preventing the development of colorectal cancer polyps. There is a very high rate of colorectal cancer among those who eat a Western Diet, heavy in meat, calories, and fat. It is well established that in Asian countries, where the diet is largely vegetarian, studies show very low rates of colon cancer. This can be attributed to the high fiber levels in plant-based diets as the fiber appears to bind the carcinogens in the bowel and prevent cancer growth. Despite what some people are led to believe, a fiber pill does not have the same effect.

As meat and cow's milk contain such a heavy protein load, the bowels usually cannot completely digest all of this protein. Undigested protein turns into carcinogens and toxins in your body. When undigested meat and its carcinogens pass through our body, they are generally stored in our rectum, which is likely why meat and dairy eaters have such high rates of rectal cancer.

Contrast that with a plant-based diet which has high fiber, low fat, and protein loads that our body can more easily digest. When fiber from plants, not pills, goes through our body and concentrates in our rectum, the fiber pulls out carcinogens over several hours. ***Think of it this way: every meal that does not consist mainly of plant-based food is a meal that has been wasted in terms of protecting ourselves against colorectal cancer.***

* Please read Dr. Allison's "Take Charge of Prostate Cancer" in the For Men Only chapter.

Fight Cancer with Nutrition

Andrea Lusser, MD

Approximately one-third of the risk factors for developing cancer are linked to nutritional deficits. By the age of 75, one-third of all people will develop some form of cancer. Since cancer is a chronic condition; we can help control the disease by nutritional factors that contain an abundance of cancer-fighting agents. Modern evidence-based scientific research recommends a balanced, plant-rich diet which can protect against cancers, heart attacks, and stroke.[1-3]

There is an established correlation between a damaged cell membrane function in cancer diseases and a copious use of unhealthy fats, which is abundant in meat-heavy diets.[4,5] Additionally, all types of sugars, including those that are "hidden" in various processed products like desserts or soft drinks are shown to feed cancer cells because they easily absorb sugars, which increases tumor growth.

On the other hand, a plant-based diet contains abundant nutritionals in a natural combination, like polyphenols, terpenes, sulfur compounds, and saponines, which have empirically demonstrated anti-cancer properties.[1] Over-acidity also plays an important role in cancer growth; since a plant-based diet is primarily alkaline, increasing the alkalinity of the body will provide yet another level of support. Plant-based proteins provide the additional advantage of a full spectrum of cancer-inhibiting phytochemical substances. These plant proteins avoid the damaging ingredients found in meat, fish, milk, and milk products such as cholesterol, arachidonic acids (which can trigger inflammation), uric acid, heavy metals, and hormones. Unsaturated fats from plant origin support

The Power of Amanita Therapy

Biologist Dr. Isolde Riede found one specific nutrient- Amanitin- found in mushrooms to be effective in treating tumors using Amanita therapy. Amanitin, the active molecule in dilutions of Amanita phalloides, work by inhibiting the growth of tumor cells. RNA-Polymerase II is utilized only in low amounts, estimated 10%, in somatic cells of adults. In contrast, tumor cells use this enzyme to the fullest amount possible. Inhibiting this enzyme leads to a direct inhibition of tumor cell growth. The immune system then recognizes and digests the tumor cells. Therapy with Amanita phalloides is shown to be well-tolerated and effective.[8-11]

Warning: *Do NOT pick and eat mushrooms in the wild. They are toxic and potentially fatal. Only conduct this therapy under medical supervision and with "Riede-approved" certified dilutions containing standardized ingredients of Amanites' active substances.*

the healthy function of the cell membrane which is essential in preventing cancer.[1,4,5] It is therefore recommended to switch to a plant-based diet as a precautionary measure against cancer and even more so when cancer has been diagnosed.

Studies have found plant-based foods to be helpful in treating tumors. For example, isolated cells of a medulloblastoma, a very aggressive brain tumor, were treated with various extracts of nutritional substances. Extracts of garlic, red beets, or certain cabbage relatives could completely stop the growth of these cells. The same mechanisms plants developed to fight damage caused by microorganisms, insects, or other parasites also play a role in our defense mechanisms against cancer. In particular vegetables such as green tea, soy, and the spice turmeric contain high levels of active cancer-fighting substances. These plants are part of a traditional daily diet in many Asian countries that have the lowest rates of cancers worldwide. Other identified cancer-fighting substances include various members of the cabbage family, garlic and onions, various berries, tomatoes, citrus fruits, red wine (in moderate amounts) and dark chocolate.[1]

When it comes to cancer, the greatest advantage of a plant-based diet is that there are no side effects, only benefits.

Andrea Lusser, MD, *studied medicine at the Albert-Ludwig-University in Freiburg/Breisgau, Germany from 1977-1983. After receiving her medical degree she specialised in natural medicine, homeopathy, and psychotherapy. Since 1986 she has been working as a general private practitioner in Freiburg/Breisgau, Germany. For the past 20 years Dr. Lusser has studied and implemented effective and well tolerated tumor therapies. Following a vegetarian/vegan diet since 1976/80 herself she emphasizes the benefits of a plant- based nutrition in prevention of disease and support of cancer treatment.For more information please visit:* www.dr-lusser.de

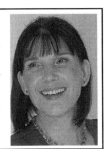

Food, Fat, and Cancer?

Michele Dodman, DO, MBA, FACOI, HPF

Most people aren't terribly surprised when they hear that fat causes high blood pressure, blocked arteries, and even diabetes, but most are quite shocked when I tell them that *fat can cause cancer!*[1] Sadly this is occurring at higher rates and in younger people.

Melissa, a 19 year old woman, was clearly frightened when her family doctor's office told her that her "liver was failing and that she needed immediate attention." As I glanced through her labs it was clear that her liver was in trouble. She was on the metabolic road to liver failure. Her blood work showed an elevation in liver chemistries (ALT of 223 nml 52 and an AST of 238 nml 45), her blood sugar was high at 156nml (should be less than 105), and her triglycerides (the fats in your blood) was 4 times the normal value, at 320. An abdominal ultrasound showed "diffuse infiltration," which means that some of the liver cells (hepatocytes) had been replaced by fat cells. Although only 19, Melissa had been steadily gaining weight through high school and now weighed 312 lbs, with a body mass index (BMI) of 41. BMI is essentially a measurement of your percent of body fat. Normal for her height and age should be 22 to 25. Melissa fortunately had the opportunity to reverse her disease and restore her liver to good health through lifestyle changes including a healthy plant-based diet, coupled with a consistent, exercise program under the supervision of her physician.

So how could a young girl, who did not drink alcohol or do drugs, have such a damaged liver? The bottom line is fat. The liver is a major recycling center, as well as manufacturing center. It 'detoxifies contaminants in the blood,' and synthesizes new proteins to help build antibodies and clotting factors that help keep us healthy.[2] Clearly we cannot live without our liver. When there's too much fat in the body, it's stored in many places in case we ever need it for energy. Some of its storages places are obvious when we try on clothes after gaining weight. What's not so obvious is that fat is also stored internally in the blood vessels going to our heart (coronary arteries) which can lead to a blockage causing a heart attack, as well as the liver which can lead to cirrhosis, cancer, and possibly death. Melissa had non-alcoholic fatty liver disease (NAFLD) which can lead to cirrhosis (liver failure), cancer and possible death. Although there was no 'immediate threat' to Melissa's liver that day, it was clearly irritated by the excess fat.

Excess fat has the ability to lead to cancer, which can end in fatality.[3] How does this happen? Our bodies break down the foods we eat and change them into a useable source of energy to fuel all of our bodily functions. We need energy to perform the millions of intricate processes that allow us to walk, think, run, panic, and even cry. This process is analogous to making gasoline from crude oil. The oil goes through numerous processes before it's sold as the gasoline that we put into our cars. Similarly, everything we eat must be changed into useable energy. When our bodies have met their 'energy demand', or it has enough 'body fuel' to perform all necessary functions, the excess energy is stored for future use.

Any excess fuel from foods is transformed into fat that functions as storage units. Fat is the richest source of fuel for our bodies. It's no wonder that our bodies store it so efficiently. Excess calories from any source, if not immediately needed by the body, are turned into fat which can be stored in our hips, arms, waist, stomach, buttocks, arteries and yes, liver.

Steatosis (excess fat in the liver) or Non-Alcoholic Fatty Liver Disease, which Melissa had, can be equally as dangerous to our bodies as heart disease. Excess fat in the liver is an irritant, much like alcohol, acetaminophen (Tylenol), hepatitis and other liver diseases.[4] Chronic irritation (like in NAFLD) over time, causes the normal liver cells (hepatocytes) to be changed and be replaced with a type of scar tissue called fibrosis.[5] Once liver cells are 'turned into scar tissue', they're no longer able to detoxify the waste products in our blood, nor are they able to make the antibodies, clotting factors, and other essential components that we need to fight infection and form blood clots. The fibrotic cells with continued irritation, take over all of the normal liver cells, and the person develops *cirrhosis of the liver*. At this point the liver is barely working, laying the foundation for cancer growth.[6]

Patients with BMI's above 35 have been shown to have a higher incidence of other types of cancers as well, including colon, breast, ovarian, pancreatic and prostate cancer. It's been well documented that most colon cancers start from growths of tissue called polyps which are found on the inside of the colon.[7] Certain types of polyps, known as adenomatous polyps, grow into colon cancer over a period of about ten years. Data is continuing to show a higher incidence of adenomatous (pre-cancerous polyps) in patients with high BMI's (again, over 35.)[8] Women with these high BMI's are at a much higher risk for breast and uterine cancer, while men with high BMI's are showing an alarming incidence of prostate cancer.[9,10]

The treatment for prevention and *reversal* of NAFLD is getting rid of excess fat.[11] This also decreases the incidence of adenomatous polyps (and subsequent colon cancer), as well as breast, ovarian, and prostate cancer not to mention coronary artery disease, stroke, and diabetes. The best, safest and most effective way to achieve and maintain ideal body weight, is to first stop ingesting more calories than your body needs in 1 day and limit fat consumption (about 30 grams a day). Most people require between 1200 to 2200 calories/day. How much is this you ask? Well, did you have an "egg muffin sandwich for breakfast" (800 cal, 14 g/fat), a burrito or some nachos for lunch (198 cal/14 g), a hamburger with fries and a shake for dinner(200 cal/ 89g/fat) your total caloric intake for those meals was about 2000 with a whooping 127grams of fat for 1 day!

Limiting fat consumption is easy following a plant based diet. Not only is a plant based diet naturally low in fat, but it's high in nutrients, minerals, vitamins, and fiber – all essential to a healthy body. Exercising as well as avoiding tobacco and alcohol is necessary for treatment and prevention.

As I shared this information with Melissa and her mother, I got a familiar look and the question, "Can't you just give her a prescription?" I looked at her mother, clearly worried about her daughter's health and glanced at the list of 13 medications this teen-ager was already taking for diabetes, depression (over her weight), anxiety, osteoarthritis she'd already developed carrying around the excess weight and a few more pills to regulate her menstrual cycles (fat can also cause menstrual irregularities).

There isn't a magic pill. It's choosing the right foods and a plant-based diet. What can happen after that is magical.

Michele Dodman, DO, MBA, *started her medical training in the military as a combat medic. She received her bachelor's degree from Oakland University, and attended medical school at the University of New England in Maine. She is board certified in gastroenterology. She earned an MBA in healthcare administration, has completed two teaching clinical fellowships, a health policy fellowship and a patient safety fellowship. She became a vegetarian at 15 and has been a vegan for 2 years.*

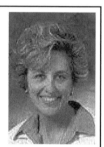

Dietary Prescription to Prevent Hormone Related Cancer

Luigi Mario Chiechi, MD

A fundamental (and neglected) aspect of nutrition is its ability to preserve health or promote disease. It is now an accepted opinion that approximately 70% of malignant cancers are related to diet, life style, or environmental factors.[1,2] One in every 2 men and 1 in every 3 women will have cancer in their lifetime[3] and about 35% of these cancers will be caused by dietary and nutritional factors.

Cancer is not a fate. Some populations such as the Hunza, have never experienced it at all. Today hormone related cancers, such as breast and prostate, have become very common. Now 1 in every 7 men has prostate cancer and 1 in every 8 women has breast cancer.[3] Why is cancer so common today?

Dietary Phytoestrogens and Hormone- Related Cancers

The main modifiable risk factors for cancers, apart from physical exercise are: 1) tobacco and alcohol, 2) diet, and 3) exogenous hormones.[4] The recent *Harvard's New Guide to Healthy Eating*[5] advises to limit milk/dairy, red meat and cheese, to avoid bacon, cold cuts and other processed meats. Instead intakes of fruit/vegetable and dietary fiber should be the increased.

Diet has enormous importance in favoring or counteracting hormone-related tumors. In particular, dietary phytoestrogens have preventive effects against hormone related cancers.

Dietary phytoestrogens are components of plant-based foods. The first scientific observation of their hormonal activity in plants was reported in 1946 by HW Bennetts, following the occurrence of the so-called "*clover disease*" in Australian sheep grazing on pastures of trifolium subterraneum, that induced infertility, abortions and other hormone-related diseases in these animals. For many years these compounds were considered plant estrogens, but this concept has changed over time and, more appropriately, they are now considered natural SERMs (Selective Estrogen Receptor Modulators).[6] In fact, they are so biochemically similar both to estrogens and to anti-estrogens such as tamoxifen, the most widely used drug in treating and preventing breast cancer. This structural similarity means they can similarly influence production, metabolism, and biological activity of sex hormones.

There are many classes of phytoestrogens, but those of concern are isoflavones and lignans. It is established that soy-isoflavones and whole grain-lignans have protective effects against breast, prostate and colon cancer.[7] *Isoflavones* are biologically more potent than lignans but present only in beans and legumes. *Lignans* are primarily present in fiber-rich foods such as seeds, whole grains, vegetables, fruits, and particularly flaxseed. These are the main components of the Asiatic and Mediterranean diets which are known as the healthiest in the world. These diets are low in animal foods, including milk. Beyond protecting against hormone related cancer, epidemiological studies have provided evidence of their importance in protecting cardiovascular diseases, osteoporosis and menopausal disturbances.[8,9]

Can a Therapy Cause Cancer?

A significant possible cause of breast cancer is postmenopausal hormonal replacement therapy (HRT), whose impact has been devastating. For the first time in 2003, instead of increasing, breast cancer significantly decreased[6], after a WHI study publication that showed HRT did more harm than good. The prescription of these hormones collapsed and so did the related cancer.

When Phytoestrogen lignans are converted by intestinal bacteria to the bioactive enterolignans enterolactone and enterodiol, they exert their positive effects via estrogen receptor-independent mechanisms, such as inhibition of tumor growth, angiogenesis, stimulation of apoptosis[10], reducing the risk of breast cancer[11,12] and in increasing the survival in postmenopausal breast cancer patients.[13] Finally it has been recently suggested that a soy isoflavone rich diet can especially benefit women at increased risk of breast cancer because of polymorphisms in genes associated with the disease, a promising evidence for a modern personalized medicine[14] based on a gene-diet interaction approach.[15]

More than 10 years ago, my collaborators and I carried out the Menfis study,[16,17,18] a randomized trial designed to evaluate the effects of a phyto-estrogen rich diet in postmenopausal women, compared with both Hormone Replacement Therapy and a control group. The results were surprising. The efficacy of plant-based diet on the biomarkers of risk for cardiovascular disease, osteoporosis and obesity were, overall, even better than that of HRT. Moreover this diet showed important positive effects on the endometrium, which can help explain the protection of soy intake against endometrial cancer.[19] The aim of the Menfis study was to use dietary phytoestrogens as an alternative to synthetic estrogens. After the large number of anthropological, ethic, and biomedical studies published, we believe that a phytoestrogen rich or plant-based diet, preferably organic and without chemical manipulation, is simply the natural diet for people and one that protects against cancer.

The Science Behind Why Phytoestrogens Work

Here's how phytoestrogens work: After ingestion, they are metabolized by intestinal bacteria to their biologically active form genistein and daidzein. Because of their structural similarity to natural estradiol, phytoestrogens are able to bind to the estrogen receptors (ERs) ERα, ERβ and possibly GPER[20], acting in a very complex manner, specific to cell types and tissues. ERα plays a major role in the uterus, vagina, mammary gland, hypothalamus. ERβ plays a role in the ovary, cardiovascular system, bones and brain. In most tissues ERα promotes cellular proliferation whereas ERβ has anti-proliferative effects balancing each other in a Ying Yang manner when present in the same organ.[21]

The final biological effect of phytoestrogens can be estrogen-agonistic and estrogen-antagonistic, meaning it can promote estrogen in one tissue and limit it another. This is exactly how the drug tamoxifen acts and is used to heal breast cancer by acting antagonist on breast tissue. Tamoxifen has, however, some detrimental side effects, such as the increase of both endometrial cancer and thromboembolic risk.[22]

Dairy Can Promote Hormone- Related Cancer Growth

While surprising to some, it makes sense that dairy is not part of healthy diet.[23] Milk and fermented dairy products increase serum growth factors GH and IGF-1 levels in humans. This follows logically as milk is the best food to promote neonatal growth, but after weaning, it is not necessary and can increase cancer risk as a consequence of the high serum IGF-1 levels.[24] In particular, high levels of galactose, a by-product of lactose in milk, is associated with an increased risk of ovarian cancer. Additionally industrial milk production which increases hormonal composition through artificial growth hormones, also increases the risk of other hormone-related cancers such as breast, prostate and ovarian.[25]

Also **egg consumption has been found to nearly triple the risk of breast cancer** and increase risk of several other cancers including colon, bladder, oropharynx, prostate, and lung.[27] The high cholesterol content in eggs increases the production of estrogens which increases breast cancer risk. Consumption of eggs should be added to the most known dietary risk factors for breast cancer, which include cheese and meat.[28]

Can Dairy Cause Less than Radiant Skin?

Western diets are rich in animal based foods and dairy-based hormones "may be the source of the androgenic and mitogenic progestin that drive acne, prostate and breast cancer."[26] Whey proteins in the milk raise insulin and IGF-1 levels which increase the risk of acne, diabetes and cancer. This is evidenced by populations, such as the Kitava islanders, who exclude sugar, grains and dairy in their diet and do not have acne.[22]

Using Phyto-Estrogens as Possible Cancer Prevention

Phytoestrogen rich, plant-based diets have been shown to prevent chronic conditions such as cancer [29] as they contain high levels of antioxidant vitamins, fiber, folic acid, carotenoids and anti-carcinogens. Phytoestrogens are extraordinary vital substances able to maintain the natural hormonal equilibrium in all the phases of the human life to ensure *health preservation.*

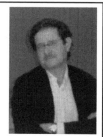

Luigi Mario Chiechi, MD, *was born in Adelfia (BA) Italy and obtained his degree in Medicine from the University of Bari and his specialization in Obstetrics and Gynecology from the same university in 1980. Dr. Chiechi served as a researcher in the Department of Bioethics, Faculty of Medicine at the University of Bari and taught Gynecological Endocrinology at the degree course in Medicine, Climacteric for the degree course in Midwifery, and Physiopathology of the Climacteric to graduate school in Obstetrics and Gynecology. He designed and carried out the randomized MENFIS study. Dr. Chiechi has participated in multiple national and European projects including the Italian unit at the European project named EUPHRATES (in The Fifth Framework Programme 1998-2002; QLG4-CT-2001-01352), and as Italian partner at the European project named PHYTOHEALTH (in The Fifth Framework Programme 1998-2002; QoL-2001-4). He is a reviewer and member of Editorial Board of national and international scientific journals and author of numerous scientific publications and chapters of scientific books. Dr. Chiechi is married, has 2 daughters and is vegan.*

ten

THE DANGERS OF DAIRY

"Under scientific scrutiny, the support for the milk myth crumbles."

-Dr. Amy Lanou

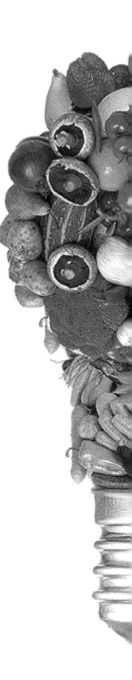

Touted as a 'superfood' for human health, we consume milk, cheese and its by-products on a massive scale based on the assumption that we are feeding our body the most perfect food for growth and development. Cow's milk is a wonderful growth food- for a baby cow. Past the point of weaning, our bodies are simply not made to process milk, and especially that of another species, evidenced in the growing number of lactose intolerance rates around the world. Dairy products rich in saturated fat, hormones, toxins, industrial pollutants and both natural and artificial growth hormones are linked to an impressive list of serious diseases including heart disease, breast cancer, prostate cancer, ovarian cancer, arthritis, allergies, acne, eczema, ear infections, Crohn's disease, multiple sclerosis, osteoporosis, and Parkinson's disease among many others.

This chapter's doctors highly recommend removing cow's milk in all its forms from our diet. Despite what we have been led to believe, the claims of dairy supporting strong bones and necessary for good health are completely unfounded. In fact, the only growth dairy is shown to be most directly associated with, is that of cancer cells. One of the most notable revelations by Dr. T. Colin Campbell in *The China Study*, reveals how casein (cow's milk protein) in a diet can subsequently turn cancer cells on. Remarkably, eliminating casein could turn the cancer cells off.[1]

The "White Lies" we have been sold as Dr. Butler states, indicate that dairy is more aptly labeled as a toxin rather than a 'perfect' food for human health.

White Lies - the Health Consequences of Consuming Cow's Milk

Justine Butler, PhD

In 2006, a report called *White Lies* described the evidence linking dairy to some of the West's biggest killers such as heart disease, diabetes, breast cancer and prostate cancer as well as osteoporosis, eczema, asthma, Crohn's disease, colic, constipation and even teenage acne. The evidence from over 300 scientific studies is overwhelming - cow's milk and dairy products are neither natural nor healthy. Although the industry has responded with a vigorous defense, the evidence continues to mount that dairy is not essential for good health but rather a leading contributing factor to our numerous chronic health conditions…

The Heart of the Matter

The saturated animal fat in whole milk, cheese, butter and dairy products can cause obesity, Type 2 diabetes and heart disease – 3 of the biggest killers in the Western world. Most health organisations now recommend avoiding or cutting down on fatty foods including egg yolks, red meat, butter, whole milk, cheese, and processed foods to reduce the intake of saturated fat.

Heart disease is the single largest cause of death in developed countries. It kills 1 in every 4 people in the US.[1] Heart disease occurs when there is a build up of fatty deposits (plaques) along the walls of the arteries that supply the heart with blood. It is known that high-fat dairy products raise both total and LDL 'bad' cholesterol levels.[2] The largest study ever conducted in the UK, comparing rates of heart disease between vegetarians and non-vegetarians, recently found that a vegetarian diet could significantly reduce people's risk of heart disease by a whopping 32%.[3] Earlier studies show that replacing saturated fat with polyunsaturated fat (found in plant foods) is more effective in lowering cholesterol and reducing the risk of heart disease than reducing the total fat consumption.[4] So it is the *type* of fat that you eat that matters and avoiding dairy and other animal foods can help.

It's not all bad news; fiber (found in fruit, vegetables, wholegrain foods and legumes) and soy protein too have all been shown to lower cholesterol. It is well-documented how following a plant-based diet can help avoid these so-called Western diseases. In 1990, Dr Dean Ornish, showed that a plant-based diet, stress management and exercise could actually reverse heart disease. Ornish treated 28 heart disease patients with diet and lifestyle changes alone. They followed a low-fat plant-based diet including unrestricted amounts of fruits, vegetables and grains. They also practiced stress management techniques and exercised regularly. After one year 82% of the test group experienced regression of their heart disease, including a 91% reduction in the frequency of heart pain compared to 165% increase in the control group.[5] No conventional drug or surgery related therapies compare with these results.[6]

Dr Caldwell Esselstyn Jr., eminent cardiologist, has also described how plant-based diets can help prevent and treat heart disease.[7] For example, after undergoing cardiac surgery in 2010, former American president Bill Clinton adopted the plant-based diet recommended by Ornish and Esselstyn, he lost more than 20 pounds and he says he's healthier than ever now. In order to protect our heart health, it is essential to drop the dairy from our diets.

Getting Abreast of the Facts

In 2003, scientists from the Medical Research Council's Dunn Human Nutrition Unit in Cambridge, UK, revealed a strong link between saturated animal fat and breast cancer.[8] They found that women who ate the most full-fat milk, butter, meat, cookies and cakes were almost twice as likely to develop breast cancer. Hot on the heels of this research, scientists from Harvard Medical School and Brigham and Women's Hospital, Boston, MA, published a study showing that young women who ate lots of full-fat dairy products and red meat also increased their chances of breast cancer.[9] More recently, a large prospective study of over 300,000 European women over 8 years also demonstrated a link between saturated fat intake and breast cancer.[10]

The raised levels of hormones in cow's milk are a source of concern to many scientists studying cancers of the breast, ovaries, colon and prostate; the so-called hormone-related cancers. Cow's milk has been shown to contain a cocktail of over 35 different hormones and 11 growth factors.[11] This is further complicated by the use of an artificial growth hormone called recombinant bovine somatotrophin or rBST, used to obtain even higher milk production from cows. The use of rBST is associated with severe welfare problems in dairy cows; increasing the incidence of lameness and mastitis (inflammation of the mammary glands). For reasons of animal health and welfare, the European Union (EU), Japan, Australia, New Zealand and Canada have banned its use. The US Food and Drug Administration (FDA) permit the use of rBST. In 2007, a USDA Dairy Survey estimated that rBST was used in over 17% of dairy cows.

Research shows that rBST increases the levels of a growth hormone called insulin-like growth factor 1 (IGF-1) in milk. IGF-1 in humans is involved in normal growth and development during childhood, but in adults it can promote abnormal growth and may lead to some cancers. This should not really come as a surprise; after all, milk is an ideal baby food – designed for infants. Cow's milk is specifically suited for the purpose of turning a small calf into a great big cow very quickly! This raises concerns about how IGF-1 from cow's milk might affect human health. Professor Samuel Epstein, an international leading authority on the causes and prevention of cancer, warns that converging lines of evidence incriminate IGF-1 in rBST milk as a potential risk factor for both breast and gastrointestinal cancers.[12] Research shows that people who drink cow's milk have more IGF-1 in their blood than those who don't.[13] Whether it is the IGF-1 in the milk (that may cross the gut wall and enter the blood), or the hormones (or peptides) in the milk that drive up production of human IGF-1, the overall concern is that IGF-1 is linked to these cancers and drinking cow's milk may increase the risk. In the laboratory, if you drop IGF-1 onto human breast cancer cells they grow uncontrollably.[14] It seems IGF-1 is turning out to be a predictor of cancer in much the same way that cholesterol is a predictor for heart disease.[15] IGF-1 is now the subject of much interest among the scientific community and we will undoubtedly be hearing more about it.

The incidence of breast cancer continues to rise. When Professor Jane Plant CBE, wrote *Your Life in Your Hands,* an account of how she overcame breast cancer by eliminating dairy, 1 in 10 UK women were affected by the disease.[16] Now, 13 years later, 1 in 9 UK women is affected. In the US, the figure is a staggering 1 in 8 women.[17]

Pus –the White Stuff!

The enormous physical demand placed on the modern dairy cow makes her susceptible to a range of ailments including mastitis or inflammation of the mammary gland in which all or part of the udder suffers from infection. The cow responds to infection by generating pus or white blood cells (somatic cells). These cells, the components of pus, and are excreted into the milk. The somatic cell count (SSC) is used as an indicator of the level of infection. One teaspoonful of milk could contain up to 2 million pus cells! The white milk moustache that features in so many dairy adverts doesn't look quite so charming now does it?

The Detrimental Health Consequences of Consuming Cow's Milk in Infants

The milk protein casein is a tough little molecule that is linked to a wide range of health problems including cow's milk allergy - the most common food allergy in young children affecting 2-5 % of infants in developed countries. As well as leading to asthma and eczema, cow's milk allergy can cause intestinal bleeding in infants, with a considerable amount of iron being lost with the blood.[18] This may affect around 40% of otherwise healthy infants.[19] This allergic reaction causes about half the cases of iron-deficiency anemia in US infants; a staggering number of children considering that over 15% of infants under 2 years suffer from this condition.[20]

Additionally not only does casein cause the intestinal bleeding as an allergic response which depletes iron sources, it also inhibits the absorption of non-heme iron. There are two types of dietary iron: heme and non-heme. Heme iron is derived primarily from hemoglobin and myoglobin in animal tissue and makes up around half the iron found in red meat, poultry and fish. Non-heme iron makes up the other half of the iron in animal tissue and all of the iron found in plant foods, dairy foods (which contain a very small amount) and eggs. Non-heme iron is the type of iron added to iron-fortified foods. Most dietary iron is non-heme. While heme iron is more easily absorbed than non-heme iron, vitamin C in fruit and vegetables can increase non-heme iron absorption considerably. But as stated above, casein can inhibit non-heme iron absorption.

The high protein, sodium, potassium, phosphorus and chloride content of cow's milk present what is called a high renal solute load; this means that the unabsorbed solutes from milk must be excreted via the kidneys. This can place a strain on immature kidneys forcing them to draw water from the body which increases the risk of dehydration. The renal solute load of infants fed cow's milk has been shown to be twice as high as that of formula fed infants.[21]

Over the past 60 years, the worldwide incidence of type 1 (juvenile onset) diabetes has been increasing by 3-5 % per year, doubling approximately every 20 years with a steep rise in the very youngest children.[22] A substantial body of evidence suggests that the early exposure to cow's milk in infancy (including cow's milk infant formula) may be a trigger for this disease in some people.[23] Casein (the main protein in milk), and/or other milk proteins can trigger an autoimmune reaction that ends with the destruction of cells in the pancreas, the cells that produce insulin. However, modifying the diet to include high-fiber low-fat content has been shown to be effective in reducing the need for treatment in both type 1 and type 2 (adult onset) diabetes.[24,25]

In 1998, concerned about the links to juvenile onset diabetes and the effects of cow's milk allergy, Dr Benjamin Spock, author of the world-famous book *Baby and Child Care*,[26] withdrew his support for cow's milk recommending that after the age of two, children avoid all dairy products stating that other calcium sources offer many advantages that dairy products do not have. This is why most health organisations and governments advise that parents do not give infants under the age of 1 'off the shelf' cow's milk.

Considering the high renal solute load that cow's milk presents on immature kidneys, the links with childhood obesity and types 1 and 2 diabetes, cow's milk is clearly an inappropriate food for infants.

Boning Up and the Calcium Paradox

The idea that dairy is essential for bone health has been drummed into us for decades. The evidence simply does not support this but rather indicates that cow's milk and dairy products are actually damaging to bones. The Harvard Nurses Health Study followed 75,000 women over 12 years and found that increasing cow's milk consumption did not protect against the risk of bone fracture, this extensive study showed that dairy products *increased* the risk of fracture.[27] Additionally a review of 58 studies on dairy products and bone health published in the journal of the American Academy of Pediatrics summarized that there was little evidence to support the association between milk consumption in childhood and stronger bones.[27]

In fact, the countries that consume the most calcium and, therefore dairy, are also where the highest levels of osteoporosis occur. The World Health Organisation calls this the *Calcium Paradox.*[28] It has been suggested this may be due to low vitamin D status and/or high animal (but not vegetable) protein intake. But why would animal protein be harmful to bone health? Animal proteins contain higher levels of sulfur than plant protein. The theory is that as animal protein is digested, acids are released into the blood and the body attempts to neutralise the acid by drawing calcium from the bones, this calcium is then excreted in the urine.[29] As the sulfur content of the diet increases so does the level of calcium excreted.

There are many plant-based sources of calcium including dark green leafy vegetables such as broccoli, kale, collard greens, cabbage, bok choy, parsley and watercress (spinach is not such a good source as it contains a substance called oxalate that binds calcium and reduces its availability), figs and dates, nuts, particularly almonds and brazilian nuts, seeds including sesame seeds, and pulses such as soy beans, kidney beans, chick peas, baked beans, lentils, peas and calcium-set tofu. A good additional source is calcium-enriched soy milk. These foods provide health promoting fiber and disease-busting antioxidants and do not contain the damaging saturated animal fat, animal protein, cholesterol, hormones, and growth factors found in cow's milk and dairy products.

The most critical determinant of bone health is physical activity, load-bearing exercise (walking, stair-climbing, dancing). The best thing we can do is exclude dairy from the diet and start exercising more.

The Bottom Line

Consider this: most people in the world do not drink milk or eat dairy products, they are lactose intolerant and cannot digest lactose (the sugar in milk). Lactose only exists in mammals' milk, including human breast milk. In order for lactose to be digested, it must be broken down in the gut by the enzyme lactase. Most infants possess lactase and can therefore digest lactose, but this ability is lost in most people after weaning (around the age of two). In the absence of lactase, lactose is fermented by bacteria in the gut, this leads to a build up of gas. Symptoms include nausea, cramps, bloating, wind and diarrhoea. The treatment is straightforward: avoid lactose. Losing the ability to digest lactose at this age is a clear indication of how humans are not designed to drink milk as adults; it is not a natural food for us. Clearly, the majority of people in the world obtain calcium from plant-based sources.

We are the only mammal that continues to drink milk beyond weaning, and not just that, the milk of another species. Really, it's an odd thing to do; would you suckle from a pregnant dog? What's the difference?

Justine Butler, PhD, *is a Senior Health Campaigner at Viva! Health. Dr. Butler holds a PhD in Molecular Biology, BSc Biochemistry and Diploma in Nutrition. As well as writing for Viva! Health, Justine has had an extensive list of articles published in health and trade journals, national and regional newspapers. She is a regular contributor to Network Health Dieticians magazine.* justine@viva.org.uk www.viva.org.uk www.vivahealth.org.uk

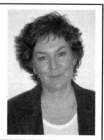

RETHINK
FOOD

Colic, Cravings, and Casomorphin

Kerrie Saunders, MS, LLP, PhD

Completely aware that I will be shedding new light on a food substance many Americans believe they love and need, let me begin by borrowing a quote from one of my favorite thought leaders, Howard Lyman: "I refuse to apologize for something that saved my life."

The elimination of cow milk from my diet literally saved my life. I was less than a month old, sick, colicky, crying and losing weight rapidly. After visits to 2 physicians, the third physician stated unequivocally he did not believe I would survive unless cow's milk was eliminated from my diet. Upon elimination, the colic stopped, the crying stopped, and my health rebounded almost instantly.

Cow's milk really is the perfect food—for a baby cow. Breast milk is the gold standard for humans,[9] but we're also supposed to wean away from baby milk and onto solid food, just like all of the other mammals on the planet. Autoimmune response, allergies, mucus formation, asthma, diabetes, attention disorders, dehydration, anemia, osteoporosis, and lactose issues are some of the conditions now linked by research literature on the human consumption of cow's milk. [1,2,3,4,5,6] In fact, there is a growing body of research demonstrating some of these ill effects in breast-fed babies caused by *mothers* who drink cow's milk. The best course of treatment is the elimination of cow's milk from the mother's diet.[7,8]

One of the earliest scientific papers to describe how cow milk can play a role in asthma and cause a mucus thickening, occurred back in the 12th century.[10] Famous physician, Moses Maimonides, called it a "humidifying effect," similar to descriptions referencing "*dampening* and *phlegm*" in traditional Chinese medicine.

In 2009, Bartley and McGlashan studied how opioid receptors in the mucus glands of the respiratory tract respond to casomorphin— a component of casein in dairy products related to addiction— and could stimulate the production and secretion of mucus.[11] In fact, many integrated physicians today, will eliminate dairy products at the first sign of chronic ear infections in children. It is well established that cow's milk produces a histamine reaction in many individuals, producing many of the symptoms of allergies, such as a rash, runny nose, or sneezing.

"Lactose intolerance" is actually a statistically normal state for humans over the age of 3 years. Lactose, the sugar in milk, requires the lactase enzyme to be present in your small intestine, liver, and kidneys to break the lactose down into glucose and galactose. When you ingest lactose with little or no lactase, it ferments and causes gas, bloating, abdominal pain, fatigue, and diarrhea. Instead of acknowledging nature's hint that we are to wean by around age 3, we develop products with non-human and fungi-based lactase additives.

Casomorphin: An Exploration of Comparison and Addiction

There are 2 main proteins in cow milk—whey and casein. Whey is a milk serum (mainly containing lactoglobulin and lactalbumin) and is the liquid remaining after milk has been curdled and strained. Once considered a by-product of cheese manufacturing, it is now sold to commercial markets and non-vegan bodybuilders, instead of being discarded. Casein is found in all mammal milk, including cow, goat, monkey, cat, and human. The casein protein breaks down into smaller amino acids. Our stomach acid and intestinal bacteria cut the casein molecular chains into casomorphins (opiates) of various lengths. One of the shorter strings, made up of just 5 amino acids, has about a tenth of the pain-killing potency of morphine. Casomorphins binds to opiate receptors in the brain, similar to the way heroin and morphine act.

But to understand cow milk casomorphin addiction theory, we need to look at some numbers.[1]

Comparison	Human Milk	Cow Milk
Average Protein, as % of Total Calories	7%	21%
Whey: Casein Ratio	70:30	20:80
Total Casein	2.5 grams per liter	27.3 grams per liter

Most important for this discussion, is to understand that the amount of casein is 10 times higher in milk designed for cows, than the milk designed for us. Since it takes 10 pounds of milk to make 1 pound of cheese, there is a concentration of casomorphin content in cheese. This is probably why some of us have heard the statement, "I stopped drinking milk years ago, but I just can't seem to give up my cheese or ice cream!" The more I listened, the more it sounded like substance dependence, complete with cravings and withdrawal symptoms.

Food opioid peptides (exorphins primarily from wheat and dairy) have been studied for decades for links associated with digestive, autistic spectrum, schizophrenia, and other disorders.[13] While science has identified 13 variants of beta casein (also used industrially in some paint, glue, condoms, and plastics), the main player in current international research is beta casomorphin-7 or b-CM7. These partially undigested peptides (b-CM7) can be absorbed by the body, bind to receptors, and cause abnormal behavioral or physiological reactions. Many researchers have noted that urine samples from people with chronic fatigue, fibromyalgia, depression, autism, celiac disease, and schizophrenia contained high amounts of the casomorphin in their urine. It appears that once casein is completely removed from the diet, it takes reportedly 3 days to 8 months, depending upon individual factors, for abnormal peptide levels to drop.

Researchers have long accepted that whatever we define as pleasurable, is tied to a more general neurotransmitter, dopamine. Neurotransmitters are chemicals that send messages to our brain and dopamine helps us feel driven toward pleasurable goals. So the more rewarding a food or drug is deemed to be, the greater the release of dopamine in the brain. In fact, positron emission tomographic (PET) imaging studies have shown that both obese individuals and drug dependent individuals have significantly lower dopamine receptor levels than controls.[17]

> ### A1 vs A2 Beta-Caseins Link to Chronic Diseases
>
> A few researchers have, honed in on genetic variants and mutations, noting the major difference between an A1 and A2 beta-casein protein. A1 has the amino acid histidine at position 67, while A2 has the amino acid proline at position 67. Human milk is more like A2 whereas A1 that has been implicated as a potential etiological factor in type 1 diabetes mellitus, ischemic heart disease, and as a modifier associated with some neurological conditions such as autism.[2,3,4,5]

While the scientific community has historically easily identified and accepted addictive components related to grains, leaves, and beans (i.e. alcohol, caffeine, nicotine, and cocaine), it curiously struggles to accept similar components in bread and dairy products. Validation studies are currently being conducted on Yale University's Food Addiction Scale.[16]

There is also a growing body of global research linking the components of cow milk to osteoporosis, asthma, diabetes, cardiovascular disease, allergies, mood and behavior disorders, and of course, obesity.[18] It is common sense that cow milk was designed for cows, cat milk for cats, goat milk for goats, and human milk for humans. I imagine if we had to lie under the cow with our mouths on her udder, the peculiarity of it all might finally become real.

Kerrie Saunders, MS, LLP, Ph.D. *is an internationally known presenter and author of The Vegan Diet as Chronic Disease Prevention. She has been featured on television and radio, and in numerous newspapers, books, and magazines, including her "Dear Dr. Kerrie," advice column for VegNews Magazine. Dr. Saunders co-stars with Ellen DeGeneres' fitness trainer, John Pierre, in When Bachelor Meets Homemaker. Dr. Saunders has worked with Physicians Committee for Responsible Medicine. She lectures frequently for hospitals and universities, and is the coordinator of the Michigan Firefighter Challenge. You can find more on her work at www.DrFood.org*

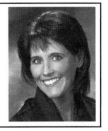

Why Milk Makes Us Sick

Gilbert Manso, MD

Just as in any typical family practice or pediatric medical office, my waiting room was normally filled with sick children. Cough, fever, runny noses, ear aches, asthma, and eczematous skin rashes make up the bulk of a pediatrician's or family doctor's patients. It took me a while to notice that kids began getting sick when they received their first immunizations and when they were weaned. The relationship between cow's milk and subsequent illness was obscured by the fact that so many babies, were on milk formula from the very start, so they seemed to be sickly from birth.

Conventional medical thinking attributes the colds, runny noses, bronchitis, asthma, and other "typical" childhood conditions to viruses and germs. These conditions are then treated with a variety of medications, principally antibiotics, antihistamines, and steroids. The results of these treatments are generally poor and patients keep coming back for relief. It takes no time at all to create an assembly line or mass production mill where, incidentally, doctors, nurses, pharmacists, hospitals, and Big Pharma profit handsomely. It seems to be a win-win situation, except, of course, for the patients. While pediatric patients and their inconvenienced parents appreciate our efforts, we continue to blame increasingly resistant germs and flu strains for their chronic illness, while the government and industry pin their hopes on discovering a new and more powerful vaccine.

So what do runny noses, sinus congestions, bronchitis, middle-ear infections, and various body discharges have in common? The answer: mucus. Mucus is an excellent growth medium for germs. Inflammation on the mucosal membranes of the nose, the bronchial linings, the intestines, and elsewhere leads to an excessive production of mucus, resulting in runny noses, and congestion. Ultimately, this leads to infection that is then treated with antibiotics and/or antihistamines. Sold by the millions, antihistamines attempt to block excessive histamine (that produces the inflammatory response) with variable success. Ultimately, they fail unless histamine consumption is controlled.

What are Histamine and Histidine?

Where does histamine come from? Histamine is a very powerful component and trigger of the inflammatory response. We do not manufacture our own histamine,—we have to ingest it. Milk and animal protein are the main sources of histamine in our systems.

This is because all animal protein is rich in histidine. Histidine converts to histamine. Milk products, especially cheese, and shellfish are particularly significant sources of histidine. The production of histamine resulting inflammation affects other areas in our bodies as well. In fact, many of the most common illnesses are associated with an inflammatory response.

The great majority of my patients, children and adults, get rid of their allergies and recurrent inflammatory mucus-produced conditions by the simple expedience of eliminating milk products from their diets. It is not uncommon in my practice to rid a patient of years of misery from allergies, eczema, and the like by just abstaining from milk for a couple of weeks.

Humans are the only known species that drinks the milk of another species, and the only known species that continues to drink milk into adulthood. Cow's milk naturally contains the large amount of hormones and protein needed to turn an 80-pound calf into a 1,000-pound cow in 1 year.

Problems and Side Effects Associated with Milk Protein Consumption[1]

General: Loss of appetite, growth retardation.

Upper gastrointestinal: Canker sores (aphthous stomatitis), irritation of tongue, lips, and mouth, tonsil enlargement, vomiting, gastroesophageal reflux disease (GERD), Sandifer's syndrome, peptic ulcer disease, colic, stomach cramps, abdominal distention, intestinal obstruction, type-1 diabetes.

Lower gastrointestinal: Bloody stools, colitis, malabsorption, diarrhea, painful defecation, fecal soiling, infantile colic, chronic constipation, infantile food protein-induced enterocolitis syndrome (FPIES), Crohn's disease, ulcerative colitis.

Respiratory: Nasal stuffiness, runny nose, otitis media (inner ear trouble), sinusitis, wheezing, asthma, and pulmonary infiltrates.

Bone and joint: Rheumatoid arthritis, juvenile rheumatoid arthritis, lupus, Beheta's disease, (possibly psoriatic arthritis and ankylosing spondylitis).

Skin: Rashes, atopic dermatitis, eczema, seborrhea, hives (urticaria)

Nervous system (behavioral): Multiple sclerosis, Parkinson's disease, autism, schizophrenia, irritability, restlessness, hyperactivity, headache, lethargy, fatigue, "allergic-tension fatigue syndrome," muscle pain, mental depression, enuresis (bed-wetting).

Blood: Abnormal blood clotting, iron deficiency anemia, low serum proteins, thrombocytopenia, and eosinophilia.

Other: Nephrotic syndrome, glomerulonephritis, anaphylactic shock and death, sudden infant death syndrome (SIDS or crib or cot death), injury to the arteries causing arteritis, and eventually, atherosclerosis.

Unfortunately, there are enormous cultural and financial forces that are vested on the consumption of milk and animal products. For generations, consumers have been bombarded by the media which, sadly, determines the behavior and opinions of the populus. I highly recommend to my patients that they let their bodies and not the media determine what is good for them.

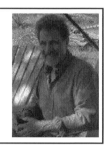

Gilbert Manso, MD *graduated from the University of Texas Medical Branch in 1969. He was an assistant professor in the faculty of UTMB and UTMS Houston for some 20 years and he has logged over 140,000 patient visits, covering the spectrum from Amoebas to Zoonosis.* www. drmanso.com

Drop the Dairy

David Ryde, MB, BS, FRCGP

As a family doctor, who is 84 years old and been vegan for the past 30 years, I have spent much time over the years advising patients on the benefits of a plant-based diet, and have built up an extensive and positive clinical experience diet in relation to both health and disease**.**

As a medical student in the late 1940s, nutrition was not part of the curriculum. It wasn't until the early 1980s I began to suspect that dairy foods might be unhealthy. Cancer cells are naturally present in our body. Whether they are expressed or not depends upon whether they are triggered. Dairy and its natural growth hormone- IGF-1 can trigger cancer cells.[1] When dairy is eliminated and a plant-based diet is adopted, the growth hormone in milk no longer triggers the cancer cells.

In 1993, my brother-in-law was also afflicted with multiple cancer deposits from prostate cancer. At my suggestion, he switched to a whole-food, plant-based diet, and within a few months all signs of disease had gone. His surgeon thought he had made a wrong diagnosis. His PSA was 111 and it gradually dropped down to less than 1. He passed away at age 87 without any evidence of cancer.

I often get asked how people get their calcium if they avoid milk. Osteoporosis is not due to a dietary lack of calcium but to a loss of calcium. Animal and dairy protein contains 5 times more sulphur than plant protein and this creates an acidic effect.[2] The body eliminates this sulphur by combining it with calcium, hence the formation of calcium sulphate stones in kidneys of meat eaters.

Reversing and Curing Disease on a Plant-Based Diet

The anatomical factors that differentiate between carnivore and herbivore digestive systems place humans firmly in the plant-based system. This is why I have suggested a nearly total vegan diet for chronic conditions such as obesity, diabetes, coronary artery disease, and high blood pressure among others with remarkable results. On a plant-based diet, patients with angina or type 2 diabetes could reverse their condition back to normal. This is because a plant diet is rich in fiber and is devoid of cholesterol. I had other patients lose as much as 140lbs in one year and lower their blood pressure, while being able to reduce or quit using their medications. One patient of mine, 48 years old, had 3 heart attacks and quadruple by-pass surgery. He was largely confined to a wheelchair. Within 6 months of becoming vegan, he was backpacking, and 5 years later he ran his first marathon. The cholesterol-free diet had enabled his heart arteries to re-open.

My Hope for the Future

In review, I see two opposing aspects in adopting a vegan lifestyle. The advantages would be an improvement in the nation's health; up to 1/3 of rural England would be available for reforestation and a growth in national parks and animal exploitation would largely cease. The opposing view would be that the national economy would be damaged because the farming industry would be largely reduced. My hope is that the country adopts a more natural and meat-free diet, that contributes to a healthy and more innovative national economy.

David Ryde MB, BS, FRCGP, *is a retired general practitioner in the UK after 40 years of clinical practice. He served as the Captain of the Royal Army Medical Corps in 1954 and is an Honorary Life Member of the British Association of Sport and Medicine. Dr. Ryde was on the Medical Sub-Committee of British Olympic Association and the medical advisor to several national sports teams. He has lectured in 6 countries and appeared on numerous radio and TV programs. Vegetarian since age 11 and vegan for over 20 years, at age 84 Dr. Ryde still keeps fit. Dr. Ryde has 4 children, 9 grandchildren and 1 great grandson.*

eleven

GET STRONG BONES AND POWER JOINTS

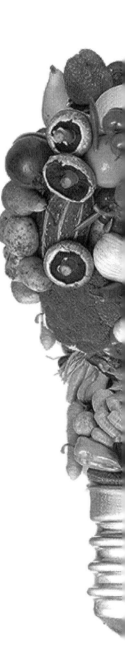

The amount of misinformation surrounding calcium and strong bones and joints, is a catastrophe. In fact, Harvard University recently declared that "Got Milk" does not translate to "Got Strong bones?"[1] While this information goes against the core principles of nutritional information in the market, science continues to evidence that dairy products are not components for healthy strong bones.

As osteoporosis has increased, the constant dietary advice has been to flood our bodies with calcium from dairy. This is one of the most damaging milk myths. As the orthopedic surgeons and dietitians in this chapter reveal, our obsession with calcium from dairy actually weakens our bones and damages our joints. Strong bones stem from exercise, Vitamin D intake, and the right sources of calcium for absorption. Contrary to popular belief, plant foods such as broccoli and kale are superior calcium sources to dairy.

Meat and cow's milk create an inflammatory environment that can promote arthritis. For patients with arthritis they are often told they will be on medication for the rest of their lives. Some of these medications such as Methotrexate, a form of chemotherapy, can have serious side effects. However, changes in diet are proving to not only lessen the pain but for some eliminate it completely. Evidenced in this chapter, the path to a pain-free life begins by removing dairy products and getting our calcium from plant-based sources.

Building a Plant Strong Body

Scott Stoll, MD

One of the underappreciated systems of the body that allows us to play and work is the musculoskeletal system, comprised of muscles, bones, joints, cartilage, and connective tissue. The musculoskeletal system is a network of living cells and therefore a plant-based diet can have positive disease prevention and reversal potential. I have witnessed these amazing benefits in the lives of my patients.

Bones 101 and Osteoporosis

All 206 of our bones are alive and continually being remodeled by cells that build bone (osteoblasts), cells that digest bone (osteoclasts), and the orchestrator cells (osteocytes) that direct bone growth both locally and in communication with distant organs. Our bone density changes over time and is influenced by our environment. The presence or absence of environmental factors such as weight bearing exercise, diet, tobacco, stress, medications, and vitamin D sends the message to either begin digesting bone or building new bone. The right signals can reverse the process of bone loss and build new bone.

Today, supplemental calcium and dairy are considered the crème de la crème of calcium sources. However, consuming more calcium, especially from dairy sources, is not the answer to building stronger bones. A Yale study analyzing 34 published studies from 16 countries casts doubt on more calcium as the solution. For instance, South Africans' daily calcium intake was 196mg (compared to the recommended 1500mg in the U.S.) and yet they were 9 times less likely to suffer hip fractures than their American counterparts who consumed more calcium.

It is a misguided belief that all calcium ingested finds a resting place in our bones. Vitamin D is a critical component in calcium absorption. When calcium reaches the stomach, the acid dissolves the calcium and prepares it for absorption in the small intestine. Individual foods have differing absorption rates. A cup of milk has only a 32% calcium absorption rate. By comparison, leafy, green vegetables, such as bok choy, produce a 40-70% absorption rate.[1] Essentially more bio-available calcium is present in green, leafy vegetables than dairy.

The Western diet high in animal protein actually promotes calcium loss and excretion. With excess dietary protein from animal products, approximately 50-100 mq of excess acid per day is produced, resulting in chronic, low-grade acidosis.[2] To buffer acidosis, the body primarily uses calcium by drawing from the bones.[3] Shifting to a plant-based diet not only stops the loss of calcium by up to 50% but also improves bone density and health.[4,5]

Eating fruits and vegetables are an extraordinary, multifaceted therapy for building stronger, healthier bones. Studies strongly suggest that antioxidants from fruit have a significant effect on bone strength and bone mass, and enable bone formation while suppressing bone resorption.[6] Similarly, phytochemicals such as isoflavones (soy), lignans (strawberries, flax seeds, and broccoli), and stilbenes (berries, grapes) conserve bone by stimulating the osteoblasts, inhibiting the osteoclasts (demolition crew) and restoring bone density.[7] Emerging studies are finding that phytochemicals and antioxidants, like quercetin from apples and myrectin from onions and berries, activate stem cells. In the presence of the right phytochemicals, stem cells differentiate into osteoblasts and promote bone growth and improve bone density.[8,9]

Understanding Musculoskeletal Disease

Every year, 30 billion doses of non-steroidal anti-inflammatories, such as ibuprofen and naproxen, are sold to unwitting consumers who are looking for a quick fix for their painful joint or aching low back. However, cortisone and lidocaine joint injections, a cornerstone of musculoskeletal care, are toxic to the cartilage cells (chondrocytes),[10,11,12] and knee and hip arthroscopic surgery can accelerate the degenerative process.[13,14]

Meat consumption greater than 1 time per week is one of the most significant proinflammatory dietary components. It is more strongly linked to rheumatoid arthritis than any other dietary factor, including sweeteners, fish, and dairy.[15,16,17] Plant-based diets, rich in antioxidants, phytochemicals, vitamins and minerals, reduce inflammation, support connective tissues, and maintain cartilage.

What is Fibromyalgia?

Fibromyalgia is a chronic, disabling condition, characterized by widespread pain and painful response to pressure. It leaves modern medicine scratching its head, and prescription pads for solutions. It has no known cure. People with fibromyalgia typically have lower levels of anti-oxidants and minerals like selenium and magnesium and higher levels of oxidative stress, which is related to consumption of animal products.

When a plant-based diet is utilized to treat rheumatoid arthritis patients, a statistically significant number reported less pain, improved function, required fewer medications and demonstrated significant improved laboratory markers for inflammation.[18,19] Several studies on fibromyalgia patients on a plant-based diet found a significant improvement in pain and function compared to omnivore subjects.[20,21] Considering potential side effects and expense of medications, a plant-based diet should be the first line intervention.

How do plants fight inflammation? Vitamin C in combination with other phytochemicals, improves cartilage repair, decreases damage, and leads to less severe arthritis.[22] Minerals such as selenium (walnuts, barley, mushrooms) and magnesium (leafy greens) decrease inflammation in joints and maintain collagen and connective tissue. Additionally beta-carotene and lycopene, phytochemicals found in leafy green vegetables and tomatoes- directly suppress the activation of the signaling molecule NF-kB molecule, which is a critical step in the inflammatory process. The NF-kB factor regulates over 400 genes involved in the inflammatory pathway.[23] NF-kB has been implicated in rheumatoid arthritis and osteoarthritis and is a target for pharmaceutical treatment.[24]

Additionally phytochemicals interact with our DNA influencing genetic expression through a process called epigenetics, a study of environmental factors that alters gene expression either protecting or exposing susceptible regions. Bite by bite our food interacts with our genes. When we drink a smoothie, the phytochemicals retard and even reverse epigenetic changes associated with chronic inflammation altering disease progression, enhancing cartilage integrity, improving quality of life and likely impacting future generations.[25, 26]

Finally, phytochemicals and antioxidants alter stem cell function. There are several types of stem cells in your body and the mesenchymal stem cell line can differentiate into the cells that grow and repair bone, cartilage, muscle, skin, and connective tissue. When you are eating a side of broccoli, the phytochemical sulforaphane and isothiocyanates activate the mesenchymal stem cells and protect them from early death or apoptosis.[27,28]

The novel research of stem cells and plant-based nutrition is just beginning and suggests what we already understand and feel after eating a delicious plant-based meal. Plants are a synergistic symphony that nourishes the body, protects against degeneration and disease, and optimizes every system from the muscle to the DNA.

Scott Stoll, MD *is a member of the Whole Foods Medical Scientific Advisory Board, Plantrician Advisory Board, Future of Health Now advisory board, team physician at Lehigh University, and department chairman of Physical Medicine and Rehabilitation at Coordinated Health. Dr. Stoll is the co-founder of the North American Plant Based Nutrition Healthcare Conference. Dr. Stoll is the author of, Alive! A Physician's Biblical and Scientific Guide to Nutrition. He was a member of the 1994 Olympic Bobsled team and now serves as a physician for the United States Bobsled and Skeleton team. Dr. Stoll resides with his wife and 6 children in Bethlehem, Pennsylvania. For more information:* FullyAliveToday.com.

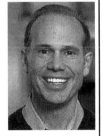

Get a Grip on Strong Joints

Stefan W. Kreuzer, MD, MS

In general terms, healthy bone has to be a combination of the right amount of calcium and the right amount of hormones that is influenced by proper diet and exercise. There is a phase of life where we build bone, and then there is a phase in life where we lose bone. Women start at a lower bone density to begin with, so when they get into this phase of losing bone they are at an increased risk of having brittle bone related fractures, such as, hip, line, and wrist fractures.[1]

Calcium absorption is as important, if not more important than calcium consumption. Although dairy products are advertised as having high calcium, it is important to have a form of calcium that is easily absorbed. Plant derived calcium is better absorbed than animal derived calcium.[2] Dairy produces an acid condition in the body, which actually causes the leeching of the calcium out of the bone to neutralize the acid instead of depositing the calcium into the bone.

Most of the patients that I see for bone issues and joint replacements can be traced back to obesity. Obesity wreaks havoc on our joints and can lead to the development of arthritis. Obesity presents a challenge to surgery because it is technically much more difficult to perform a surgery in an obese patient, than a non-obese patient. Even though we might be successful doing the operation, the ability of the implant is ultimately limited because of excess weight.

A plant-based diet is optimal for weight-loss because the ratio of nutrition per calorie is much higher. If you walk thru a grocery store, it is easy to see what is high in nutrition. Most people understand that vegetables, fruits, and whole grains are the most nutritious of foods. However, it is just as important to understand that meat and dairy products are caloric dense but not as nutrient dense.

Despite the constant promotion of fad diets, there is no such thing as a diet that works. As an orthopedic surgeon, I am flabbergasted by how little primary care physicians and cardiologists talk to their patients about the relationship between our food choices and excess weight. About 60% of my patients state that their primary care physicians have never talked to them about their excess weight. Unfortunately, by the time these patients are referred to me, they have major joint problems, such as arthritis, that could have been prevented through plant-based dietary choices that promote weight-loss. As the rate of childhood obesity is frightening, it is time we start educating ourselves about the importance of proper nutrition and weight loss.

I had 2 weeks of nutrition in my medical school, which is virtually nothing. However, it is amazing how appreciative patients are when they are empowered with the knowledge to take control of their health and their weight. We are providing them with real hope, not just another fad diet.

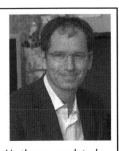

Stefan W. Kreuzer, MD, MS *is a Board-Certified and Fellowship-Trained Joint Replacement Surgeon that has pioneered the development in Minimally Invasive and Computer Assisted hip and knee replacement surgery. He is actively involved in training and has been invited to lecture and demonstrate his surgical techniques for surgeons throughout the United States, Asia and Europe. Dr. Kreuzer is currently on multiple design teams for the development of the next generation of knee and hip implants. He also serves on several medical advisory boards, is the Director of Education for the anterior hip collaborative, and is 1 of 5 board members of DASH (Direct Anterior Society of the Hip). A native of Switzerland, Dr. Kreuzer moved to the United States in 1983. He graduated from medical school at the University of Texas in San Antonio in 1995, and went to Galveston, Texas for his orthopedic residency. He then completed a Fellowship in Adult Joint Reconstruction at the Baylor College of Medicine in Houston, Texas in 2001. Currently he is a Faculty member with the University of Texas Physicians in Houston, Texas.*

Beyond Calcium: Building Bone Vitality Without Dairy

Amy Joy Lanou, PhD

Osteoporosis is responsible for more than 8.9 million fractures each year. This means a fracture occurs roughly every 3 seconds.[1] In the US, 1 in every 6 women (17%) fractures a hip during her lifetime. Interestingly, 4 worldwide epidemiological surveys conducted by different research teams over 20 years agree that the countries that consume the most calcium (the U.S., Western Europe, Australia, and New Zealand) have the highest rates of hip fracture. Meanwhile, countries that consume little or no milk, dairy, and calcium supplements (much of Asia and Africa) have fracture rates 50% to 70% *lower* than those in the U.S.[2] The World Health Organization calls this the "calcium paradox".

In doing research over the past 10 years on how we can best take care of our bones, I've learned 4 really important things about how to promote bone vitality.

1) Milk, dairy products, and calcium supplements do not prevent fractures. Of the 86 human trials testing whether milk, dairy, or calcium pills by themselves or in any combination reduce fracture risk, 62 studies (72%) offer no support for the conventional wisdom. In fact, some show that as milk and dairy intake increases, fractures become *more likely*.

The same is true for children's bones. A review of dairy and bone health in youth found that of 37 studies of dairy or dietary calcium intake, 28 studies found no relationship between dairy or dietary calcium intake and measures of bone health.[3] Pouring more calcium into the body in the form of milk or supplements is not having the intended effect. **So if dairy is not recommended, where will we get our calcium?**

Calcium Absorption Rates	
Brussels Sprouts	64%
Mustard Greens	58%
Broccoli	53%
Turnip Greens	52%
Kale	40-59%
Fortified Orange Juice	36-38%
Milk	32%
Calcium Supplements	28-32%

What does matter is keeping calcium in the bones. We do need some calcium but plant foods are better sources of calcium because they tend to have high calcium absorption and are alkaline forming. Beans and the greens are the best. In fact, 1 cup of cooked kale has the same amount of absorbable calcium as a cup of cow's milk, without all the excess calories.[4] We need to be thinking about the overall dietary pattern rather than just calcium intake.

2). Eating a low-acid diet key to osteoporosis prevention. Research shows that a low-acid diet high in fruits and vegetables and low in high-protein foods like meats, poultry, fish, milk, and dairy, helps keep calcium in bones. Why? Osteoporosis prevention begins in the bloodstream. For good health, the blood must maintain its pH (relative acidity or alkalinity) within a very narrow range. As the body digests high-protein foods, the blood becomes more acidic. To neutralize excess acid in the bloodstream, the body draws on the calcium compounds in bone, eventually weakening bone and causing osteoporosis. Neutralizing excess blood acidity releases calcium, which eventually leaves the body in urine.

Osteoporosis is caused by an *imbalance of calcium and other nutrients, not calcium deficiency*. Simply put: as animal protein intake increases, so does the rate of hip fracture. Meanwhile, as consumption of protein from fruits and vegetables rises, the rate of hip fracture falls.[2]

3) Eat fruits, vegetables, and legumes and spend time in the sunshine. Strong, healthy, fracture-resistant bones require 17 nutrients. Consuming lots of calcium without enough of the other 16 nutrients is like building a brick wall with no mortar. The richest sources are fruits and vegetables. Black, red, and pinto beans are good sources of bone strengthening nutrients such as Vitamin 6, calcium, magnesium, and zinc. Vitamin D deserves special mention as it helps absorb calcium from the digestive tract, and more importantly helps move calcium and other nutrients from the blood stream into bone. Our main source of Vitamin D is produced in our skin in response to sunlight

4) Exercise gives bones a reason to become and stay strong. Just as exercise improves muscle strength, exercise also strengthens bones. Out of the 86 studies on exercise and fracture risk, 87% show a positive benefit.[5]

The calcium theory is bankrupt. The best approach is a diet very low in or devoid of animal foods and high in fruits and vegetables, combined with walking or equivalent exercise for 30 to 60 minutes a day, every day. That's the safe, simple, scientific prescription for osteoporosis prevention—and for optimal health and longevity.—

> **Know Your Food pH**
>
> **Very Alkaline:** Typical serving of fruits/vegetables
>
> **Close to Neutral:** Typical serving of beans, soymilk, pasta, bread
>
> **Moderately Acid:** Typical serving of rice, milk, yogurt, egg
>
> **Highly Acid:** Typical serving of fish, poultry, meat
>
> **Very highly Acid:** Cheese (made from mammalian milks)

Amy Joy Lanou, PhD, *is the Associate Professor in the Department of Health and Wellness at the University of North Carolina, Asheville. She is Consulting Senior Nutrition Scientist for the Physicians Committee for Responsible Medicine and co-author of "Building Bone Vitality" with Michael Castleman.*

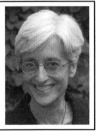

Miracle Medicine

Alpa Yagnik, M.Sc M.Phil, BAMS, India

Our inner environment plays a major role in the onset of any disease. Generally, arthritis can stem from dietary choices consisting of fast food, junk food and lots of dairy products. Observational studies indicate that high intake of dairy, sugary, and refined products disturb the acid-alkali balance of the body. To remain healthy, the blood pH should be around 7.4 or slightly alkaline. When our pH is disturbed due to over consumption of acid-producing food, it can lay the foundation for onset of disease. When the acid circulates through the blood, it gets deposited in the joints where it can cause inflammation. "Itis" means inflammation. Any disease with suffix "itis" reveals that the excess acid generated caused the inflammatory reaction in that particular organ. Examples: arthritis, dermatitis, gastritis, colitis, and sinusitis.

A young patient of mine was diagnosed with severe Rheumatoid arthritis, considered an auto immune disease in which the immune system mistakenly attacks and destroys healthy body tissues. It can be triggered by genetic susceptibility, environmental or biological infection, allergic reaction, or hormonal changes. This patient's joints were so painful and swollen that he could barely move. All of the Rheumatologists he visited prescribed high doses of pain killers and even steroids which had lots of side effects. Within 6 months of switching to a plant-based diet, the patient's health tests were absolutely normal and his pain and swellings had been eliminated. As his energy level increased, his immunity increased and he has not since suffered from any secondary infections.

The human body functions as a single unit. This means if one organ is affected then the whole body is disturbed and balance needs to be restored. The excess acid needs to be neutralised. Our body is very smart so if no alkaline is available the body will start depleting the alkaline reserves by leaching calcium and magnesium from our bones and teeth. Thus weakening our bones and contributing to the onset of osteoporosis. Vegetables and fruits are the best alkalisers needed by our body. Among them, green leafy vegetable are the best as they have the optimal sources of all minerals.

Today we rely on expensive medications to cure our ailments and chronic conditions. As the following testimonial reveals, there can be a much simpler solution when we take dietary factors into consideration.

Three Aspects of 'OrthoWellness'

Dennis Gates, MD

As a board certified orthopedic surgeon for over 40 years as well as an integrative medicine physician, my patients come to me with 3 main questions:

1. How can we avoid breaking bones and getting osteoporosis as we get older?

2. How can we treat our arthritis without taking all those medicines?

3. How can we get the best result from this total hip or total knee replacement?

There is the same, simple answer to each of these questions: an anti-inflammatory or plant- based eating program combined with an exercise/ activity program.

How to Avoid Osteoporosis

Osteoporosis occurs when your body excretes more calcium than it absorbs. Our bones are constantly being remodeled. This is a natural healthy cycle, which helps repair minor damage. In order to keep our bones strong we have to maintain and enhance the calcium in our bones and strengthen the matrix that forms bone. Calcium has to be received in a natural way to maintain it. When the balance changes, and calcium is lost, small holes, like a broken spider web, begin to appear. As more calcium crystals are pulled out, the bones begin to crumble. A simple fall shatters a hip. A cough can crack a rib.

Aging is one cause, genetics is another, diet is a third, and disuse is the fourth.[1,2] We can't stop aging but we can affect the integrity of our genes, enhance our diet, and avoid disuse. We affect our genes by decreasing our 'toxic load.[3] US beef and chicken and other meat products contain numerous toxins including growth hormones, sex hormones, antibiotics, pesticides, sugar, and many other chemicals, which directly affect our genetic activity. Toxins can turn on a bad gene that leads to diseases.[3] Since osteoporosis is also genetically activated, removing the toxin can allow a gene to heal and reverse the disease. The toxins can also prevent proper absorption of nutrients, thus further putting us at risk.

We enhance our diet by increasing those foods that provide the nutrition our bones need and eliminating the foods that do not. The high fat content, and the high trans

Vitamin D and Keys to Strong Bones

Vitamin D, obtained from sunlight and leafy green vegetables, is essential to proper calcium absorption. Vitamin D is really the only supplement that we really need to take for strong bones. Other nutrients such as- magnesium, boron, zinc, copper and Vitamin K, which interact with and enhance the metabolism of calcium, can all obtained from plant-based foods. Every adult American should have their Vitamin D level measured, and be taking a supplement of about 1000 to 2000 units per day.

Osteoporosis is also related to our OVER consumption of salt, animal protein, soft drinks, caffeine, refined carbohydrates, alcohol, and smoking. All of the above leach calcium and other nutrients out of our bones as well as decrease calcium absorption.

Key to strong bones:
- Stop adding salt to your food.
- Eliminate animal protein, or at least markedly restrict it.
- Eliminate soft drinks which are just sugar and toxins. Try club soda with a twist of lemon.
- Decrease your caffeine.
- Stop eating refined carbs, which are simply metabolized quickly into sugar.
- Decrease alcohol. It is essentially sugar.
- Stop smoking. Nothing good comes from it.

fat content of the standard American diet is detrimental to the absorption of the little calcium we ingest.[4] **Going on a plant-based eating program, which means no meat, no chicken, and especially NO dairy, will strengthen your bones more than any medication.[5]** Along with a plant-based diet, exercise is essential to bone health and strength.[6]

What about calcium from milk? The discussion of cow's milk and bones provides an interesting dilemma. Despite the health claims from advertisements about milk and calcium, not much of the calcium in the cow's milk that you ingest makes it into your bones. Rather, the opposite happens as the calcium in milk actually causes calcium to leach out of the bones.[7] Hard to believe, but true. This phenomenon is related to the acid-base ratio of our bodies. Calcium acts a neutralizer because dairy is acidic (pH 6.5) and our body likes to stay in a more alkaline state. This relationship is well known among orthopedic surgeons, who have previously protested the presence of dairy advertisements and promotion at international orthopedic conventions.[8]

How to Prevent and Reverse Arthritis

The most common type of arthritis I see is osteoarthritis, also known as degenerative arthritis. Arthritis is the deterioration of the ends of bones or the joints where the cartilage begins to wear away thru micro fragmentation. Each time these micro fragments break, they cause inflammation and pain, resulting in swelling, tenderness, stiffness, and even deformity over time. When the cartilage wears away completely, a total joint replacement or arthroplasty is required.

Although patients with arthritis generally come in complaining of joint pain they attribute to an injury in the past, (which holds some truth), the real causes of osteoarthritis are either genetic, the result of repetitive trauma, or chronic inflammation. All three of these can be related to the nutritional inflammation from eating the Standard American Diet (SAD). To date, there is no direct proof diet directly causes arthritis BUT there is a strong relationship. Most humans, if accurately tested are allergic to the non human protein in milk (casein) and to the sugar (fructose) in milk to some degree. Allergies cause inflammation and low grade long term inflammation in the body affects our joints.[9]

All animal products, including fish, have a component called omega 6, which produces inflammation. Although we hear about omegas all the time, the two are not created equal. omega 3s, inhibit inflammation, as opposed to the 6's, which promote inflammation. Both are needed, but the ratio of omega 3 to omega 6 should be about 2:1. In the SAD diet, it is about 1:20 or 1:30. While fish are notoriously promoted for their omega 3 content, the problem with all fish is that they also contain a plethora of toxins ingested from the river beds from pollution.

Since arthritis is an inflammation of the joints, it is important to eat an anti-inflammatory diet, which means eliminating all animal products from our diet. The anti inflammatory diet is based on vegetables, such as broccoli, spinach, greens, and fruits such as apricots, apples, cantaloupe, peaches, all contain antioxidants which are needed to decrease inflammation.[10] Additionally a plant-based diet can aid in weight-loss which is an important step in preventing and reversing osteoarthritis.[11] Following an anti inflammatory diet along with exercise and stretching programs will markedly decrease arthritic and bone pain. As it takes time for the bone metabolism to change, significant improvement generally occurs around 3 months time.

Maximizing Results from Total Joint Replacements

Having performed over 3,000 hip replacements and 2,000 knee replacements as well as having had both my hips and knees replaced, this subject is close to my heart. Why does someone need a total joint replacement? Essentially a joint wears out when the cartilage surface of the joint, the smooth glistening lining that moves so effortlessly in the average person loses its moisture content and becomes inflamed. We use the expression 'bone on bone,' meaning the adjoining bones are rubbing against each other without any cartilage left. The joint becomes extremely painful, swollen, and eventually one cannot walk or use the joint.

Why does this happen? The same reasons that promote arthritis, (i.e. inflammation from foods and repetitive trauma) are the same reasons joints wear away to the point of no return. We don't know if it is possible to avoid surgery completely, but we do know we can delay the process and aid in a smooth recovery. The path to healthy bones, joints and 'orthowellness' begins with simple steps: an anti-inflammatory plant-based diet and exercise.[12]

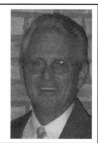

Dennis J. Gates, MD *graduated of Loyola Stritch Medical School, and did his orthopedic residency at Northwestern University in Chicago. He has a fellowship in Integrative Medicine from the University of Arizona. He spent his 37 year career as an Orthopedic Surgeon at Mercy Hospital and Rush University Hospital in Chicago. Dr. Gates conducts workshops on Optimum Health for Cancer Patients and works with World Orthopedic Concern overseas. He just returned from working in Ethiopia, and traveled to Haiti on 6 mission trips after the earthquake with his wife, Lois and their 5 children.*

Plant-Based Diets: A 'Joint Effort' in the Fight Against Arthritis

Rick Weissinger, MS, RD, LDN

The term 'Arthritis' comes from a combination of two words: *arthro* (joint) and *itis* (inflammation).[1] Osteoarthritis (OA) is the most common form of this disease in the United States, and the incidence is increasing[2] while the incidence of rheumatoid arthritis is fairly equal across different populations.[3] A Western diet can increase the risk for arthritis by promoting obesity and inflammation while plant-based diets may help to reduce the severity of arthritis and slow its progression.

Osteoarthritis and Obesity

Obesity is one of the main risk factors for osteoarthritis, and is involved in its progression.[2] The 'wear and tear' concept explains osteoarthritis as a disease in which joints made to handle a certain weight have to cope with greater stressors than they were made for, resulting in irreversible damage over time that eventually requires joint replacement.

Inflammation has recently been added to explain how osteoarthritis progresses. Our body fat (adipose tissue) releases inflammatory chemicals ('adipokines'), (include *leptin, adiponectin, tumor necrosis factor* (TNF-α) and *interleukin-6* (IL-6)), which participate in most inflammation-related diseases, and are architects of the joint destruction seen in osteoarthritis.[4-6] Not surprisingly, losing excess weight improves both hip and knee osteoarthritis.[7]

Given the importance of obesity in arthritis, what *should* people be eating to attain a healthy weight? Meat, eggs, and dairy products represent unnecessary sources of calories. Animal protein is more likely to play a role in obesity than plant protein, because it is the chief dietary stimulus for insulin-like growth factor-1 (IGF-1).[8] IGF-1 has been shown to promote weight gain by triggering the development of pre-adipocytes (immature fat cells) into mature fat cells.[9] Animal protein is also the only dietary source of an omega-6 fat (arachidonic acid, AA), which promotes fat storage through increasing appetite and food intake.[10] In contrast, eating higher amounts of whole grains, fruits, vegetables, and legumes has been shown to help with weight loss as well as reduce inflammation.[11,12]

Western Diets, Inflammation, and Arthritis

Western diets are pro-inflammatory. A higher meat intake has been associated with rheumatoid arthritis in ecologic studies[13], and in the European Prospective Investigation of Cancer in Norfolk [EPIC-Norfolk]) study, higher intakes of meat and total protein were linked with inflammatory polyarthritis.[14] Meat, eggs, and dairy products promote inflammation through the saturated fat,[15] cholesterol,[16] oxidized cholesterol, [17] advanced glycation end products (i.e., 'glycotoxins'),[18]and arachidonic acid (AA)[19] they contain. Arachidonic acid provides the raw material needed for the body to manufacture *tumor necrosis factor* (TNF-α)[20], one of a number of proteins called *cytokines* that are involved in increasing inflammation in rheumatic diseases especially. Cytokines are the targets of the latest generation of drugs for rheumatoid arthritis; several types, including TNF-α, prompt immune cells to fire off oxygen free radicals that damage joint tissue, a condition known as 'oxidative' stress.[22]

Diet, Oxidative Stress, and Arthritis

Western diets cause a degree of 'oxidative' stress[23], characterized by the release of free radicals by immune cells. In turn, these cause the age-related damage seen in the joints of arthritis patients, as well as interfering with joint healing.[24] Oxidative stress turns on a 'master regulator' of inflammation (NF B) that in turn increases production of TNF- and other cytokines.[25] Oxidative stress also activates a class of enzymes called *matrix metalloproteinases* (MMPs),protein-munching enzymes implicated in degrading collagen and in causing irreversible joint erosion.[26]

The Benefits of Plant-Based Diets for Arthritis Patients

Eliminating animal fats from the diet leaves room for the intake of unsaturated fats that also affect inflammation.[27] For example, the omega-6 fat linoleic acid, found in nuts, seeds, and vegetable oils, is metabolized to gammalinolenic acid (GLA) and dihomo-gammalinolenic acid (DGLA), both of which suppress inflammation.[5,27] In addition, certain micronutrients (e.g., magnesium, boron, and vitamins K and C) and phytochemicals (e.g., carotenoids, flavonoids, polyphenols, and many others) found in higher amounts in plant-based diets appear to be important for the maintenance of joint health and the prevention of arthritis.

Micronutrients and Arthritis

Magnesium may be a critical nutrient for preventing and treating osteoarthritis as it has an important role in cartilage development. The majority of high-magnesium foods are plant-based. Low magnesium intakes are associated with inflammation and inflammation-related diseases[28], and studies have found an association between magnesium intake and knee osteoarthritis in certain populations.[29]

Plant-based diets are also higher in vitamin K and boron than Western diets, and both may be critical for osteoarthritis prevention and treatment.[30] For example, vitamin K may retard arthritis by limiting an increase in certain cells (fibroblast-like synoviocytes) involved in the progression of RA.[31]Studies have also shown a lower risk for rheumatoid arthritis in persons who eat higher amounts of foods high in vitamin C and certain carotenoids (e.g., -cryptoxanthin, found in mandarin oranges, persimmons, oranges, papayas, pumpkin, and red sweet peppers).[31]

Apart from the important vitamins and minerals found in plant-based diets, the phytochemicals in these diets have the ability to affect osteoarthritis risk through their antioxidant and anti-inflammatory effects. One of these involves suppressing a key enzyme found in all body tissues that is involved in inflammation (cycloxygenase, or COX). Another involves down-regulation of NF B.[32-34] Certain phytochemicals can also keep osteoarthritis from getting worse by slowing the protein-degrading enzymes (MMPs) involved in joint erosion.[35]

Connections between Plant-Based Diets, the Gastrointestinal Tract, and RA

Plant-based diets may also affect rheumatoid arthritis through the *microbiome* (the balance of good and bad bacteria).[36] For example, the bacteria *Proteus mirabilis* is suspected of contributing to joint damage and inflammation in rheumatoid arthritis as anti-*Proteus mirabilis* antibodies have been found in patients with rheumatoid arthritis.[37]Studies indicate a decrease in disease activity in patients with rheumatoid arthritis eating uncooked vegan diets, purportedly through a change in the balance of friendly vs. pathogenic bacteria.[38,39]   Diet may also affect RA and other autoimmune diseases through an effect on the integrity of the gut lining. When the integrity of this lining is altered, bacteria may be transported into the blood circulation, thereby triggering inflammation. This process is dependent upon *zonulin*, the only known modulator of the 'tight junctions' between cells lining the intestinal wall. Zonulin, affected by diet and particularly fiber, disassembles these junctions, and is thereby involved in trafficking of large molecules from the gut into the bloodstream.[40] Therefore an important benefit of plant-based diets in rheumatoid arthritis may be derived through their higher fiber content.

Conclusion

Both osteoarthritis and rheumatoid arthritis are intimately tied to diet. Plant-based diets are also a low cost option; in fact, patients are able to spend far less on groceries by eliminating animal foods from their diets. In contrast, state-of-the-art drugs for rheumatoid arthritis such as etanercept (Enbrel) cost $20,000 per year and are associated with numerous side effects. Whether plant-based diets work at the level of the gut, the immune system, the rheumatic joint itself or by other mechanisms yet undiscovered (these are not mutually exclusive) is academic; the existing evidence is enough to suggest patients try a plant-based diet to treat their arthritis, whether as a primary or as an adjunctive treatment.

Rick Weissinger, MS, RD, CPT *is a Registered, Licensed Dietitian/Nutritionist. Rick co-authored a number of publications, including a handbook for medical students (Nutrition Guide for Clinicians); a book on diet and cancer risk (What the Experts Say About Food and Cancer) and education programs for other Nutritionists (The Psychology of Weight Control). His next book (Excuse Me, Your Brain is On Fire) focuses on the cutting-edge evidence that foods have a dramatic ability to impact mood. He currently works as a Nutritionist in Maryland, in private practice in Northern Virginia, and as a long-term care consultant.*

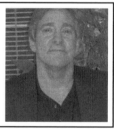

twelve

A HEALTHY GI PASSAGEWAY FOR SMOOTH SAILING

Since about 70% of our immune system exists in the lining of our stomach, the saying "go with your gut" takes on a whole new meaning. We have billions of gut microbes and bacteria in our stomachs that regulate our internal environment by producing necessary hormones and enzymes, disease-fighting antioxidants, and immune boosting properties. Our internal environment is in a constant tug of war between good and bad bacteria. Bad bacteria thrive on animal fat and processed food products whereas good bacteria feed on fiber. Fiber, only found in plant-based foods, is critical to removing excess toxins and fat from our bodies.

As this chapter's experts attest, the most influential factors to a healthy gut flora are our food choices. Meat and dairy products profoundly change our gut environment and introduce harmful bacteria that disrupt the proper functioning of our system. When our gut's balance is thrown off it allows these harmful bacteria to break through and "leak" into our blood stream. Poor food choices can lead to a host of common gastrointestinal and renal problems such as kidney failure, fatty liver, acid reflux, and autoimmune conditions such as Crohn's disease and irritable bowel syndrome. As some health problems like kidney failure are irreversible, making the right food choices is imperative.

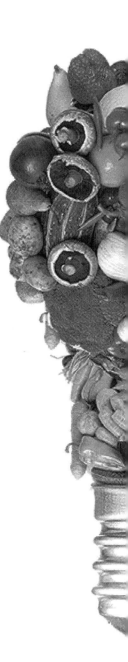

The Forgotten Two: The Kidneys

Lauren Graf, MS, RD

We are bombarded with information on the importance of lifestyle and diet for weight control, bone health, and preventing heart disease, cancer, etc. We often don't think or hear about the way our diet impacts the health of our kidneys. In fact, most of us take this pair of organs for granted, not realizing how much vital work they do to keep us alive and well. Kidney disease seems to sneak up on us so suddenly because it develops slowly over time. It is a silent disease, and the harmful effects of the Western diet often manifest in high blood pressure or diabetes, which slowly but surely damages the filtering units of the kidney.

The kidneys (most of us have 2 but you can actually live perfectly well with just one) are one of the main detoxifying organs in the body. These small, bean-shaped organs located in the middle of your back filter about 200 quarts of blood daily to remove wastes and toxins, which are excreted in the urine. Each kidney has about a million delicate filtering units called nephrons. Nephrons have the complicated job of filtering out waste and excess fluid. Without kidneys, harmful toxins build up in the body and your blood would become chemically unbalanced which would impede your ability to pee. When kidneys completely shut down, as in end-stage kidney disease, they are no longer able to make urine.

Think about what would happen if your pipes stopped working in your home—your sink and shower would not drain unless you got buckets to dump out all the excess. Well, when your kidneys don't work, fluid and waste products (breakdown of protein, etc.) remain trapped in the body until a machine (called a dialysis machine) is able to remove it. Many of the toxins that build up in the bloodstream of patients with kidney failure (ammonia, urea and uric acid) are produced from protein metabolism. Sophisticated advances in medicine can keep us alive if our kidneys don't work, but this is not the best quality of life or healthiest way to live. In fact, being on dialysis for a long period of time significantly shortens a person's lifespan.

Kidney failure has many different causes, but the 2 most common are uncontrolled diabetes and high blood pressure. Currently 26 million Americans have kidney disease and millions more are at risk of developing it.[1] Alarmingly, the incidence of kidney disease has risen greatly not only in the United States but also worldwide.[2,3] This is largely the result of the toxic Western diet which coincides with the rise in obesity. Consumption of excess protein in and of itself places more stress on the kidneys and can lead to damage over time. Despite the slow progression of this disease, the consequences are no less devastating and painful.

The good news is that most kidney disease can be prevented, or the progression of the disease drastically slowed. One of the most powerful things you can do to protect your kidneys is to change your diet. The Western diet, high in animal protein and refined carbohydrates (think white bread, most commercial cereals, and soda), dramatically increase our risk of type-2 diabetes, and high blood pressure. Although some causes of kidney disease are beyond our control, consuming a plant-based diet can slow the progression of and drastically and improve overall health and quality of life of kidney transplant recipients.[4,5,6] If you already have kidney disease, don't feel helpless! Taking control of your lifestyle will empower you to live healthier and stronger than ever before.

Prevent or Slow Chronic Kidney Disease Progression with a Plant-Based Diet

Whole food, plant-based diets are naturally rich in fiber, vitamins and minerals, anti-oxidants, and phytochemicals that help protect our bodies against heart disease, high blood pressure, and diabetes. Much of the mainstream diet information advises limiting carbohydrates and opting for a heavier animal-protein diet, especially for diabetics. Many people are taught to manage their diabetes by tallying up grams of carbohydrate without regard for much else. When we think about food in terms of a single component (calories, carbohydrates, sodium, etc.), as we are often taught to do, we lose sight of the big picture. However, it's the junk food carbohydrates that wreak havoc on our blood glucose and insulin, not high-fiber whole foods. A meal of quinoa, lentils, and veggies will have a very different effect on the body than the same amount of calories and carbohydrates grams from a hamburger on a white bun and a soda.

One study compared a low-fat vegan diet with a diet based on the American Diabetes Association (ADA) guidelines. The ADA nutrition guidelines emphasis portion control, and encourage fruits and vegetables but they also recommend animal protein (lean meat, poultry, fish and dairy) with meals.[7] Not only did participants on the low-fat vegan diet have improvements in blood sugar control, they also were able to reduce their medication much more than those on the American Diabetes Association Diet.[8] Other studies have consistently found that vegetarians have a significantly lower risk of developing type 2 diabetes than non-vegetarians.[9,10,11]

Diabetic patients may indeed be able to keep blood sugar controlled by strictly limiting carbohydrates and increasing protein. Unlike carbohydrates and fat, the body cannot store excess protein. It is the job of the kidneys to eliminate the toxic waste products of protein metabolism and this places more stress on these delicate organs. Shifting to a heavier animal protein diet in an effort to keep their blood sugar low can actually damage the kidneys.[12] This kidney damage can be detected in the very early stages in a simple urine test—long before a person experiences any symptoms. The microalbumin urine test can detect very small amounts of the protein albumin. When kidneys are damaged, proteins such as albumin leak into the urine. One study found that when diabetic patients switched from a omnivorous diet to a diet lower in animal protein and higher in plant-protein, the amount of albumin in the urine decreased by 50%.[1] Other studies comparing a diet high in animal protein to a diet of primarily plant protein have found similar protective effects (decrease in proteinuria).[14,15,16,17,18,19] The less protein we eat, particularly animal protein, the lower the workload on our kidneys. In patients with more advanced kidney disease, vegan diets have shown promise in slowing down the disease process and keeping the cardiovascular system healthy.[20,21,22]

The way our bodies digest and absorb food is far too complex and multi-factorial to be reduced to numbers. Take carb counting for example; one third cup of lentils would be considered equivalent to a slice of white bread. But there are dramatic differences between these 2 foods including the fiber content, type of carbohydrates, antioxidants, protein, and the body processes these foods very differently. It's no wonder there is so much confusion surrounding what to eat.

What If I Already Have Kidney Disease?

Unfortunately, some forms of kidney disease are not preventable even with the most careful attention to diet and lifestyle. There are congenital causes of kidney disease, as well as genetic and autoimmune causes. The great news is that people with kidney disease can live long, fulfilling lives with advancement in medicine coupled with optimal nutrition. Throughout my years working in nephrology, I have seen many patients transition from dialysis to transplant with a wonderfully working kidney. If you already have kidney disease, are on dialysis or have an organ transplant, adopting a plant-based diet can have major health and longevity benefits as it can protect your heart and bones and decrease the risk of other chronic diseases such as cancer.

However, far too many patients develop other serious problems such as cardiovascular disease, heart attack or bone fractures early in life that could have been largely prevented if their diet had been healthier leading up to their transplant. The number one cause of death in people with kidney disease is heart disease.[23,24] This is true even in young patients. Many of the risk factors are completely within our control. Knowledge is power and it's time to get in the driver's seat of your own health. It's important that patients be informed of their disease and how they can to participate in their health care.

The kidneys and heart work together to control blood pressure, cholesterol, and inflammation. As is the case with the general population, much of the traditional diet advice given to patients with chronic or end-stage kidney disease may be putting them on a path towards cardiovascular disease. **Yes—the nutritional information you're likely to receive from mainstream clinicians is often downright harmful.**

Perhaps the most serious harm of a diet high in animal protein is that it promotes inflammation as well as heart and blood vessel disease.[25,26,27] This process is aggravated by kidney disease. If you have severe kidney disease, you may have been told to restrict the minerals potassium and phosphorus in the diet. Healthy kidneys excrete excess potassium and phosphorus easily, but if your kidneys are not working well or at all, you are forced to limit them in the diet, otherwise these minerals can build up to dangerous levels in the blood. When damaging levels of phosphorus builds up in the blood it can pull calcium out of the bones, which weakens them. Phosphorus binds with the calcium and form deposits in your blood vessels, eyes and heart. Having high blood phosphorus levels over a period of time can dramatically increase your risk of heart attack and stroke. Whole-food plant-based diets can help you maintain normal blood levels of phosphorus, which will dramatically reduce your risk of cardiovascular disease.[28]

The phosphorus that ends up in blood vessels comes directly from the foods we eat. The largest contributors to dietary phosphorus are animal protein and processed foods with phosphate additives. The phosphorus from meat and dairy products is readily absorbed by the body and increases blood levels. Unprocessed plant-based foods such as nuts and beans are relatively high in phosphorus as well, but it is not absorbed nearly as well as the phosphorus from animal foods.[29,30] Plant foods naturally contain phytates, the storage form of phosphorus, which is not digestible to humans. Therefore much of the phosphorus from plant foods passes through us undigested rather than ending up in blood vessels. Both animal and human studies comparing meat-based diets with vegetarian diets in kidney disease have found significantly lower phosphorus levels in people on a vegetarian diet.[28,30]

While animal protein exacerbates heart disease and inflammation, dietary fiber, which is present only in plant foods, has the reverse effect.[29,30] Most of us are familiar with the fact that a high fiber intake protects the heart and decreases our risk for a number of diseases. Fiber has an even more dramatic protective effect in patients with kidney disease. A recent study found that those people with chronic kidney disease that consumed the most fiber (i.e. plant foods) had significantly lower markers of inflammation and risk of death compared to those consuming the least fiber.[30] In another clinical trial comparing vegan diets to a conventional meat based diet in patients with severe kidney disease, those on the vegan diet had lower levels of inflammation, improved blood lipid profile and a better antioxidant status.[22]

People on dialysis are often told they need more protein, particularly animal protein, because it has traditionally been considered superior to plant protein. Animal protein contains all the essential amino acids and the thinking was that once you are on dialysis, your body needs more protein to maintain muscle. Plus, your kidneys have already failed, so the extra protein won't cause any damage, right? Wrong. People on dialysis still have hearts and blood vessels and bones they need to keep healthy. Animal protein puts more strain on the heart by increasing inflammation, acid levels, and uremic toxins in the body.[31] Studies have found that plant-based diets reduce markers of inflammation, improve the lipid profile, maintain bone density, and decrease risk of death from heart disease.[8,22,25,26,28] While people on dialysis need slightly more protein to account for the losses in dialysis, it is minimal and can easily be met with a whole food, plant-based diet.[34,35]

People with kidney disease are also at high risk for acidosis because the failing kidneys are unable to remove enough acid from the body. Vegan diets rich in fruits and vegetables are alkaline forming in the body, while animal protein and processed food tends to be acid forming. Acid base balance is crucial to preventing bone loss, maintaining muscle mass and reducing inflammation. Studies have found that diets rich in vegetables and fruit lower acid levels and reduce kidney injury (slowing the progression of disease) and helps improve blood pressure in patients with chronic kidney disease.[34,36,37,38]

The positive findings of plant-based diets for people with kidney disease are not surprising given the overwhelming evidence that this diet is protective in the general population. Diet is one of the most vital components of health and well being, and it plays a crucial role in the management and progression of kidney disease. Sadly, most clinicians do not promote this dietary lifestyle to their patients so it is important to play an active role in your health care. You should question and analyze the nutrition advice your health care professionals provide, including the source of and scientific basis for such advice. Fortunately, you are in control of the foods you eat, and it is easy and inexpensive to adopt a plant-based diet.

My Personal Experience

Living and eating well with kidney disease has been near to my heart on a more personal level. As a teenager, I was diagnosed with a kidney disorder called minimal change nephrotic syndrome. Nephrotic syndrome is a disorder where you have large amounts of protein in the urine. This protein, called albumin is lost through the glomeruli of the kidneys. This results in swelling throughout the body, high cholesterol and a weakened immune system. Fortunately, I completely recovered and have not had a relapse. I believe that medication along with lasting dietary changes played a major role in my recovery. I was also lucky to have a pediatric nephrologist who recognized the impact of nutrition on health and kidney disease. Looking back on the experience 16 years later, I realize he was ahead of his time.

Although having an illness as an adolescent was a difficult experience, it also inspired me to choose a career in healthcare. It was at that time that I realized how fascinating the connection is between nutrition and health. I hope I can inspire you to experiment with more plant-based meals and understand more clearly how nutrition impacts your health. The choice is yours.

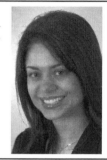

Lauren Graf, MS, RD, *is the nutritionist for the Montefiore-Einstein Cardiac Wellness Program. She received her BS and RD degree from the University of Connecticut and completed her dietetic internship at the UConn Health Center. She received her master's degree in clinical nutrition from New York University. In addition to counseling patients on nutrition, Lauren has written articles for a variety of academic and professional publications including journals such as Advances in Chronic Kidney Disease and US Nephrology, and quoted in numerous publications including Women's Health Magazine and The Wall Street Journal. Ms. Graf has also appeared on WABC TV news and BronxNet news discussing nutrition and heart health.*

Save Your Kidneys With a Plant-Based Diet

Phillip Tuso, MD

A plant-based diet may be able to prevent End Stage Renal Disease (ESRD). ESRD is when a significant portion of the kidney has been damaged to the point that your kidneys cannot perform their natural functions to support life. Unfortunately once the damage is done the scarring is irreversible. This is why emphasis on prevention through diet is so important. Preventing vascular disease and occlusion of blood vessels is the most effective treatment and prevention of kidney disease. It is also the most effective treatment and prevention for heart disease, stroke, high blood pressure, and diabetes.

We are born with 2 kidneys located in the middle of your back on either side of the spine. Each kidney is about the size of your fist. The kidneys are vascular organs that receive blood from the heart. The kidneys' basic function is to clean the blood and remove excess water and waste, which is excreted as urine. The kidneys also play a role in producing Vitamin D, important to calcium absorption, as well as the hormone that regulates red blood cell production. Kidney Disease and Renal Failure is the loss of the kidneys ability to adequately perform these critical functions. Most kidney diseases destroy both kidneys simultaneously and the damage can occur slowly over many years. As the process is usually asymptomatic, most people do not know they have kidney disease.

How Does Kidney Disease Develop?

We can think of the blood vessels in the body and our kidneys as a plumbing system. As the pipes get clogged, the flow of water through the pipes gets disrupted. This may result in a decrease in water pressure or even a leak that requires re-piping. Diseases like diabetes mellitus, high blood pressure, high cholesterol, obesity, and injury from tobacco products affect our bodies plumbing system causing blood vessels to get clogged and injured. Over time, if these diseases are not treated, the blood vessels going to our vital organs (brain, heart, and kidneys) get occluded and damage the organ they are supplying blood. Therefore, to protect our kidney from damage and to prevent further loss of kidney function we must control blood pressure, control blood sugar (if you have diabetes mellitus), avoid obesity, control blood cholesterol, avoid kidney toxins, and stop smoking.

There are 2 dietary issues when you look at kidneys, one in purveying the injury and the other is ensuring no further injury. Today, the standard Western Diet consists of animal-based and processed foods that are high in sugar, salt, and endothelial cell toxins. Red meat consumption is the main issue. The initial injury mainly comes from L-Carnitine found in red meat. L-Carnitine produces trimethylamine-*N*-oxide (TMAO), which promotes atherosclerosis.[1] Cholesterol then promotes the injury as it tries to heal the endothelial cells by "patching" up the arteries. Omnivorous human subjects were found to produce more TMAO than did vegans or vegetarians following ingestion of L-carnitine. Similarly, studies indicate polyphenols found in vegetables might have a role in the prevention of several chronic diseases.[2] Researchers found that polyphenols were is an independent risk factor for mortality and concluded that high dietary intake of polyphenols may be associated with longevity.

As kidney function is lost through vascular cell injury the kidneys lose the ability to excrete phosphorus and acid. Meat (made up of amino acids) and dairy products (containing large amounts of animal protein and phosphorus) can overwhelm the kidneys ability to maintain a healthy acid base balance. To buffer the acid in our bodies, the bones will release calcium and phosphorus. In kidney disease, elevated levels of phosphorus can cause additional injury to blood vessels and remaining kidney cells. In order to neutralize the acid, your body pulls the calcium from the bone as a buffer. As renal failure patients cannot excrete acid, this increases the risk of renal osteodystrophy.

A plant-based diet can be preventative because it does not contain toxins that damage the endothelial layer, it is lower in salt, leading to lower blood pressure, and lower in sugar. In 2013, researchers found mortality rates for diabetes and renal disease were significantly lower for vegetarians than non-vegetarians.[3] This data strongly suggests that individuals at risk for renal disease would benefit significantly from a whole food plant based diet. My hope for the future is that by educating our patients about the benefits of whole food plant based diet we will be able to make health more affordable, prevent preventable disease, and substantially improve patient lives.

The views expressed here are those of the author and do not represent the official views of his employers.

Phillip Tuso, MD, *is the Kaiser Permanente Care Management Institute National Physician Lead for Total Health and the Southern California Permanente Medical Group Physician Lead for Complete Care. He is a board certified Nephrologist and Fellow of the American College of Physicians. Dr. Tuso has authored more than 40 scientific publications as well 4 books for lay readers. Dr. Tuso is a co-founder of the Foundation to Improve Nutrition a non-profit organization, and has received many honors for his community service. Dr. Tuso has been married for over 30 years and has 4 children. In his spare time he enjoys running half marathons and volunteering at his local church.*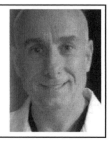

Real People ~ Real Food ~ Real Results

Kerrie Saunders, MS, LLP, PhD

At the age of 35, Ross was literally in a fight for his life. He had been diagnosed with a Stage III kidney disease called Focal Segmental Glomerulosclerosis (FSGS), placing him at risk for a kidney transplant, or possible premature death.

In normal functioning kidneys, millions of tiny glomeruli filters process about 200 quarts of blood, sorting out 2 quarts of waste products and water to be excreted as urine every single day. In FSGS, sections of the glomeruli filters become rigid or sclerotic, with lesions and scarring rendering them unable to sort excess proteins and toxins, which then build up in the bloodstream. FSGS, confirmed via kidney biopsy, typically also presents with hypertension and excessive fluid retention.

When Ross and I began working, he had high cholesterol, high blood pressure, and years of lab levels indicating chronic kidney failure. Ross had reduced his alcohol intake to zero, and he had stopped smoking. A well-planned, whole food, plant-based diet was the clear choice for us to help preserve and protect his kidney function. Moving to a plant-based diet and protein sources (i.e. beans, peas, lentils, sprouts, quinoa), naturally achieves a zero cholesterol and increased fiber and nutrient intake. The zero cholesterol, higher quality and easier protein load necessary for organ support are key benefits of a vegan diet. Vegan diets are also typically superior in nutrient density over the Standard American Diet (SAD), making it desirable for optimal performance and disease prevention. However, with FSGS, potassium, phosphorous, sodium (and even water intake at times) require close monitoring. Although potassium can be specifically recommended to help stabilize blood pressure, potassium can also reach a life-threatening toxicity in the presence of FSGS.

Working as part of his integrated team, my goal was to shorten his list of supplements, medications, vitamins, minerals and Chinese herbs as much as possible, in an effort to lessen any unnecessary burden on his liver and kidneys. Ross' physician-approved nutritional strategy:

- A whole food, plant-based diet
- 40+ grams of fiber per day, & 55-70 grams of plant based protein per day
- Zero intake of nicotine, non-prescription drugs, alcohol, trans fats, animal products, soda pop
- Zero intake of his identified Serum IgG food allergens
- Monitored potassium (Under 1 cup total daily of: edamame, durian, tomato paste,

apricots, beet greens, noor dates, chia seeds, quinoa, parsley, radish, chives, peppers, melon, rhubarb, papaya, lemon, guava)
- Monitored phosphorous (Under 1 cup total daily of: chia seeds, chives, rice bran, quinoa, soy, peanuts, oat bran, rye, squash seeds, sunflower seeds)
- Closely monitored sodium intake
- Low to moderate fat intake
- Daily omega-3 from a list of varied sources

Although this program may look daunting at first glance, we designed a lifestyle Ross found exciting and delicious, from the amazing variety of available plant foods.

The real test came when Ross saw Dr. Jeffrey Kopp, MD, a globally-known expert on FSGS from Cornell University, now working at the National Institutes of Health. An overview of Ross's lab values since the beginning of the year included normal values of sodium, potassium, chloride, glucose, albumin, and BUN. Further, his creatinine was at 1.9 mg/dl (down from 2.4), and his total cholesterol was at 155 mg/dl (down from 340). His urine protein was at 1100 mg/day (down from 4000), and just 5 months after his meeting, his urine protein had dropped to 570 mg/day. Ross's commitment to his health translated to remarkable results, and he was successfully staving off the need and criteria for a kidney transplant.

Dr. Kopp approved of the nutrition plan and stated he had tried to get others with kidney disease to eat a similar low protein, sodium, potassium and phosphorous nutritional model, but without much compliance. I believe that compliance would increase if the protein sources in the study were solely from plants (rather than animal), essentially offering patients a wider variety of foods for patients to choose from.

Although every situation is unique, it is my hope that Ross's story inspires others to celebrate food, fitness and other therapeutic lifestyle changes, as part of their own integrated medical and wellness approach.

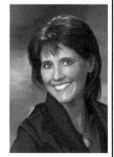

Dr. Kerrie Saunders, MS, LLP, PhD *is an internationally known presenter and bestselling author of The Vegan Diet as Chronic Disease Prevention. Dr. Saunders also co-stars with Ellen Degeneres' fitness trainer, John Pierre in their Food Demo DVD series, When Bachelor Meets Homemaker. Dr. Saunder's work is featured numerous newspapers, books and magazines, including her "Dear Dr. Kerrie," advice column for VegNews Magazine. Dr. Saunders has worked in both diabetes and cancer prevention for the Physicians Committee for Responsible Medicine. She lectures frequently for hospitals and universities, and is the Coordinator of the Michigan Firefighter Challenge. Dr. Saunders earned her Doctoral degree in Natural Health after post-graduate coursework at the University of Michigan, Miami University and Clayton College. You can find more on her work at www.DrFood.org*

Skip the Emergency Room Lines

Lino Guedes Pires, MD

Eating animal protein contributes to the most prevalent diseases I face in the emergency room which include: acute gastroenteritis, diarrhea, indigestion, irritable bowel syndrome and allergic colitis. These diseases are the starting point to more serious illnesses such as acute abdomen, appendicitis, diverticular disease and even cancer. Many, many people come to me due to horrible abdominal cramping because they ate meat, fish, eggs, or poultry. Such sources of protein can generate terrible cramps and pain.

Many of our most common problems begin within our guts. While most people think we need to get our protein from animal sources, the best sources of protein actually come from our own digestive system. Articles indicate that the bacteria in our guts can be divided into fermentative and putrefactive.[1] Fermentative and putrefactive bacteria do not mix well together. When you eat a piece of meat, poultry, fish or eggs it causes putrefaction and putrefactive bacteria growth. This bacterium kills the fermentative ones which arise thanks to carbohydrates of vegetables, similar to what happens when we produce beer or wine. When we eat whole or plant- based foods such as green leaves, cereals, fruits and roots, the fermentative bacteria will die. When the bacteria dies it releases within our intestines and produces amino acids that we need to build our own individual proteins. Unfortunately, not many patients know this information and therefore suffer from common gastrointestinal issues, such as diarrhea up to the most devastating forms of cancer. While diarrhea doesn't seem serious to most, if it is not treated correctly with water and salts, people do not recover properly and anti-spasmodic drugs have to be prescribed. Simple problems such as diarrhea can then turn into nightmares.

Another common emergency room condition related to diet is kidney stones. Kidney stones are an extremely painful condition that is generally due to lack of water and magnesium in the diet. Magnesium is the mineral that gives vegetables their green color and is often an overlooked mineral by many doctors. Magnesium plays a vital role in our metabolism, prevents calcium from being lost in our urine, and helps fix calcium to our bones. Magnesium is also responsible in the formation of Adenosine Triphosphate or ATP, the molecule that releases energy in our cells. Without magnesium we have little or no energy which detracts from our ability to solve problems. Processed foods and fast foods in general significantly lack micronutrients and magnesium. Yet this is what most people consume. When we go to the grocery store we need to be cognizant of products that are falsely advertised as being healthy for us. So many foods today are created to appeal to our sugar, fat, protein, and salt cravings but these processed products do not contain the micronutrients we need. **We can avoid many of these common emergency room afflictions by simply eating a diet rich in unprocessed starch and completely void of animal protein.**

The problem with the current healthcare system and prevalence of illnesses commonly treated with antibiotics like the gastrointestinal problems mentioned above, is that we are reaching the end of the antibiotic era. It is common sense that within 20 years, our present antibiotics will no longer be effective against common bacteria. Since the probability of new antibiotics being developed in time due to cost and regulations is low, it seems we will be facing a whole new set of problems. A whole foods, plant-based diet can significantly aid in fighting infections as well as an understanding of how to hydrate, how to make use of herbs, what foods to avoid, acupuncture and daily exercise, items present in age old medicine from India and China. The problem is there is no money in prevention or nutrition.

Each of us has the power to improve our behavior, diet and implement preventative measures. Look inside and give yourself the freedom to improve yourself and habits and in doing so you are giving yourself the right to lead a happy life and be a source of inspiration to others.

Lino Guedes Pires, MD *is an emergency room physician practicing in Brazil. Dr. Pires received his medical degree from UFRJ (Universidade Federal do Rio de Janeiro) and currently works at 2 hospitals in Rio de Janeiro.*

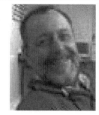

A Plant-Based Diet to Soothe the Stomach

Ira Michaelson, MD

I never set out to become a vegan doctor. I ate meat and chicken on a daily basis and had ice cream several times a week. My idea of a good Saturday-night snack was pizza, French fries, or onion rings. However, about 6 years ago I was overweight, out of shape, and I wanted to do something about it. Although I knew I should be eating less and exercising more, I wasn't getting anywhere. Several of my physician colleagues were in a similar predicament. Over a period of 2 years, 10 of my colleagues suffered major coronary events, including heart attacks, coronary bypass surgeries, and stents. A few of them died.

When my colleague Jerry, a picture of fitness and health, had emergency coronary bypass surgery, I became even more motivated to change. Apparently, he had never paid much attention to diet and his cholesterol had been high for years. He suffered a fate similar to his father's. My own father, also a physician, had died from a sudden myocardial infarction at the young age of 55, and I was sure it would only be a matter of time until it would happen to me.

As I researched my options, I came across the renowned Dr. Caldwell Esselstyn Jr. at the Cleveland Clinic, and was amazed by his program for reversing coronary artery disease through a whole food, plant-based diet. Over a period of time, I adopted a plant-based lifestyle and shared it with many of my patients to help with their various conditions. Several of my patients have been able to reverse their type 2 diabetes and come off medication, as well as ameliorate their gastrointestinal conditions.

If we look at societies where chronic conditions like coronary artery disease, type 2 diabetes, and obesity are rare and compare them to America in the last few decades, a common thread arises. Our highly processed, high-fat diet is clearly playing a big role. Where chronic diseases are rare (evidenced in rural China, Northwestern Mexico Tarahumara Indians, and the Papau, New Guinea Highlanders), diets are low in cholesterol and saturated fat, the building blocks of chronic conditions. The plant-based diet free of cholesterol, low in saturated fat and high in fiber, prevents these conditions from developing and in some cases, can arrest and reverse them.

As a practicing gastroenterologist, I frequently see conditions such as acid reflux esophagitis, Barrett's esophagus, fatty liver, diverticulosis, and peptic ulcer disease that are often due to poor dietary habits. Let's take acid reflux disease, diverticulosis, and fatty liver as examples.

Acid Reflux Disease, according to some estimates, affects about 1 in 4 Americans. Acid reflux happens when acid comes up into the esophagus or swallowing tube where it doesn't belong. Reflux requires two basic components: excess stomach acid and abnormal relaxation of the sphincter muscle of the esophagus (a one-way valve when it is working.) Common symptoms include heartburn, nausea, and pain in the abdomen or chest even by coughing or wheezing.

All too often, patients are just given medication to limit acid production. Acid-blocking medications, such as Tagamet and Zantac, and the newer proton pump inhibitors (Prilosec), generate billions in sales every year.[1] These acid blockers have significant side effects. The proton pump inhibitors such as Prilosic have been known to interfere with medications like Plavix, taken to keep coronary stents open. Prilosec can cause the Plavix to be less active; resulting in occlusion of the stents and heart attacks.[2] A new study from Methodist Hospital in Houston[3] found that the proton pump inhibitors may increase the risk of major adverse cardiovascular events. This is because the proton pump inhibitors increase the amount of ADA (asymmetric dimethyl arginine), a chemical known to inhibit the amount of nitric oxide, a major vasodilator in the body. It makes sense to do everything we can to treat reflux with as little medication as possible, to avoid these side effects. Also, I often see patients unresponsive to medications. When medications produce little relief, it is often because the patient is continuing to eat a highly acidic diet.

Meat and dairy products are not only high in fat but also are highly acidic—adding to acid production in the body. By following a lean plant-based diet, there is less stimulation of the acid-making (parietal) cells in the stomach. This in turn means there is less acid available for reflux. Many of my patients have been able to eliminate the need for medication altogether by following a largely plant-based diet.

Calm Your Stomach's Irritability

Irritable bowel Syndrome (IBS) is an all too common condition with many manifestations, including diarrhea, constipation, abdominal pain, and bloating. IBS can be ameliorated by avoiding dairy and removing sweets and other carbohydrates, in the form of cookies, candies, and soda. A high fiber, plant-based diet sets patients on the road to recovery.

Diverticulosis is a common condition marked by the presence of pouches or diverticula in the bowel. It is accompanied by various symptoms including pain, infection, and sometimes diarrhea. Acute diverticulitis can be manifested by nausea, vomiting, and fever, which can require the patient to be hospitalized and treated with intravenous antibiotics. It may sometimes progress to perforation or a hole in the bowel, which requires surgery.

The development of diverticulosis is related to insufficient dietary fiber.[4] Foods rich in fiber include vegetables, fruits, whole grain breads, pastas and rice, as well as beans (legumes).[5] Meat and dairy contain absolutely zero fiber and yet make up most of what people consume today. It's interesting that in the 1950s and the 1960s this condition was seen only in patients 60 years of age and older. In more recent years, with the adoption of a high-fat, low-fiber diet, diverticulosis is now seen in much younger patients not only in their 40's and 30's, but even patients in their 20's. Treatment includes implementing a high-fiber diet and avoiding refined foods as well as meat and dairy products. I highly recommend green vegetables such as spinach, broccoli, and kale. A plant-based high fiber treatment impedes diverticulitis from recurring and eliminates the need for antibiotics and hospitalization.

Fatty Liver now affects about 1 in 3 Americans today.[6] When I started out in practice more than 30 years ago I never heard of or saw this problem. Now I see it multiple times a day in patients who also have diabetes, obesity, elevated cholesterol, and heart disease. Fatty liver occurs when fat slowly accumulates in the liver over a period of time, and is an insidious problem. Left untreated, it may silently progress to chronic inflammation, which can lead to cirrhosis or severe scarring of the liver. Cirrhosis is very serious and shortens a person's life expectancy by several decades.

The onset of fatty liver develops in conjunction with diabetes and insulin resistance, and is associated with a high-fat diet rich in meat and dairy products.[7] In particular, the consumption of processed foods, which includes high fructose corn syrup (HFCS), plays an important role. HFCS has many names—high fructose corn syrup, corn sugar, crystalline fructose, corn syrup. It is found in everything from soda to cotton candy, soft and hard candies, cookies, breakfast cereals, yogurt, and health food bars. HFCS causes fat to accumulate and is reported to be contaminated with mercury.[8-10] It has been associated with gout, progression of chronic kidney disease, and it may promote colon, breast, and pancreatic cancer growth.[11-15] By eliminating processed foods as well as meat and dairy foods from their diet, a number of my patients have successfully reversed their fatty liver on a plant-based diet.

The Way Forward

As a nation, we are now struggling with health problems. According to estimates, all males over 60 and all females over 70 have coronary artery disease whether symptomatic or not.[16] Because more drugs and procedures will never cure these diseases, we should be looking into prevention and reversal. We are currently devoting 15% of the gross national product to healthcare.[16] Does it look like more of the same will work?

As practicing physicians, it is our duty to relieve suffering by any means possible and that means we must not limit ourselves to drugs and surgery. We should have the courage to tell our patients that their nutrition is a contributing cause of their illness. By taking away the building blocks of chronic disease—animal fats and proteins, unnatural sugars (high fructose corn syrup), and excess salt—we can prevent and reverse many of the conditions that plague our society and begin to live healthier lives. Our patients want to get better and we can empower them to do so. If there is an alternative that it is more powerful than drugs and surgery, what are we waiting for?

Ira Michaelson, MD, *is a board certified gastroenterologist practicing at Mystic Gastroenterology in Medford Massachusetts. Dr. Michaelson is the proud husband of Shari and father of four fantastic children. Recently at his daughter's wedding the entire reception for 250 people was plant-based.*

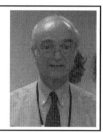

Stop the Burn: A Dietary Answer to Acid Reflux

Adam Weinstein, D.O.

Ever experience a squeezing or burning in your chest or back after a meal? Most of us have experienced GERD (Gastro-Esophageal Reflux Disease), known as acid reflux at some point. Reflux is one of the most common complaints seen in a general practice and gastroenterology offices every day and costs over $10 billion dollars on medication annually. Almost half of the adult population in the U.S. reports suffering from heartburn or reflux.

The symptoms of reflux occur when the acidic stomach contents pass backwards up into the esophagus, throat and mouth. This may or may not be accompanied by vomiting. This is NOT how it was designed to happen. Normally, the valve separating the stomach and esophagus (the lower esophageal sphincter a.k.a. LES) prevents the acidic stomach contents from flowing backwards.

In most cases, acid reflux is a self-inflicted disease. That's right; it is a disease, not just a symptom because it has several serious long-term consequences. GERD may lead to esophagitis (inflammation and bleeding of the swallowing tube). As your body tries to repair the esophagitis, the result can be a stricture of the esophagus (narrowing of the swallowing tube), often necessitating an invasive procedure to open up the stricture. Barrett's Esophagus, which is a pre-cancerous transformation of the esophageal lining, often leads to cancer of the esophagus.

Acid refluxing into the throat may result in laryngitis (hoarseness), cough, sore throat or asthma. Long term refluxing into the throat and lungs can lead to pneumonitis and fibrosis of the lungs resulting in permanent lung damage. It is powerful to think that one digestive problem can lead to so many chronic long-term symptoms and complications.

There are substantial economic and medical consequences associated with the "gold standard" therapy, acid blocking medications such as PPIs (proton pump inhibitors ex: Nexium, Prevacid and Prilosec) and H2 blockers (Pepcid and Zantac). Patients spent $6.3 billion dollars on Nexium alone in 2011. The cost of Nexium and other PPIs is not limited to financial cost. The FDA has issued multiple warnings regarding the health consequences of chronically using these medications which include:

- reduced absorption of vitamin B12 and iron leading to anemia (ironically B12 deficiency is one of the carnivores most frequent arguments against plant based diets)

- reduced absorption of calcium leading to osteoporosis (again, one of the chief arguments levied against those that follow a plant based diet is "where do you get calcium if you don't drink milk")
- reduced effectiveness of blood thinners like Plavix which are used to treat cardiovascular disease (cardiovascular disease is strongly linked to meat and dairy consumption)

The majority of GERD cases are food related, as discomfort after eating is the frequent symptom. Although in some cases certain diseases can cause reflux, our lifestyle choices such as smoking, alcohol, caffeine and fatty foods such as meats and dairy are more associated with reflux occurrence. Studies in the U.S. and Asia correlate increased symptoms with increased meat in the diet. Additionally, diets high in meat and dairy are directly linked to obesity, which is an independent risk factor for reflux as worldwide studies throughout link obesity with increased chances of GERD. Diets high in fruits, vegetables, grains and legumes is associated with lower obesity rates and a decreased risk of reflux.

Three major food related causes of GERD are 1) obesity 2) saturated fat and 3) dairy intolerance/lactose intolerance -which does not cause GERD but is frequently mistaken for GERD. This leads to unnecessary medications and testing when it doesn't even exist.

Obesity causes GERD both directly and indirectly. Diets high in animal protein are directly linked to obesity. Various studies confirm that higher BMI (Body Mass Index) correlates with higher rates of GERD, and lower BMI correlates with less GERD. The mechanisms in which obesity predisposes to GERD are three fold. There is diminished lower esophageal sphincter pressure, leading to backflow of acid into the esophagus. Increased development of hiatal hernias leads to lower esophageal sphincter malfunction, and increased intra-gastric pressure forcing acid backwards through the lower esophageal sphincter. Science confirms that those that eat primarily

Case Study: Eliminating GERD with Diet

E.S. was a 39-year-old man with no medical history other than being overweight. His reason for visiting was listed on his new patient questionnaire: cough, chest pain, and heartburn. His problem was GERD brought on by diet. E.S. was a self-proclaimed "meat and potatoes" man. I explained that if he ate smaller portions in general, minimized processed food, eliminated dairy and followed a plant based diet, I was confident he would a) not have GERD anymore; b) feel better overall; c) lose weight; and d) minimize his risk of chronic diseases and cancer in his life. Six weeks later, E.S. returned 12 pounds lighter with a big smile on his face. He had been faithful to my instructions and did not have one single episode of cough, chest pain or heartburn associated with food since his first visit. All of this was accomplished without any over the counter or prescription medications.

plant-based diets (vegetarians and vegans) are less likely to be obese. Therefore, by following a plant-based diet, you can achieve a significantly lower BMI leading to less GERD.

Saturated fat is found in copious amounts in dairy, eggs and all fatty meats. There are very few plant sources of saturated fat (coconut milk, coconut oil, palm oil) and they are not common elements of most plant-based diets. Several recent studies draw a direct correlation between these saturated fats found mostly in dairy, eggs and meat with the symptoms and complications of GERD.[1-5] Saturated fats cause the lower esophageal sphincter to be dysfunctional, allowing acid to backflow into the esophagus. Many people can instantly improve or eliminate GERD by removing the meat, dairy, and eggs from your diet.

Lastly but importantly, dairy/lactose intolerance can mimic and exacerbate GERD. The bloating, heartburn, and belching associated with each disease process can be indistinguishable. The human body in many cases is incapable of digesting lactose, one of the sugars found in all dairy. When the body cannot digest lactose it proceeds into the intestines where the normal bacterial flora begins to dine on the sugar, leading to the production of voluminous intra-abdominal gas. This distends the intestine and can cause the inability of the lower esophageal sphincter to completely close, leading to GERD once again. However, the inability to digest the dairy/lactose often leads to gastrointestinal discomfort not due to GERD, but often mistaken for it. Removal of dairy from the diet can immediately resolve many digestive issues mistaken for or related to GERD.

Fortunately, the medical and scientific community have gathered enough evidence supporting the health of plant-based diets, that in 2009 the American Dietetic Association declared, "It is the position of the American Dietetic Association that appropriately planned vegetarian diets, including total vegetarian or vegan diets, are healthful, nutritionally adequate and may provide health benefits in the PREVENTION and TREATMENT of certain diseases..."[6] If we all follow a plant-based diet, there will be increased health, decreased healthcare costs, much less GERD.

Adam Weinstein, D.O., *attended Baylor College of Medicine. Dr. Weinstein is a Board Certified Internist taking care of patients and teaching medical students at the University of Texas Health Science Center in Houston, TX. Dr. Weinstein combines the latest in modern medicine with traditional values, providing patients with optimal personalized healthcare and promoting wellness and longevity with an emphasis on diet and nutrition.*

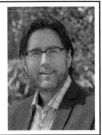

What Can Diet Do For Inflammatory Bowel Disease?

Lilli Link, MD, MS

Do you find yourself sitting doubled over on the toilet thinking, "Why me?" On the surface, the question might seem like mere self-pity, but it's actually a great question. Understanding why this is happening to you will give you a better idea of how to stop it. Perhaps you've heard that Inflammatory Bowel Disease (IBD) is an autoimmune disease where the body's own immune system attacks itself and the reason is not really known. Yet recent studies offer insight into why people develop IBD and there are even some studies that shed light on what *you* can do about it.

Inflammatory bowel disease is just that – an inflammation of the bowel. It happens when the immune system's white blood cells are mistakenly called to attack some area(s) of the GI track. IBD refers mainly to Crohn's disease and ulcerative colitis. (This is not to be confused with Irritable Bowel Syndrome (IBS) – they are not the same disease.) In both Crohn's disease and ulcerative colitis, there is inflammation of the gastrointestinal tract causing symptoms such as abdominal cramping, bloating, diarrhea, and the passing of blood and mucous. The simplest distinction is that Crohn's disease can occur anywhere along the digestive tract, from the mouth to the anus, while ulcerative colitis occurs only in the large intestines.

These diseases occur in the greatest numbers in the most developed areas, specifically northern Europe, the United Kingdom and North America. There are about 1.4 million cases of IBD in the US. Until recently, IBD was rare in less industrialized regions, like southern and central Europe, Asia, Africa and Latin America. As these places have become more

Six Factors Associated with IBD:

1. Smoking: While it increases the risk for Crohn's disease, it curiously and for unclear reasons, decreases the risk for ulcerative colitis.

2. Antibiotics: It is associated with an increased risk for both Crohn's disease and ulcerative colitis, presumably because it changes the balance of microbes in our GI tracts.

3. NSAIDS, such as ibuprofen, make the GI tract more porous and easier for large proteins to leak through.[1]

4. Hormones (i.e., estrogen and progesterone) may increase IBD risk.[2]

5. GI infections, like salmonella, can increase risk.[3]

6. Diet: Inflammatory foods effect and influence the types of microbes living in the gut.

westernized the incidence of ulcerative colitis and Crohn's disease have started to rise.[4]

When looking at the incidence of disease within families, only 10% of IBD patients have a family history of the disease. Identical twins are born with the same DNA, so if genetics were the only factor in determining who develops IBD, both twins would either have, or not have, the disease. Among identical twins, only 10-20% has ulcerative colitis and 50-60% has Crohn's disease in both siblings.[5] Clearly there are significant non-genetic factors at play.

Go With Your Gut

There are an estimated 100 trillion bacteria in each of our GI tracts. That is 10 times more cells than we have in our entire body! Bacteria make up the vast majority of the organisms in the gut, but viruses, fungi, phage (viruses that live inside bacteria), archaea (a relatively recently discovered type of microbe) and parasites also contribute to the make-up of the gut microbiome.[6] These microbes begin inhabiting our bodies as we exit the uterus at birth and different factors influence our microbiome. For instance, breast feeding contributes different microbes compared with bottle-feeding. The microorganisms in the body are affected, for better or for worse, by all types of foods, antibiotics, probiotics and hygiene. One study which changed healthy participant's diets to either a low-fiber/high-fat diet or low-fat/high-fiber diet found that within one day of altering their diets, their gut microbiomes began to change.

A key part of developing IBD revolves around the gut microbiome. Our bodies have not only learned to live with these microbes, we've also come to rely on them for good health. They help with digestion, produce vitamin K, regulate the turnover of cells that line the intestines, assist in keeping the intestines from becoming 'leaky' or porous, and help our immune systems develop and protect us from pathogens (disease-causing organisms).[7,8]

As unhealthy bugs overpopulate it, the lining of the intestines becomes porous and can no longer effectively protect the barrier between the gut and blood stream. Large proteins and microorganisms leak through into the blood stream setting off an immune response to these 'invaders.' This is an important step in the development of autoimmune diseases. Although the interplay between the gut microbiome and the development of IBD isn't completely worked out, the evidence supports a strong and direct connection. For example, IBD occurs most often in the small and large intestines,

> **A Healthy Gut**
>
> *Ruediger Dahlke, MD,*
> *author of "Peace Food",*
> *Germany*
>
> Scientific studies find that animal protein and fat can wreck havoc on the immune system. Probiotics from vegetables and fruits can return the gut to a healthy balance, which plays a direct role in a properly functioning and responsive immune system.

the areas of the GI tract with the most microbes. Also, people with IBD have different types and amounts of microbes compared to those with healthy GI tracts.[9]

Diet's Role in IBD

Epidemiologic studies of dietary changes show that avoiding red meat, processed meat, dairy, and simple carbohydrates is linked to a decreased risk for IBD. These foods affect inflammation in the gut and impact the microbiome. For instance, in 2010, a large study spanning 10 years and including more than 67,000 middle-aged French women, found that those women who ate the most animal protein (i.e. red meat, poultry, fish, dairy and eggs) were about 3 times more likely to develop ulcerative colitis or Crohn's disease compared with the women who ate the least amount of animal protein. Eating vegetable protein was not related to IBD risk.[10]

Additionally a study of children found that the girls who ate a diet high in meat, fatty foods, and desserts had higher incidences of Crohn's disease, while boys and girls who ate vegetables, fruits, olive oil, fish, grains, and nuts were less likely to get IBD.[11] A study of Japanese adults who ate bread for breakfast, butter, margarine, cheese, meat, ham and sausage also had a higher risk for developing ulcerative colitis.[12] Additionally one study followed 191 patients who were in remission for ulcerative colitis to determine which foods were associated with a relapse.[13] The worst offenders were meat, particularly red and processed meat, eggs, and alcohol.

Meat, in particular, has a number of attributes that make it unhealthy for intestinal health including heme irone, which is pro-oxidants (the opposite of anti-oxidants); and high in omega-6 fatty acids which increase inflammation, make the intestines more porous, and allow unwanted molecules to enter the blood stream. Meat contains large amounts of the bacteria, *Yersinia*, which may, independently contribute to the development of Crohn's disease. Meat can also be tainted with antibiotics often used in its production which will alter the intestinal microbiome.

Most types of fat, except DHA, a type of omega-3 fatty acid found in fish and some algae, show an increased risk of IBD. The two studies that looked at DHA both showed it decreased risk for ulcerative colitis.[14] However, another study of omega-3 supplements (including DHA) did not prove helpful.[15] Other contributors to IBD include dairy and gluten. Like any food that is not well-digested, it has the opportunity to ferment in the GI tract and contribute to the imbalance of microbes.[16]

By contrast, fruits are generally associated with a decreased risk of Crohn's disease, and studies of vegetables suggest they are protective against ulcerative colitis.[17] The theory behind why they could help avoid developing IBD is because bacteria in the colon ferment fiber, which forms short-chain fatty acids. One short-chain fatty acid in particular, butyrate, is known to reduce inflammation in the gut, as do the many anti-oxidants in fiber-rich foods. These short-chain fatty acids improve the balance of beneficial and harmful organisms in the gut. They also contain healthy phytochemicals, like flavonoids, which help keep the intestines' cells tightly connected so harmful bacteria and food do not pass through into the blood stream.[18]

There is still much research to be done to find a clear answer for IBD patients. Research endeavors such as the Human Microbiome Project of the National Institute of Health, which attempts to identify all of the different microbes in the gut as well as other parts of the body and determine their genetic coding, could help elucidate which combinations of organisms are ideal and perhaps help determine a cure for IBD in the future. In the meantime, paying attention to what you eat can make a world of difference.

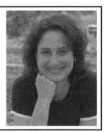

Lilli B. Link, MD, MS, *is a board-certified internist currently practicing as a nutrition specialist in New York City. She has Masters of Science degree in epidemiology and health services research. Dr. Link uses an integrative approach to nutrition and lifestyle modification to help people with chronic diseases and those who want to lose weight.*

Push Constipation Away

Eric Slywitch, MD

What Causes Constipation?

Constipation is a change in the bowel habits that results in decreasing the number of bowel movements and changes in the consistency of our waste. While some diseases and medication can lead to constipation, the most common causes are improper habits, such as nutritional habits. The simplest and most efficient way to eliminate constipation is the adoption of a vegan diet composed exclusively of natural foods and whole grains.

When you put food in your mouth, the digestive process begins. This food travels through the entire 9 meter digestive tract composed of 25 cm of the esophagus, 25 cm of the stomach, 7 meters of the small intestines (important point for the absorption of nutrients) and 1.5 meters of the large intestine.

The large intestines are important because this is where our waste is formed to eliminate toxins from our body. The large intestines are a powerful place for de-watering the material that is inside it. The large intestines are capable of absorbing 5 to 7 liters of water per day. The longer a person does not evacuate, the more water is extracted from the stool. With this, the content becomes dried and hardened. Thus, the decrease in stool volume makes for a greater effort to go to the bathroom, leading to constipation.

Implement Healthy Habits

1) **Move:** Physical activity is very important to strengthen the abdominal muscles and activate peristalsis (bowel movement). This is why bedridden elderly people tend to be constipated.

2) **Drink Water:** Hydration is key factor as the large intestines remove water from the feces. With lower liquid intake, more water is drawn from the stool and it becomes dry. Hydration can be in the form of water, juice or tea.

3) **Eat Fiber:** Fiber intake is essential for proper bowel function because bacteria in our gut use fiber to create glucose that slows fluid loss. This means stools are larger, moister and softer. In comparison to animal products which has zero fiber,

fruits and vegetables are high in fiber. Specifically, black plums (fresh, dried, or in juice form) contain an acid called dihydroxifinil isotina, which stimulates bowel movement. The most effective grains to use are, the whole rye and barley, because they have 5 times more fiber than brown rice.   The rule is simple: use what is natural and whole. Remove whatever is refined and processed. Refined foods, which are present in many foods, are poor choices for those who have constipation.

4) **Keep your Gut Healthy:** Healthy bacteria in the gut keep the body as whole healthy. Compounds found in plant origin such as inulin, are important for the beneficial bacteria in the gut to remain in good quantity. Foods such as endive, leeks, artichokes and green banana (cooked or in the form of flour) are great for providing this compound.

Please read Dr. Slywitch's "Insulin Resistance as a Source of Chronic Diseases" in Diabetes chapter, You Deceive Me

The Spark of Life: A Proper Sodium-Potassium Ratio Can Change Your Life

Thomas Sult, MD

first met Kaitlyn in my office when she was 24 years old. She had extreme exhaustion, irritable bowel syndrome (IBS), and multiple joint and muscle pains. In high school, Kaitlyn had been a star player on the girls' basketball team. She'd had endless energy, been a straight-A student, and in college she continued her academic and athletic career, studying and playing basketball all 4 years. When she started to feel tired during her sophomore year, she attributed this to her heavy basketball and academic schedule, but over the years, her energy levels never improved. In fact, they slowly got worse.

Unfortunately, it wasn't so easy to convince Kaitlyn that her diet was problematic. Throughout high school Kaitlyn said she had survived on cereal, jelly sandwiches, Ding Dongs, and Ho Hos. Even fortified flour is processed as fortification strips the fiber and many of the nutrients from wholesome, natural food, bleaches the food white, and then adds back a few vitamins. Now it's fortified!

Sugary foods and other sources of simple carbohydrates, generally packed with sodium, do not have the nutrition needed for digestion from natural wholesome foods, packed with potassium, so the body must draw upon its nutrition stores to digest them. By doing a urine test to measure sodium and potassium, we can get a sense of the balance of unhealthy and healthy foods. A healthy person typically has between 3 and 5 times more potassium than sodium, meaning that a healthy sodium-to-potassium ratio is between 1:3 and 1:5. Being closer to 1:5 is probably better. Kaitlyn's ratio was 1:1, meaning she was in an extremely depleted state.

Kaitlyn's body had depleted its stores of nutrients and couldn't make adequate amounts of neurotransmitters, resulting in depression, and Irritable Bowel Syndrome (IBS), since the same neurotransmitters that regulate mood also regulate your gut. She became unable to repair and maintain her muscle tissue, ligaments, and tendons, at which point she developed chronic muscle and joint pain. Finally, this depleted state resulted in the inefficient manufacture of adenosine triphosphate (ATP), the basic currency of energy used by every single cell of the body.

The Spark of Life

We are electric beings, and our "spark of life" is the *sodium-potassium ATPase pump.*

This pump is what creates the electrical potential across our cell membranes. The spark of life- which we would die without- is absolutely dependent on the balance of sodium and potassium in the body.

The body expends a tremendous amount of energy in the form of ATP in order to keep this electrical charge present across the cell membranes. It is this electrical charge that allows our neurons to fire and our muscles to contract. This "spark of life" also gives us the mental clarity and concentration we need, especially in our fast paced world today.

This "spark of life" is also imperative for every type of communication between cells in our body. The electrical gradient across the cell membrane is called the *action potential*, and it is required in every cell-to-cell communication event in your body. Action potentials are involved in hormone function, nerve function, muscle movement, detoxification, assimilation, and nearly every other activity of the body. When every type of communication event is being negatively affected by a skewed ratio that suppresses our spark of life, it hurts the communication between body and spirit. Probably not good things, right?

Kaitlyn is not alone in struggling with this compounding set of problems caused by imbalance. The crucial sodium-potassium ratio has been significantly thrown off in many of us by changes in the Western diet over the past fifty years, and it's causing widespread problems. Depletion of nutrients and interference with the spark of life can result in conditions as disparate as ADHD, anxiety, depression, IBS, heart-rhythm problems, and chronic fatigue.[1,2]

The solution, of course, is to get more nutrients. People often ask what nutrient they should take for a specific disease. What vitamin is best for depression? What herb is best for arthritis? However, it is the opposite question that is more useful: What nutrient do I need to be truly well? **Wellness is *not* the absence of disease; it is disease that is the absence of wellness. With vibrant wellness in place, disease cannot flourish.** Vibrant wellness comes from a balance between a person's lifestyle and genes. A plant-strong vegan who's a type-A workaholic will not be well for long. And a meditating monk on Kaitlyn's diet will not be well for long, either. It's all about balance.

Finding Balance and Achieving Wellness

Eating a plant-based diet is one of the best first steps you can take toward achieving balance, optimizing communication, and promoting wellness.

Let's take broccoli as an example to see some of the nutrients found in a single vegetable. Broccoli is a cruciferous vegetable rich in vitamins A and C, folic acid, and calcium. Vitamin A is essential for vision, gene transcription, skin health, and is an important antioxidant. Vitamin C is critical for the production of collagen, which is widely known for its ability to prevent wrinkles on your face and is used in multiple enzyme systems related to hydroxylation, helps form carnitine, a nutrient essential for converting fatty acids into energy, and it supports the immune system as a powerful antioxidant. Folic acid prevents neural tube defects in the fetus which prevents birth defects, is essential for the proper formation of sperm and can reduce the risk of heart disease and stroke by lowering homocysteine levels.[3] Proper amounts of it reduce the risk of metabolic syndrome in children.

More importantly, broccoli is a rich source of both soluble and insoluble fiber. Fiber performs three basic actions in our body: bulking, viscosity, and fermentation. The least understood and probably most important aspect of fiber is fermentation. The probiotic bacteria in our gut act on the indigestible fibers in our diet to form short-chain fatty acids (SCFA). These SCFA are an important source of energy (food) for enterocytes, the cells that line your gut and when absorbed they have anti-inflammatory and energy-producing properties.[4]

Short-chain fatty acids help keep the gut lining intact and prevent it from being "leaky." This is vital as 70% of the immune system exists in the lining of the gut. If the gut becomes leaky, abnormal interactions between the content of the gut lumen and the immune system occur which can result in food sensitivities, allergies, and even autoimmune diseases like autoimmune thyroiditis and arthritis.[5] Since bacteria, fungi, food particles, and other particles that live in the gut lumen have "coevolved" with us, in a healthy gut lining, these particles remain unseen because our immune system is protected by the intact gut lining. As the gut becomes leaky, these once unseen particles are more easily recognized by the immune system, which reacts by making antibodies against them. These antibodies can cross-react with our tissue, resulting in "auto-antibodies" or autoimmune disease.

Broccoli also contains phytonutrients- indoles and thiocyanates that are established to have potent anti-carcinogenic, antioxidant, and anti-atherogenic effects. I3C's anti-cancer effects appear to be related to its ability to improve the way estrogens are detoxified in the body. There are two major pathways to dispose of used estrogens, the 2-estrone pathway and the 16-OH-estrone pathwayI3C favors the 2-estrone pathway, resulting in fewer active metabolites, lower risk of cancer, and fewer symptoms associated with PMS.[6]

Sulforaphane, a thiocyanates phytonutrient, is derived from glucoraphanin in broccoli. Hundreds of scientific studies conducted on sulforaphane document its powerful antioxidant, detoxification, cellular metabolism, and cell-life regulation effects.[7] The antioxidant effect of sulforaphane is longer acting than antioxidant vitamins- lasting up to 72 hours. Sulforaphane activates several key detoxification enzyme systems and is crucial in maintaining a healthy gastrointestinal flora, which improves response to inflammation, and a healthier immune, eye, and cardiovascular system. Sulforaphane also inhibits abnormal DNA activation- promoting normal gene regulation and cytokine balance, which are body-made chemicals, that influence and balance inflammation and oxidative stress.

Just 3 months after adopting a plant-based diet, Kaitlyn was her old self again. Simply adjusting Kaitlyn's urine sodium to potassium ratio through a plant-based diet was enough to return this shell of a young woman to a state of vibrant wellbeing.

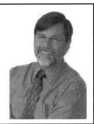

Thomas Sult, MD, *practices functional medicine in Willmar, Minnesota. His book, "Just Be Well", is available at all online retailers. Dr. Sult is on the faculty of the Institute for Functional Medicine, where he teaches the week long introductory class "Applying Functional Medicine in Clinical Practice" and the advanced module on gastrointestinal health. He is board certified in family medicine and in integrative holistic medicine. For more information visit: justbewell.info.*

thirteen

FOR WOMEN ONLY

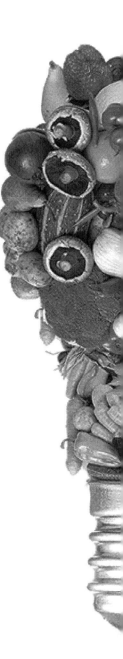

Ladies, whether we plan to get pregnant or not, our food choices significantly impact our reproductive organs and the health of our baby, both in and out of the womb. Maintaining hormonal balance is critical to women's health. Meat and dairy products, however, contain both natural and artificial hormones. Consuming a basket of hormones, especially from another species, disrupts our body's fine-tuned balance and can directly cause female cancers, fertility issues, menstrual cycle irregularity, and fibroid development, to name a few.

Food choices become even more important when "Moms To Be" are eating for two. Avoiding meat and dairy is just as important while pregnant to protect the growing baby from exposures to toxins and unneeded hormones. While most women avoid fish because of the potential harm to the unborn child from mercury poisoning, doesn't this indicate that fish consumption is harmful to everyone all the time? Toxins accumulate in the adipose or fatty tissue in animals and we ingest these toxins when we consume animal products. Remember, ladies, everything we eat, the baby eats. The rise in toxin levels, researchers are finding could be a leading contributor to the spike in developmental problems in children and the growing presence of autistic children.

As the following obstetricians indicate, plant-based diets provide the most nutritious foods for a growing baby, pregnant mother, and women's health.

The Importance of a Pregnant Mother's Nutrition

Chelsea M. Clinton, MD

The female body has the amazing ability to generate an approximately 7 ½ pound human out of very few supplies (i.e. egg and sperm). It is up to mom to provide the building blocks to do this. These building blocks can be provided by hot dog and sugar cravings or by thoughtful consumption of organic whole foods. Does it really make a difference?

Food Choices Can Affect Fertility

When a woman is contemplating pregnancy, she is already in a position to improve her and her baby's health during pregnancy and beyond. The Harvard Women's Health Study of over 18,000 women[1] showed that increasing consumption of plant proteins and complex carbohydrates (brown rice, pasta, dark bread) as well as regular exercise can improve fertility. By contrast, consumption of trans fats and animal protein can promote ovulatory infertility. An article in Newsweek titled "Fat, Carbs, and the Science of Conception"[2] discussed that infertility was 39% more likely in women with the highest intake of animal protein than in those with the lowest. Even after controlling for total calories, adding just 1 serving a day of red meat, chicken or turkey led to a nearly one-third increase in infertility risk. Comparatively, women with the highest intake of plant protein were substantially less likely to have had ovulatory infertility than women with the lowest plant protein intake. It was also found that women who consumed 2 or more servings per day of low-fat dairy products had 1.85 times the risk for infertility. Whole milk products are unfortunately far from a health food as it is a concentrated source of saturated fat and cholesterol.[3]

How Weight and Nutrition Can Affect Pregnancy and Delivery

Our food choices play an integral role in weight and optimizing weight prior to and during pregnancy is of utmost importance for a healthy baby.

The risk of neural tube defects (problems with forming the fetal spine) is approximately doubled in pregnancies complicated by maternal obesity.[4] Studies have also shown a correlation with increasing BMI and risk for stillbirth[5] as well as increased risk of having a baby with fetal growth restriction.[6] According to ACOG, "If you are overweight or obese, you will need to pay close attention to how much you eat during pregnancy. Smaller amounts of weight gain or even a small weight loss may be recommended to ensure a safe pregnancy and a healthy baby."

However, population studies show that vegetarians are 3 times less likely to be obese than meat-eaters and vegans are 9 times less likely to be obese than meat-eaters! Adult vegans are typically 10 to 20 pounds lighter than adult meat-eaters. And vegan and vegetarian diets can also improve pregnancy outcomes independent of weight loss. "The Farm" is a vegan community in Summertown, Tennessee and maternity records of 775 vegan mothers found only one case that met the clinical criteria of pre-eclampsia, a high blood pressure disorder that can lead to seizures in the mother and problems with baby including growth restriction and early delivery.[7] It is clear that vegan and vegetarian diets are a sustainable and healthy method of weight managements and loss and can make a big difference for moms and their babies.

It is Healthier to be Plant- Based While Pregnant

Surprisingly, the amount of food you eat during pregnancy does not have to change drastically.

Just to reinforce this point, let's run through a list of what you want to be sure you're getting as well as how a plant-based diet can adequately fulfill these needs.

- Fiber: Plant- based foods are packed with fiber. In addition to the many health benefits of fiber such as helping in weight loss, studies have also shown that increased fiber intake may decrease the risk of pre-eclampsia.[8]

- Protein: Pregnant women need approximately 25 grams more of protein per day, for a total of approximately 70 grams per day. Vegan foods that provide protein include beans, grains, nuts, seeds, nut butter, seed butters, vegetables, soy foods, meat analogues, and seitan. However, protein should not be a high concern. When we eat excess protein our body converts it into fat.

- Iron: The daily recommended intake during pregnancy is 27 mg/day.[9] Vegan sources include iron-fortified cereals and energy bars, oatmeal, cream of wheat, tofu, soybeans, dark chocolate, legumes, nuts, seeds, dark green leafy vegetables, and blackstrap molasses. Vitamin C can help your body absorb iron. Approximately half of all pregnant women develop iron-deficiency anemia, but studies have shown there is no increased incidence of iron-deficiency anemia in vegans.[10]

- Calcium: The recommended daily intake is the same as pre-pregnancy: 1000 mg/day. It is easy to get this much calcium on a whole foods plant- based diet. Pregnancy actually increases the body's calcium absorption and absorption from plant-based foods is often better than that of dairy products. Vegan sources of calcium include tofu, soy beans, dark green leafy vegetables, broccoli, calcium fortified non-dairy milk, turnip greens, bok choy, and blackstrap molasses.

- Vitamin D: The daily recommendation is also the same as pre-pregnancy: 600 IU. Vitamin D helps the body absorb calcium. Vegan sources include mushrooms, fortified non-dairy milks, fortified cereals and juices, and of course the sun! All it takes is 5-10 minutes a few times per week on your face and arms without sunscreen.

- Folic acid: Protects against neural tube defects. Vegan sources include leafy vegetables, beans, oranges, and peanuts.

- DHA (an essential omega-3 fatty acid): is important for fetal neurodevelopment. Research is emerging with several other benefits including increased visual acuity and neurocognitive development for baby, as well as decreased incidence of childhood asthma. Less than 2% of pregnant and lactating women have adequate DHA levels.[11] Be sure to use plant-based sources of DHA as fatty acids from fish oils are unstable and can release free radicals when decomposing, whereas omega-3 fatty acids found in plant-based sources are much more stable. Vegan sources of alpha-linoleic acid (ALA), which is converted into DHA and EPA, include flaxseeds, flaxseed oil, canola oil, hemp seeds, hemp seed oil, walnut oil, and walnuts.

- B12, Zinc, and Iodine: will be found in most prenatal vitamins.

Foods to Avoid While Pregnant

Animal based products, alcohol, tobacco, soda, sugar, and highly processed junk foods are major foods to avoid. They actually cause the body to excrete vital vitamins and minerals mom and baby need. Animal foods in particular, are essentially devoid of fiber, have added saturated fats, cholesterol, and inflammatory proteins as well as are often contaminated with pesticides and toxins that bio-accumulate. These foods, such as meat, fish and eggs, are also often the foods that trigger morning sickness. It is thought that this is our body's protective mechanism against harm as these are often the foods that carry a risk of contamination. For example, Listeriosis is a bacteria that can infect unpasteurized milk and soft cheese, raw or undercooked meats (including poultry and shellfish) as well as prepared meats such as hot dogs or deli meats unless heated until steaming hot. Listeriosis can cause miscarriage and stillbirth. Finally, large fish including shark, kingfish, tilefish, and mackerel can contain high levels of mercury and should be avoided.

Dairy Products are Toxic for Your Baby

Milk is packed with contaminants from growth hormones to antibiotics to pesticides and it is well understood that these chemicals can readily cross the placenta to reach a developing fetus. Physicians Committee for Responsible Medicine (pcrm.org) states that "pesticides, polychlorinated biphenyls (PCBs), and dioxins are examples of contaminants found in milk. These toxins do not readily leave the body and can eventually build to harmful levels that may affect the immune and reproductive systems. Even the central nervous system can be affected. Moreover, PCBs and dioxins have also been linked to cancer."[12] Studies find that vegetarian women have been shown to have much lower levels of environmental contaminants in their milk than non-vegetarians.[13] Finally, there are allowable limits for the amount of pus and blood allowed in cows' milk. Pus cannot be boiled, steamed or frozen out of milk.

If you are having a hard time making the switch to vegan, remember that the more you replace meat and dairy with fruits, vegetables, and whole grains, the better off you and your baby will be during pregnancy and beyond.

Chelsea M. Clinton, MD *is a resident OB/GYN at New York Presbyterian Weill-Cornell Hospital in New York City. She recently coauthored the book, "Waist Away". She is interested in pursuing a career in high risk obstetrics and continuing research on how diet affects health status, particularly during pregnancy.*

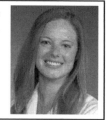

Baby, Drop the Cow's Milk

Victor Khayat, MD

As an obstetrician, I have found that pregnant women who eat a healthy diet are likely to have a more healthy pregnancy. Diets rich in fruits and vegetables have helped keep a number of my patients' vitamin and mineral levels in the normal range. By contrast, I have found that pregnant women who have diets high in meat and dairy tend to have more issues with acid reflux, and some have also had increased gall bladder issues. In those patients that have gallbladder issues, reducing or eliminating fried, greasy foods, and meat and dairy products, seem to help alleviate their symptoms significantly.

After deliveries, I have noticed some babies experience colic-like symptoms. The word *colic* is used broadly by parents, clinicians, and researchers in Western cultures to refer to infants who cry for no apparent reason during the first 3 months of life. Some theories are that babies with colic have symptoms that are caused at least in part by an allergy to either casein or whey, which are components of cow milk. These infants have a significant reduction in symptoms within a few days after removing dairy and initiating a hypoallergenic diet. Some children develop significant allergies to cow's milk when they stop breast or formula feeding. One theory is that the body develops antibodies to the milk and thus creates an immune response that presents as eczema-like lesions, asthma symptoms, and even more serious anaphylaxis, which can be life threatening. Some of these allergies do resolve in later childhood, but others can persist even into adulthood.

It is important to understand human physiology and how certain foods can augment the body's functions, and others can interfere and harm those same functions. I discovered the link between diet and health about 8 years ago when I was diagnosed with high cholesterol. My family practitioner placed me on a cholesterol-lowering statin drug but I began experiencing side effects such as muscle pain and elevation of my liver enzymes, when he increased my dose to combat my still high cholesterol. I began doing research into the area of nutrition after reading articles written by physicians from Harvard, the Mayo Clinic, the Cleveland Clinic, and many large population studies, I noticed a pattern: The people in the trials who were eating more vegetarian diets appeared to be doing better than those who were not eating vegetarian diets.

Based on what I learned, I made a conscious decision to eliminate all meat from my diet and restricted my dairy intake. Within 12 weeks of making these changes, I noticed that my elevated cholesterol levels had fallen to normal. I stopped taking my cholesterol lowering statin medications and was surprised by how fast my levels came down to normal. I did not think I would have normal levels after merely 12 weeks but they have stayed that way since. In the process of converting to a plant-based diet, I lost about 9 to 10 pounds and my energy levels significantly improved. This is extremely important as my work requires me being up at all hours of the night delivering babies and performing emergency surgeries.

Diet plays such a vital role in the function of the human body. Children should be taught at a young age about nutrition and how it will impact them and their health. We as physicians need to educate our patients on the benefits of a healthy plant-based diet to ensure that we can help prevent many of the preventable diseases in medicine. However, each individual it is up to the individual to make these changes. "An ounce of prevention is worth a pound of cure," should hold true to how we try and live our lives and how we practice medicine.

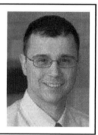

Victor Khayat, MD. *is a Board Certified Obstetrician and Gynecologist. He is a Fellow of the American Congress of Obstetricians and Gynecologists and a Lieutenant Colonel in the United States Army Medical Corps. He has spent over 8 years in the military as a physician and surgeon, and volunteered on medical missions outside the United States. Dr. Khayat received his Bachelor of Science degree from Emory and Medical degree from University of College Dublin Medical School. He completed his residency in obstetrics and gynecology at the Western Pennsylvania Hospital in Pittsburgh, Pennsylvania, where he was the chief resident. Dr. Khayat currently practices in New Ulm, Minnesota.*

A Beautiful Vegan Pregnancy

Lisa Bazzett-Matabele, MD, OB/GYN Cancer Specialist

Often people wonder about the implications of following a plant-based diet while pregnant. When I did my research on the safety of a vegan pregnancy, I only found positive information. In reality, you do not eat much differently as a pregnant versus non-pregnant vegan. I simply increased my calorie intake as is recommended in any pregnancy to support my growing baby. It gave me the opportunity to eat more healthy fats like nuts and avocados, which I really enjoy. My pregnancy was probably one of the most healthful times in my life. I just felt great!

If you are over 35 when pregnant, as I was, it puts you at additional risk for pregnancy- induced diabetes, high blood pressure and a list of other potential complications. I did not have a single one of these problems. My blood pressure was normal and never rose during pregnancy, my diabetic screen was one of the best my obstetrician had ever seen, and I never once had blood sugar problems.

So where do you get your protein and calcium? On a whole food, plant-based diet getting sufficient protein and calcium should never be a problem. We get protein from plants as well as from tofu, beans, grains, and seeds. People think that you need milk for calcium, but calcium from animal milk and dairy is harder for our body to absorb because milk is acidic. I ate my usual plant-based diet and never had any nutritional deficiencies. Our daughter is now a beautiful vegan toddler.

*Please read Dr. Bazzett-Matabele's article in Chapter 9, Plant-Based Diet and Cancer: The Open Secret."

Ladies, Eat Your Veggies!

Deborah Wilson, MD

As a Gynecologist, I see many patients with painful periods, fibroids (benign tumors of the uterus), endometriosis, troublesome ovarian cysts, and reproductive cancers every day. There is no doubt in my mind that meat and dairy intake are huge contributors to many of these issues that ail my patients.

Fibroids are benign muscle tumors that affect 60% of women in the United States.[1] Fibroids generally begin to cause problems, such as heavy bleeding, pelvic pain, pressure on other organs, and painful intercourse, in a woman's 40's, but can show up much earlier. It is also a myth that fibroids regress and cease to cause problems after menopause as I often see bleeding issues after menopause that can be directly attributed to fibroids. When fibroids occur in a woman's 20's or 30's infertility can be the result. If a pregnancy is achieved, fibroids can complicate the pregnancy by causing preterm labor and delivery.

According to the U.S. Department of Health and Human Services, eating red meat and ham are associated with an increased risk of fibroids. Red meat consumption may increase your exposure to xenoestrogens -- industrially made substances with estrogenic properties -- which are stored in fatty tissue where they alter the body's natural hormone levels and increase the risk of fibroids. Additionally excessive Insulin-like growth factor (IGF-1) levels are a risk factor for fibroids as well as breast cancer, colon cancer, and prostate cancer. Recombinant Bovine Growth Hormone, which contains high levels of a growth factor known as Insulin-like growth factor 1(IGF-1), is found in genetically engineered milk and meat.

A plant- based diet low in fat and high in fiber has the ability to modulate blood hormone concentrations and reduce levels of growth factors. This may be why studies indicate that women who eat red meat and are overweight have more fibroids. In fact, women who eat more than one serving of red meat per day have a 70% greater risk of fibroids. However, increasing your consumption of green vegetables can reduce fibroids. Evidence indicates that green vegetables may protect women from developing fibroids.[2]

Dysmenorrhea, or painful periods, is the most common gynecologic complaint we hear. Dysmenorrhea is related to the release of prostaglandins during menstruation, resulting in pain. Dysmenorrhea can also be caused by fibroids, endometriosis, infection, pelvic adhesions, and cervical stenosis.

A plant- based diet is associated with reduced blood estrogen concentrations and may reduce symptoms of dysmenorrhea. Low fat vegan diets are shown to increase a substance found in blood that binds estrogen. Since high levels of estrogen in the blood cause more pain, the pain is reduced. Vegetarian diets also contain more omega-3 fatty acids and fewer omega-6 fatty acids, thus reducing prostaglandin formation and consequently reducing menstrual pain.

As a plant-based risk reduces risk of fibroids and endometriosis, it generally reduces the likelihood of suffering with cramps.

Uterine Cancer involves the uterine lining cells or the muscle of the uterus. Studies have found a 50% greater risk for uterine lining cancer (endometrial cancer) among women who eat processed meat and fish often.[3] The same holds true for women who eat red meat, eggs, and a high fat diet.

Obese and overweight women have 2 to 4 times the risk of developing this disease than women of a normal weight, regardless of menopausal status.[4] A vegan diet helps maintain and lose weight, thus exposing the uterus to fewer hormones and decreasing the risk of uterine cancer significantly.

Ovarian Cancer is the leading cause of death from gynecologic cancer in the United States[5] and is usually diagnosed in an advanced stage because the symptoms are subtle. Symptoms include bloating, pelvic pressure, swelling, low back pain and indigestion. High intakes of saturated fat increase the chance of developing ovarian cancer. In particular, meat, eggs and whole milk are implicated. Animal fat, especially from animals given Bovine Growth Hormone which increases the IGF-1, leads to a higher incidence of ovarian cancer. Milk consumption, including skim milk, places women at higher risk for ovarian cancer due to the IGF-1 and a toxic effect that the milk sugar galactose has on the ovaries. Obesity also increases the risk of ovarian cancer, particularly if a woman is obese as a teenager.

A woman with ovarian cancer can, after appropriate treatment, increase her chances of survival by altering her diet to include only plant-based foods, particularly organic cruciferous vegetables such as broccoli, cauliflower, and cabbage.[6]

As a well advertised vegan, I attract other vegans to my practice. By comparison, my vegan patients have fewer reproductive problems than my meat eating patients. When patients do embark on a plant-based diet their reports and results are stunning from weight loss, freedom from pelvic pain, reduction in menstrual bleeding, and general improvement in well being.

Deborah Wilson, MD, *practices Gynecology and Advanced Laparoscopic Surgery. Dr. Wilson is the director of Feathers Foundation and Circle L Ranch. www.drwilsonobgyn.com; http://www.circlel.org*

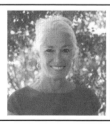

fourteen

FEEDING KIDS RIGHT

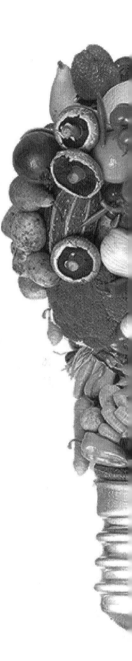

Every parent aims to provide the best for their kids; yet conflicting information on nutrition leaves most confused as to what to feed them. This confusion along with the growing number of fast and packaged foods has contributed to the escalating rates of obesity, and simultaneous global epidemic of childhood health problems. Our children are developing food allergens at unparalleled rates, developmental problems such as autism and dyslexia are increasingly more common, and the incidence of type 2 diabetes, autoimmune diseases, and cancer are beyond alarming. What is happening to our children?

Much media attention has been devoted to the plethora of sugary drinks and processed snack foods on children's restaurant and lunch menus. A report by the Center for Science and Public Interest stated that 97% of the children's menus at major restaurant chains were deemed unhealthy. However, the percentage of unhealthy children's menus is probably closer to 100% as "healthy" foods included grilled chicken, a roast beef sub, and 1% milk.[1]

The following doctors in the chapter discuss how meat and dairy are NOT at all healthy for our children. Laden with antibiotics, toxic chemicals, and poisonous additives, preservatives and growth hormones, the meat and dairy in our children's meals and snacks are contributing to sad rather than happy meals for their health. These doctors testify to the amazing protective qualities of a plant-based diet and how these nutrient rich food choices plant seeds of wellness instead of disease.

Dairy is Not For Children

Yamileth Cazorla-Lancaster, DO, MPH, MS

Milk does the body good, right? I disagree. As a pediatrician, I often see that dairy consumption causes more problems than benefits. Dairy is one of the foods that I spend much time counseling families to significantly decrease or eliminate from their children's diets. Even as a young pediatrician, I have witnessed the negative effects of dairy beginning from birth and continuing through adulthood.

Dairy Allergies in Infants

Cow's milk protein is one of the top allergens. Cow's milk protein allergy develops in the first few days or weeks of life and can manifest itself in a variety of ways, but it often leads to colicky, fussy babies that spit up frequently. In extreme cases, it can cause malabsorption so that neonates have vomiting and diarrhea, and cannot gain weight.

This allergy is not only seen in babies who are drinking formula made from cow's milk, but also in infants who are breastfed by mothers who consume dairy. The cow's milk protein is transferred from the mother's breast milk to the baby and causes the symptoms in the affected infant. Dairy is so prevalent in the standard American diet and the dairy addiction so strong, that I've seen mothers who would rather switch their babies to a soy- based formula than adhere to a dairy-free diet while breastfeeding.

Common Health Complications in Young Children

The list of health risks for our children associated with milk consumption is long. It includes obesity, constipation, anemia, bone fractures, recurrent ear infections, allergies, and malnutrition. There have also been several studies linking milk consumption to an increased risk of developing type I diabetes in children who are genetically susceptible.[1]

The dairy consumed by children in the United States is often high in fat, protein, and calories. As a society, we have long believed that higher protein in our diets is beneficial. However, we are seeing that children are now growing faster, getting larger (both in height and weight) and reaching puberty earlier.[2] This may be partially caused by the increased protein in our diets and it is likely not the advantage that we hoped for.

As standard infant formula is made from cow's milk, formula-fed babies are at higher risk for obesity and abnormal weight gain, and are also more likely to suffer from constipation. Dairy consumption combined with the usual low-fiber American diet is a leading cause of constipation in children. Infants who develop this condition often suffer from chronic constipation if they continue to consume dairy throughout their lives. Constipation is a very common cause of chronic abdominal pain, bloating, painful defecation and rectal bleeding. It can also lead to a loss in appetite in children and at its most extreme, leakage of stool. Constipation is very frustrating to parents because they often seek a temporary cure without realizing that they never eliminated the cause of the problem.

In children with the highest milk consumption, the anemia can be severe and insidious, and I have seen cases that required hospitalization. The reason is that dairy tends to displace other foods that have iron as well as cause microscopic bleeding in the gut resulting in a slow loss of iron over time.

Additionally because some children become so attached (and likely addicted) to milk, they have little interest in other foods, leading to malnutrition. Because so many parents believe that milk is healthy, they allow this heavy milk consumption because they fear their children are not eating enough. This contributes to a vicious cycle and a greater number of children can become overweight and obese as well as lack vital nutrients for proper growth and development.

Children are our future and we want them to be healthy and strong. We can support this healthy growth and development by eliminating or greatly reducing their dairy consumption and starting them on a path of success for a vibrant, active life.

Yamileth (Yami) Cazorla-Lancaster, DO, MPH, MS *attended University of North Texas Health Science Center in Fort Worth, where she earned multiple degrees – Master of Science in Clinical Research and Education, Master of Public Health and Doctor of Osteopathic Medicine. She most recently completed her Pediatric Residency at Cincinnati Children's Hospital Medical Center. Receiving a scholarship through the National Health Service Corps, she is committed to serving the medically underserved as a primary care pediatrician.*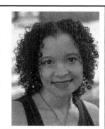

Disease-Proof Your Child Through Nutritional Excellence

Joel Fuhrman, MD

As parents, we want what is best for our children. We would never intentionally harm them. In fact, we make sure to get them the best care we know, read to them at bedtime and insist they wear their seatbelts, but when it comes to children and food, somehow we don't know what is the best thing to do. Our children seem finicky and only eat cheese, pasta, chicken fingers or milk and cookies. At the same time, we notice that they are frequently ill. They suffer from recurring ear infections, runny noses, stomachaches and headaches. We note their symptoms and haul them in to the doctor, who prescribes yet another round of antibiotics. All this is normal for children —right? **Wrong!**

This scenario may be "normal" for kids today, but it is not normal if we feed our children the high-nutrient foods designed by nature to properly fuel them. Scientific research has demonstrated that humans have a powerful immune system, even stronger than other animals. Our bodies are self-repairing, self-defending organisms, which have the innate ability to defend themselves against microbes and prevent chronic illnesses. This can only happen if we give our bodies the correct raw materials. When we don't supply the young body with its nutritional requirements, we see bizarre diseases occur. We even witness the increasing appearance of cancers that were unheard of in prior human history.

Over the past two decades convincing evidence has emerged which links autoimmune illnesses, such as Crohn's Disease, lupus and later-life cancers with precise dietary factors from the first 10 years of life. This means that we now know what factors help to create an environment in our bodies which is favorable for cancers to surface later in life, and we understand the precise dietary factors that can prevent cancer in our child's future. The worst part is that **parents haven't been informed that what their children eat in the first 10 years of life has such a profound effect on their entire lives.** Without the necessary knowledge, detailing the dietary style that can prevent later life cancers, many parents are unfortunately feeding their children dangerous, cancer-provoking diets.

The standard American diet has begun to do its damage on our children, placing them at much higher risk of chronic diseases than previous generations. New studies found that 49% of overweight teenagers and 37% of normal-weight teenagers had one or more risk factors for cardiovascular disease, including diabetes, high LDL cholesterol, and hypertension. Twenty-three percent of teens are pre-diabetic or diabetic – this number has more doubled in the past 10 years. Twenty-two percent of teens have high or borderline high LDL cholesterol levels. Fourteen percent of teens have hypertension or prehypertension.[1]

Today, it is known that both children of American descent and from developed countries consume less than 2% of their diet from natural plant foods such as fruits and vegetables. American children move into adulthood eating 90% of their calories from dairy products, white flour, sugar and oil. Amazingly, about 25% of toddlers between ages 1 and 2 eat no fruits and vegetables at all. By 15 months, French fries are the most common vegetable consumed in America! Have parents gone crazy?

Humans, like other primates, are designed to consume a diet predominating in natural plant foods with their symphony of essential phytochemicals. Fresh fruits, vegetables, beans, raw nuts and seeds should form the foundation of normal nutrition. Food preferences and tastes are formed early in life and children learn to eat the diets eaten by their parents.

When you have a child, you have the unique opportunity to mold a developing person. One of your greatest gifts to them can be a disease resistant body created from excellent food choices beginning at youth. Ear infections, strep throats, allergies, attention deficit hyperactivity disorders (ADD or ADHD), and even autoimmune diseases can be prevented by sound nutritional practices early in life. Common childhood illnesses are not only avoidable, but they're more effectively managed by incorporating nutritional excellence into one's diet. This is far superior to the dependence on drugs to which we are accustomed. No parent would disagree that our children deserve only the best.

This is an approved excerpt from "Disease-Proof Your Child" by Dr. Joel Fuhrman

Joel Fuhrman, MD *is a board-certified family physician, New York Times best-selling author of "Eat to Live", "Disease-Proof Your Child", "Super Immunity", "Eat for Health", "Fasting and Eating for Health" and "The End of Diabetes", and nutritional researcher who specializes in preventing and reversing disease through nutritional and natural methods. Dr. Fuhrman is an internationally recognized expert on nutrition and natural healing, and has appeared on hundreds of radio and television shows including The Dr. Oz show, The Today Show, Good Morning America, and Live with Kelly. Dr. Fuhrman's own hugely successful PBS television shows, 3 Steps to Incredible Health and Dr. Fuhrman's Immunity Solution bring nutritional science to homes all across America.*

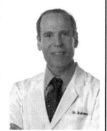

The Evidence Against Dairy

Thomas M. Campbell, II, MD

Instructor of Clinical Family Medicine at University of Rochester School of Medicine and Dentistry
Executive Director, T. Colin Campbell Center for Nutritional Studies.

"Unfortunately, we learn as medical doctors to encourage dairy foods with religious fervor. However, we don't learn about any of the evidence behind this. If we looked, we might find that those countries with the highest calcium intakes have the highest fracture rates. We might find that those populations with the highest animal protein intake have the highest fracture rates. High animal protein intake, prominent in American diets, increases calcium excretion from the kidneys and increases acid production in the kidneys, both of which may contribute to increased risk of fracture over time. We might find that the evidence linking dairy foods to fracture rates to be woefully inadequate. We might find experimental animal evidence showing dairy protein to be linked to high cholesterol and accelerated cancer promotion. And finally, we might find dairy to be the most allergenic, poorly tolerated food of all foods.

So if you love the age old wisdom advocating for dairy as nature's most perfect food, by all means don't look at the evidence. Humans are the only species to continue to 'nurse' past the age of weaning and we use another species' milk to do it. If you're sitting in front of me with your child at a wellness check-up, I do not recommend that your child drink cow's milk any more than I recommend that your child drink cat's milk. Get your vegetables and calcium, yes, but cow's milk, no."

Childhood and Adolescence: A Window of Opportunity for Cancer Prevention

Divya-Devi Joshi, MD, MMM, CPE

Have you ever asked yourself if there is something you could do to make your child's life better and longer? For the first time in history, the life expectancy of today's children will be shorter than their parents'. Evidence is mounting that childhood and adolescence is the time when the risk for adult-onset cancers starts to accumulate.

The latest figures from the World Cancer Research Fund and the American Institute for Cancer Research show that a third of the most common cancers in the world could be prevented by a healthy diet, being physically active, and maintaining a healthy body weight. Only smoking tobacco has a higher risk of causing cancer. Every parent tries to prevent their child from smoking; shouldn't we also try to influence their dietary choices?

The following 3 large studies reveal very concerning news:

1. Large American studies involving up to half a million people have reported an increased risk for early death among people who eat a diet high in red and processed meat. The consumption of processed and red meat leads to increased death rates in particular due to cardiovascular diseases, but also to cancer.[1]

2. It is estimated that up to 60% of cancers are to some extent diet related. In February 2013 a study of 96,469 North American Seventh Day Adventists clearly indicated that people who had eliminated meat from their diets lived significantly longer than those who ate meat. Most of these early deaths were linked to cardiovascular disease, but eating a meatless diet significantly reduced risks of female-specific and gastrointestinal cancers. The study showed significant evidence that red meat increases the risk for colorectal cancer.[2]

3. In March 2013, the European Prospective Investigation into Cancer and Nutrition conducted a study of 448,568 men and women. They confirmed that a high consumption of processed meat was related to increased mortality, in particular due to cardiovascular diseases but also to cancer.[3]

The evidence is clear: eating meat increases the risk of dying earlier.

Animal-Based Foods in Childhood Increase Cancer Risk

The risk of developing cancer starts in childhood. As a child's cells divide and their organs and body grow, damage done by various toxic substances accumulates over the years. The habits a child learns, including dietary choices, will greatly impact their health as adults. The American Institute for Cancer Research warned in 2007 that bad habits in childhood can lead to cancer later in life. Growing evidence links childhood and adolescent lifestyle (including diet) to subsequent risk of adult cancers.[4]

St. Jude Children's Research Hospital emphasizes in a recent article how plant-based foods, including fruit, vegetables, and whole grains (in addition to having a healthy body weight) have a protective effect against cancer, and warns that dietary changes will have to occur in childhood to be effective in adulthood.[5]

Remember that cancer takes time to develop and the damage that leads to adult cancers likely starts in childhood.

Let me reassure you: all the articles and research studies quoted in this chapter stating meat and dairy are related to cancer growth and plant-based foods have a protecting effect against cancer come from renowned institutions such as the National Cancer Institute, World Cancer Research Fund, American Cancer Society, American Institute for Cancer Research, Harvard, St. Jude Children's Research Hospital, and from peer-reviewed medical journals. (A peer-reviewed journal is one in which each article is critically reviewed and approved by national experts in the field.)

Why Doesn't My Child's Physician Tell Me About This?

1. It takes around 7 years for research data to be sufficiently validated to be accepted by the medical community. A lot of the research I mention here is relatively new.

2. Traditions and habits take a long time to change. We live in a culture that still largely sees meat as important for a healthy diet. This tradition gets handed down to us as we grow up. It is hard to question something you grew up with and that you believe is true. Not that long ago, doctors encouraged patients to smoke cigarettes to relax.

3. Entire industries would face significant financial losses if dietary habits were to change on a large scale. People are influenced by advertisements, and the ads for cow's milk are certainly well funded.

Cancer-Causing Foods

Red, Barbecued, and Grilled Meat

The National Institute of Health states that red meat increases the risk of cancers of the esophagus, colon, rectum, liver, and lung by 20 to 60%.[6] However, even when red

Your Juicy Steak is Cancer-Causing

Heme iron, a molecule found in blood, is what makes red meat red. When the heme iron from red meat is broken down in our gut it forms N-nitroso compounds. These have been found to cause DNA damage. DNA damage is the first step towards cancer. N-nitroso compounds play a known role in the development of colon cancer. If you combine the formation of toxic N-nitroso compounds with prolonged transit times in the gut, it explains the association between a high meat diet and colorectal cancer risk.

or processed meat is eaten in moderation, a Duke University cancer survivorship study showed that the risk still exists. Women who ate large amounts of red meat were more than twice as likely to suffer hormone-related breast cancer. The growth hormones given to cattle are found in their meat. They may promote the growth of hormone-sensitive breast cancer.

Cooked meats are the predominant dietary source of cell mutations. Mutations can lead to cancer. Well-validated studies by the National Cancer Institute as well as by Japanese and European scientists found that cooking meat at the required high temperatures produces carcinogens called heterocyclic amines. There are 17 different heterocyclic amines produced from cooking or grilling meats that may pose human cancer risk. They can cause mutations in the cells, which in turn can cause cancerous cells to form.

Dairy

Milk, butter, and cheese are implicated in higher rates of hormone-dependent cancers. US study that compared state-by-state data on dairy use and breast cancer risk found that the more dairy (particularly milk and cheese) a state consumed, the greater the risk their population had of dying from breast cancer. A study comparing diet and cancer rates in 42 counties showed that milk and cheese consumption was strongly correlated with the incidence of testicular cancer among men aged 20 to 39. Dairy accounts for 60-80% of estrogens consumed by humans. About 75% of American children under 12 consume dairy every day. An Australian 65-year follow-up study shows that a large amount of dairy during childhood is also associated with adult colorectal cancer.[7]

In the US, recombinant growth hormone is given to cows to increase milk production. The American Cancer Society and the National Cancer Institute are concerned that milk from growth hormone-treated cows has higher levels of insulin-like growth hormone 1. Circulating insulin-like growth hormone 1 in the bloodstream has been associated with breast-cancer risk. For this reason, other Western countries such as the European Union and Canada do not permit the use of growth hormone for cows. Among authorities that advise caution, most say that children before puberty are at greatest risk.

Fish

The World Cancer Research Fund and American Institute for Cancer Research conclude that there is limited evidence that consuming fish protects against some cancers. Children and pregnant women should avoid certain fish, because they can contain high levels of heavy metals and other contaminants.

Cancer-Protective Foods

A child's diet is one of the most *modifiable* risk factors for cancer. Studies have shown that the cancer risk can be influenced by the consumption of fruit and vegetables. In one study, British children who ate a lot of fruit during childhood had a much lower incidence of cancer 60 years later, and a lower chance of dying from cancer.[8]

Phytochemicals are naturally occurring plant chemicals. The Fred Hutchinson Cancer Research Center in Seattle has described how phytochemicals can alter the likelihood of cancer formation at almost every stage of cancer development.[9,10] Cruciferous vegetables (cauliflower, cabbage, broccoli) contain glucosinolates, which can not only inhibit the growth of blood vessels that feed an enlarging tumor, but also inhibit cancer cell growth, promote cancer cell death, and prevent DNA damage. Antioxidants in fruit and vegetables protect against free radical damage to DNA (American Institute for Cancer Research). Beans as well as berries are one of the best sources of dietary antioxidants.

A Few Myths About a Purely Plant-Based Diet for Children

Will my child get enough protein? Most Americans eat more protein than they need; excess protein is actually harmful as it leads to obesity and osteoporosis. The Centers for Disease Control state that it is very rare for someone who is healthy and eating a varied diet to not get enough protein.

Protein in the human diet can be animal-based or plant-based. Certain foods contain all the essential amino acids and don't need to be combined with other foods to make complete protein. This is true for meat, but also soy and quinoa. So-called incomplete proteins are low in one or more essential amino acid and must be complemented by other foods. This is easily accomplished with a balanced diet.

Will my child get enough calcium? Nowadays, many daily staples are fortified with calcium, such as breakfast cereals and orange juice. Dark-green leafy vegetables (collard, turnip, and mustard greens) contain calcium.

Setting the Right Example

Did you know that Albert Einstein, Leonardo da Vinci, Isaac Newton, Charles Darwin, Benjamin Franklin, Henry Ford, Thomas Edison, Albert Schweitzer, Gandhi, and Mark Twain ate a plant-based diet?

Childhood and adolescence represents a window of opportunity for cancer prevention and prolongation of a healthy life. Children and even adolescents follow their parents' example. Provide a variety of vegetables, fruits, whole grains, and beans. Make your child's meals and snacks brightly colored with red apples, blueberries, green peas, carrots, bananas…. differently colored foods have different beneficial compounds! Pick strongly flavored vegetables and fruits, as they are often the best sources of cancer-protective phytochemicals. Gradually eliminate processed meats and decrease red meat and milk. You do not have to be perfect in a day!

The main thing is to eat mindfully. It does not necessarily mean more time consuming or expensive. Small compromises now will pay off handsomely in the future.

Divya-Devi Joshi, MD, MMM, CPE, is the Chief Medical Officer at Miller Children's Hospital Long Beach, the nation's 9th largest children's hospital. Dr. Joshi is responsible for the operations of the Miller Children's Outpatient Specialty Clinics and satellite centers throughout Long Beach, South Bay and Orange County. Dr. Joshi attended medical school at the University of Vienna in Austria and completed both her residency and fellowship at the Mayo Clinic in Rochester, MN. She is board certified in Pediatric Hematology/Oncology and in Pediatric and Adolescent Medicine. Dr. Joshi also obtained an MMM (Master's of Medical Management) from Carnegie Mellon University. For 5 years she was the Director of the Pediatric Residency Program and an Attending Physician of Pediatric Hematology/Oncology at the Marshfield Clinic and St. Joseph's Children's Hospital in Wisconsin. Most recently, Dr. Joshi has served as the Chief Medical Officer of the Torrance Hospital Independent Practice Association (THIPA). Dr. Joshi is fluent in 3 languages (English, German and French) and loves traveling internationally, literature and the arts, long distance running, scuba diving and skiing.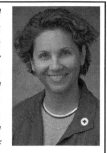

Baby, It's All About The Breast

Leila Masson, MD, MPH, FRACP, DTMH, IBCLC

My goal as a pediatrician is to start children out on a trajectory of optimal health from the moment they are born. This begins with understanding the importance of breast milk as well as a mother's food choices while breastfeeding to a child's development.

As mammals we have evolved over millions of years to drink the milk of our mothers. Artificial baby milk has been around for just a little longer than 100 years, and despite the attempt of the formula industry to make us believe that it is very similar to human breast milk it is simply NOT close.

Breast milk is produced by the mother in just the right amount, with the right composition and perfect mix of immune cells, hormones, growth factors and cytokines for her baby to grow and develop. Formula is a mixture of cow's milk proteins, sugar, and oils – some have added vitamins and fatty acids, but it is a dead liquid, not able to withstand comparison with the live breastmilk freshly produced by the mother specifically for her child.

The US Agency for Healthcare Research review of all breastfeeding studies for the US Department of Health and Human Services,[1] has once again made it clear that compared to those who are breastfed, infants fed artificial baby milk have a higher risk of allergies, asthma, eczema, type 1 and 2 diabetes, diarrhea, ear infections, inflammatory bowel disease, Crohn's disease, and SIDS or post-natal death.

Some of the health benefits for children who are breastfed as babies last a lifetime. For example they have lower blood pressure and lower bad cholesterol (LDL) as adults, which can prevent heart attacks. Studies show that breastfed children have a significantly higher IQ.

Even one bottle of non-human milk has a major impact on the infant's gut and immune system: a single feed of artificial baby milk changes the gut flora from the beneficial bacteria of the breastfed child to one with pathogenic E. coli, streptococci, and clostridia. It takes 4-6 weeks of exclusive breastfeeding to reverse this effect. This change in the gut increases the risk for diarrhea as well as the likelihood of developing a cow's milk allergy and even type 1 diabetes mellitus. Why take the risk?

These choices are not only beneficial for the baby but also for the mother. Mothers who breastfeed and eat a plant-based diet have a lower risk of diabetes, breast and ovarian cancers, post natal depression, rheumatoid arthritis and a higher survival rate.

Food Choices Matter for Breastfeeding Mothers

Although breast milk is superior to formula, it is vital for the mother to remember that her food choices affect her baby. Many of the same health problems caused by formula feeding can also come directly from a mother consuming meat and dairy while breast-feeding. For example, older children prefer to eat foods they were exposed to through the breast milk. If a mother eats a healthy diet with plenty of fruits and vegetables during her pregnancy and while breastfeeding, her children will eat those foods later in life. What an easy way to prime children to eat their vegetables! A mother can also expose her baby to the toxins in meat and dairy through breast milk, which can lead to health complications.

Dairy is the most common allergy in infants. About 2-5% of infants develop an allergy to cow's milk protein and this can present as eczema, reflux or colic. When I see a baby with any of these problems in my practice, I first recommend that the mother stops consuming any dairy products. In about 80% of cases, the eczema clears, the reflux stops and the baby is calmer, happier and healthier. Vegan mothers and babies do not have this problem. There are no species-foreign proteins in their breast milk as the mother does not have these in her diet. In omnivores, the protein from meat and dairy is absorbed into the bloodstream and then excreted into the breast milk – potentially affecting the baby's health.

Meat and dairy can contain added toxins and pesticides that can be passed through breastfeeding. A woman begins to accumulate pesticides, heavy metals and fat soluble toxins in her fat tissues from puberty. The toxins a woman accumulates over the years are excreted into the blood stream during her pregnancy and even more so during breastfeeding. As mothers lose weight during breastfeeding, the fat cells with the toxins are released into her metabolism and via breast milk into the child.

In food, toxins accumulate as you move up the food chain: they are found in non-organically grown fruits and vegetables and in higher amounts in dairy and meat as toxins concentrate in fat. Organochlorin pesticides are much lower in those who eat an organic plant-based diet as they do not consume the toxins accumulated in meat, fish, and dairy or those from commercially grown fruits and vegetables. Epidemiological studies have shown that pre-natal and post-natal exposure to pollutants are associated with higher levels of autism, ADHD and developmental problems in children, as well as increasing the risk of asthma and allergies.

Mothers who consume meat, dairy and eggs expose themselves and their baby to antibiotics. More than half of all antibiotics used in the world are given to animals, to make them grow faster and bigger in order to increase profit. The European Union outlawed this practice in 2006, but in the US and many other countries this is still common practice. This unnecessary use of antibiotics causes high rates of resistance to antibiotics as bacteria can adapt and change. This is a major concern, as all classes of antibiotics are used in animals and we are running out of antibiotics to use in humans with severe bacterial infections.

Additionally antibiotics affect the mother's gut flora. The gut flora consists of hundreds of different strains of bacteria that affect our health. We have 10 times as many bacteria in and on our bodies as we have cells in our bodies. We have co-evolved with these bacteria and would not survive without them. An abnormal gut flora has been associated with wide-ranging health problems including inflammatory bowel disease (Crohn's and ulcerative colitis), autism, chronic fatigue, and allergies.

Our children are our future. In order to provide them with the optimal chance for excellent health and protection against complications, mothers should be conscientious of their food choices and breastfeed their babies.

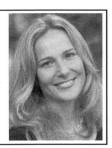

Leila Masson, MD, MPH, FRACP, DTMH, IBCLC, *is a pediatrician and lactation consultant in Auckland, New Zealand.*

Our Children Need Carrots Not Cows

Marge Peppercorn, MD, FAAP

"**F**inish your meat and drink your milk." This was a familiar refrain at my house when I was growing up as I suspect it was in the homes of most people. I grew up thinking that meat and milk were essential for a healthy diet and Medical School did nothing to change that view. I graduated from Harvard Medical School in the 70's and our only nutrition education dealt with vitamin deficiencies. Nothing at all was said about the possible role of our diets in affecting our health during school or even during my training in pediatrics at the Children's National Medical Center in Washington. Checking with other physicians has shown that this was the case at most medical schools around the country. It's no surprise then that most current practitioners know little if anything about the pros and cons of a meat versus plant- based diet.

Initially, I naively advised my patients when to start their babies on milk and meat according to the traditional way that I had been taught. Over the years, however, I become aware that farming methods had changed drastically and that an overwhelming majority of our animal products now came from huge so-called "factory farms." On factory farms animals are kept under severely overcrowded conditions, exposing them to increased risk of illness so they are routinely given antibiotics and various growth promoting hormones. This made me question my previous blind faith in the necessity of eating meat and dairy and whether or not consuming such products was in fact as healthy as I had always thought.

When I started studying nutrition on my own, I quickly realized that there were many reasons to avoid meat and dairy and that the standard American diet was misguided and most likely the root cause of many of our chronic serious illnesses. Genetic predisposition to these diseases is of course very important but studies show that diet can often modify those risks. I became convinced, that not only do we need to eat MORE fruits, vegetables, and whole grains, but that the healthiest diet would be one of ONLY fruits, vegetables, and whole grains. Even the age old maxim that drinking milk was necessary for building strong bones has been called into question by scientists who have noted increased excretion of calcium and increased bone fractures in people with increased intake of dairy and other animal proteins.[1,2,3] As it can take many years for any ill effects of an animal- based diet to develop, it is crucially important for families to instill plant-based eating habits in their children as soon they start to introduce solid foods.

Pediatric Concerns Associated with Animal Products

Over my 35 years as a community pediatrician I've listened to the concerns of many parents and watched hundreds of infants and children grow. During that time I've observed that when solid food is first introduced, most babies like fruits and cereals, at least some vegetables, and almost none like meats. As they grow older, most start liking meats and disliking the vegetables and I've often wondered why. It seems clear that if we capitalized on a child's initial natural dislike of meat and their innate fascination with animals, we could easily raise them to have a lifelong habit of a nutritious vegan diet and to thereby live longer, healthier lives.

Many people used to be skeptical about the healthiness of a vegan diet and thought that those who didn't eat meat or drink milk were extremists who were putting themselves at risk of malnutrition. Many felt that imposing such a diet on one's children would border on criminal. These people have been proven to be completely and utterly wrong. All the major nutritional committees and health boards such as the American Dietary Association as well as the Academy of Pediatrics now acknowledge the healthiness of vegan diets.[4] In fact the well respected pediatrician Dr Benjamin Spock clearly states in his last copy of *Baby and Child Care* that, "children who grow up getting nutrition from plant foods rather than meat have a tremendous health advantage-- they are less likely to develop weight problems, diabetes, high blood pressure, and some forms of cancer."[5]

This association is problematic as the seeds of diseases are sown early. Children who eat meat and dairy consume the harmful hormones given to food animals as well as the pesticides used on their feed. Of particular concern are dairy products, which in addition to artificial hormone supplements also contain naturally occurring bovine hormones. Hormone and pesticide exposure from animal products have been questioned as being among the many possible factors leading to an earlier onset of puberty. Early onset puberty is a potential problem for children because of the frequent psychological

The End of Antibiotics?

A growing problem in caring for children is the increasing emergence of antibiotic resistant bacteria and the frequent need to use newer and stronger antibiotics. For example, years ago almost all ear infections were cured by a short course of low dose amoxicillin. Now physicians are usually forced to use much higher doses and often the newer and more expensive antibiotics like Augmentin and Ceftin. The problem is even more serious with dangerous infections like meningitis and sepsis. Antibiotic resistance occurs because many bacteria are capable of developing defenses to antibiotics after prolonged exposure. The problem affects adults as well as children and has been directly linked to the vast amounts of antibiotics routinely given to farm animals merely to increase growth as well as to prevent or treat illness. It has been calculated that over 80% of the antibiotics used in this country are used for farm animals.[10] This is now recognized to be a major public health concern and could be ameliorated by reducing if not eliminating our consumption of animal products.

problems of hormonal change at a time of emotional immaturity. Early puberty also can increase the risk of breast cancer[6] and worsen acne in teens who consume dairy products. Childhood dairy consumption has also been questioned as possibly increasing the risk of breast and prostate cancer independent of its affect on puberty.[7,8] For example countries like Japan where less dairy is consumed have less breast cancer. Recent studies have similarly linked high dairy intake in adolescence with an increased incidence of adult prostate cancer.[9]

While nutritionists all generally agree on the nutrients that are needed for healthy growth and development, what is less well known is that these nutrients can be very easily obtained by a meatless vegan diet (supplemented with vitamins B12 and sometimes D). A plant-based diet likely contains less risk of and exposure to pesticide residue, bacterial contamination, unnatural hormones, less saturated fat, and caloric excess. It follows logically and been documented that vegans generally lead healthier longer lives.[10]

Marge Peppercorn, MD, *was a practicing pediatrician for over 35 years before retiring 5 years ago. Dr. Peppercorn graduated from Harvard Medical School.*

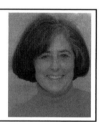

Preparing Children for a Healthy Future

Roberta S. Gray, MD, FAAP
Former Instructor and Assistant Professor of Pediatrics at Duke University Medical School
Current Private Consultant in Asheville, North Carolina

As a pediatric sub-specialist treating chronic childhood kidney and endocrine disorders, I am alarmed and disheartened to see the catastrophic deterioration in our children's health. The childhood obesity epidemic has resulted in diseases once almost unheard of in children before, such as type 2 diabetes, hypertension, high cholesterol, and kidney sclerosis, which are now commonplace in all pediatric practices. Not only are these youngsters unwell during their early years; they are destined to have devastating morbidity in adulthood and face early death.

The good news is that these serious childhood maladies are preventable with improved nutrition, particularly from a plant- based diet beginning in infancy. It has been shown that vegan/vegetarian children have excellent growth, adequate protein intake, strong bones, competitive physical strength, better cholesterol levels, and a drastically reduced prevalence of obesity compared to their peers who consume large amounts of meat and dairy products. They are spared the devastating consequences of obesity such as type 2 diabetes, with attendant cardiovascular and kidney disease.

It is not uncommon for pediatricians to discourage parents from providing their children a plant-based diet, largely because of ignorance. As a great service to our children, all pediatric healthcare providers should acquire the knowledge to effectively counsel families about the compelling lifelong health benefits of a plant- based diet.

fifteen

PROCESSED PEOPLE

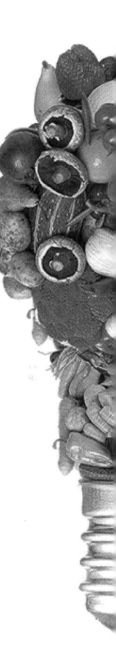

Since the 1950s our food production has vastly changed- putting chemicals, pesticides, genetically modified foods and toxins into our food system in order to make "cheap" food for more people. Along with our steady rise in meat and dairy consumption, our grocery store shelves have become far removed from the healthy, whole, nutritious foods our body needs. Our boxed and preserved foods are mere chemical concoctions designed to stimulate the "pleasure" areas of our brain. Yet, processed foods are as dangerous for our health as meat and dairy products and are directly implicated in the leading diseases today. Our body has no history of processing these chemicals. More worrisome is their true impact on our health which remains to be seen.

A huge amount of food today is overly processed and is mere fragments of the whole food it once was, as nature intended. The convenience mindset for our busy lifestyles means many of us compromise on fast food and processed food, feeling a sense of acceptance as these foods completely saturate our market-place.

As the following experts evidence, it is not enough to merely eat vegan. The advent of veganism has also brought an onslaught of unhealthy processed plant-based foods that also are not good for us. To be truly healthy and avoid becoming 'processed people' we need to select meals that are solely comprised of whole grains, nuts, fruits, legumes and vegetables.

The Pleasure Trap

Doug Lisle, PhD

The most widespread and destructive addiction in America today is junk food. Fast, cheap, oily, sugary, salty, rich, and unnatural – the foods of our time are terrible for our health. Never before have so many people had such easy access to cheap food products so brilliantly designed to artificially hyper-stimulate the pleasure centers in the brain.

The obvious result of our modern dietary environment is a population gorging itself on meat, fish, fowl, eggs, dairy products, refined carbohydrates, typically laden with oil and salt. The consequence is the epidemic of obesity, heart disease, diabetes, cancer, and dysfunction that we can easily observe on a daily basis. We also see the struggle of people trying to eat a bit more healthfully, and we see them try and generally fail. The reason for their failure is that their instinctual system is telling them "the food that tastes the best IS the best" – and it can be very hard to act against this innate signal. Like moths to the light, they get caught in a junk food pleasure trap.

The less-obvious outcome of this dilemma is psychological. It isn't merely the physical problems but also the emotional toll. People trying to lose weight, feel better, get healthier, and wanting to live their life to the fullest extent have to daily face their own internal critic who asks "Why don't you *just do it right*?!" Taken together, the mental and physical cost of the trap is great.

Since the 1990s, neuroscientists have been piecing together the story of food addiction. During that time, it was becoming increasingly apparent that there were two major neurochemical factors in addictive processes. Major drugs like cocaine, amphetamine, heroin, alcohol, and nicotine were all found to work in very similar ways – by creating an artificially excited euphoria, or a relaxed euphoria. These experiences were the result of the hyper-stimulation of the brain's pleasure pathways, via dopamine or the endorphin system. Some drugs primarily work by stimulation (like cocaine) and others by relaxation (like morphine and other opiates), and some drugs will do both. The super-normal experiences of either excited pleasure or relaxed pleasure from the use of these substances are the psychological basis of addiction.

It turns out that modern junk food works exactly the same way as drug addiction. People – and all other creatures – are designed to sense the degree of pleasure that an experience brings, and code that assessment in memory so as to prioritize the seeking of that stimulus in the future. If your mother-in-law feeds you some soup that tastes terrible to you, then you probably won't be craving it anytime soon. But if it tastes great, you will.

Now we can predict pretty accurately whether that soup will taste great to most people. All that is required is to make sure the soup tastes great is a supernormal stimulus. We would need to make sure that it hyper-stimulates the pleasure pathways of the brain, and that means we need to add artificially high concentrations of sugar, fat, and salt. Just look in your average grocery store, and observe what's there: some 60,000 products packed with sugar, salt and fat, nearly all of which were carefully designed as supernormal stimuli.

It should be no surprise that the result is an entire population that has been raised on supernormal unnatural food, and addicted to it. As the research evidence rolls in, it is becoming increasingly obvious that the artificial concentrations of sugar, fat, and salt in the modern food supply have caused an epidemic of food addiction. If there was any doubt about this before, surely there can be none now.

Every day, millions of people vow to eat less junk food, lose weight, and look and feel better. Some attempt to starve themselves, while others have their stomachs mutilated, and still others use a variety of drugs (appetite "suppressants") to fight back. Yet these solutions repeatedly fail, and the victims find themselves back at the trough, seeking the intense stimulation of drug-like food. The collective price of this situation, physically and psychologically, is staggering.

The good news is – there is absolutely a way out. The better educated you become; the better your prospects will be at defeating the most subtle thief of our modern wellbeing- unnatural foods. It takes just a few weeks of diligent effort to get out of the trap. You don't have to be perfect, but you have to be good. You have to go against your instincts, your cravings, and your habits for long enough to allow your body and mind to return to normal. For drug addiction, that process can take many months or even years. For the dietary pleasure trap, fortunately, chemical senses studies show that the escape is much shorter and easier. In a matter of a few weeks, you can be well on your way to enjoying your food as it was supposed to be enjoyed, and having the health and the life that you deserve.

Once you get the hang of it – once you know what it feels like to feel really good…you will know that healthy living is one of the best gifts you can ever give to yourself.

Douglas J. Lisle, PhD, *is the psychologist for The McDougall Program. He is the co-author of "The Pleasure Trap: Mastering the Hidden Force that Undermines Health and Happiness". Dr. Lisle also serves as the Director of Research for TrueNorth Health Center in Santa Rosa, California.*

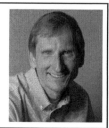

Avoiding the Road to Processville

John Pierre

The glorious nutrient-rich staples of a vegan diet I've grown accustomed to seeing decades ago have slowly metamorphosed into edibles one hardly recognizes today. An immense assortment of processed foods never before available in the past has begun to dominate and dictate our meals. These include vegan processed foods such as vegan soy burgers, veggie hot dogs, vegan pizza, cookies, donuts, brownies, pies, canned goods, and marshmallows, which have snatched plate space away from fresh fruits, vegetables, whole grains, raw nuts and seeds, potatoes, and legumes. As a result, we're beginning to see vegans suffer from predictable health consequences previously reserved only for individuals partaking in the Standard American Diet (S.A.D).

One of the reasons I'm seeing increased weight gain, higher blood pressure, cognitive decline, and lethargy in some individuals who switch to or follow a vegan diet is because a large portion of their meals revolve around vegan processed foods. These packaged, canned, and boxed items are often filled with sugar, salt, and oil. The more processed foods individuals eat, the less room remains in the stomach for wholesome, unprocessed plant foods. They get caught up in a situation I coined in my book The Pillars of Health as "Living in Processville."

The road to "Processville" often begins in childhood when we're introduced to chemically altered "foods" such as baby formula, salted and sugar-filled canned goods, and other concentrated, chemically modified products. Since we naturally gravitate toward sweet, salty, and fatty foods, processed foods become our preferred dietary choices. There's a biological reasons for this: hunger dominated much of human history and since energy-dense foods were scarce, nature programmed our brain to release opioids as rewards for eating certain types of foods. Consuming high-calorie, sweet, or salty foods triggered an opioid release that provided us with feelings of relaxation or stimulation, helping us feel better. These responses ensured we'd continue to seek out these types of foods in the future to stay alive.

Today, we no longer have a physical need to forage for our meals. Supermarkets are open around the clock, brimming with every imaginable type of food. Our brain, however, still continues to provide us with pleasant responses when we eat concentrated food products. This is why many of us continue to make processed foods the center of our menu plan.

Processed Food Problems

Just because a vegan processed food lacks animal ingredients does not necessarily mean that it's healthy. Refining a whole food condenses hundreds of calories into small, unsatisfying portions which can be consumed very quickly. When we eat fatty and sugary mixtures not normally found in nature, the natural mechanisms that signal our brain when we've had enough to eat become confused, and this can lead to overeating.

One of the biggest problems (among many) with processed foods is their lack of water content. If we put an apple into a juicer, we'd get apple juice as a result, but if we put seven bagels into a juicer, we certainly wouldn't get "bagel juice." When processed foods are consumed, they "suck" the water out of our system much like a sponge would, leading to dehydration.

Our bloodstream is about 92% water when it's healthy. Live blood, sometimes referred to as "the river of life," can become hypovolemic (thick) when we consume processed items. As the blood becomes thicker, the cells stop carrying oxygen efficiently. This is one reason why some people suffer from cerebral vascular insufficiency (not enough blood flow to the brain) which can cause them to not think clearly.

The high fat content of many processed foods causes a "wave" of fat to enter the bloodstream, which can last up to several hours. Compounding this problem, fat from a previous meal may not have fully cleared out of the bloodstream before the next wave of fat is eaten. This cycle can go on all day long–impeding oxygenation and the immune system, compromising healthy blood flow and zapping our energy.

Additionally many processed foods are filled with pro-oxidants. Pro-oxidants cause premature aging and harm the body and brain. Eating processed foods daily causes oxidation to accelerate all day long. In the last decade, I've seen premature cognitive and physical aging as some of the most common ailments affecting my clients.

What we need to do is gravitate towards foods with high water and antioxidant content such as fresh fruits and vegetables. These foods keep the bloodstream clean and healthy. The antioxidants found in fresh fruits and vegetables also act as the "body guards" to our brain and body to protect them from free radicals. Free radicals are rouge-like molecules that cause cellular damage. They can originate from various sources such as pollution, toxic heavy metals, and excess stress, and from dietary components such as preservatives, food colorings, and additives, among others. Since our brain is 60% fat by weight and free radicals are highly attracted to attacking fatty tissue, we need the power of antioxidants to help protect the brain and body. For example, if we cut an apple in half, it will start to turn brown or oxidize. But if we squeeze some fresh lemon juice onto the exposed apple tissue, it will stay fresher looking for a longer period because the antioxidants contained in the lemon juice act as natural protectors. Similarly, ingesting high-antioxidant foods (fruits and vegetables) accomplishes the same important achievements in our body.

As people transition from the Standard American Diet (S.A.D.) toward a plant-based diet, processed vegan foods can sometimes be initially helpful. They should be thought of as transitional foods; foods that help one make an easier switch from animal products to plant-based items. When we offer a child a baby blanket, we don't expect it to be carried to a job interview 20 years later. Similarly, vegan processed foods are not meant to be eaten forever.

I encourage my clients to wean themselves away from processed products. The key is to get back to the whole food, plant based diet we were eating decades ago. A whole foods plant-based diet is the best choice to make for superior health and the wellbeing of our planet. Avoid the road to "Processville" and get on track to a route that leads back to these whole, nutrient brimming foods.

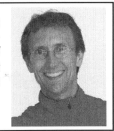

John Pierre *is a renowned nutrition and fitness consultant and is often referred to as a "Trainer to the Stars." John trains a wide range of clientele, including military personnel, hardcore athletes, Hollywood celebrities, rock-stars, and Fortune 500 executives. He is credited as being one of the first pioneers in the U.S. to create "brain-building" classes that enhance cognitive fitness in our geriatrics community as well as a pioneer in the area of geriatrics. John is the author of "The Pillars of Health". Visit www.johnpierre.com*

How to Avoid Becoming Processed People

Alan Goldhamer, DC, DO

We know that smoking, heroin, and cocaine are addictive, and that alcohol can be addictive. But we don't often think about how artificially concentrated foods packed with added sugar, oil, and salt can act just like drugs and over-stimulate the reward centers in our brains. Large food processing companies understand how this works, and they put a lot of effort into designing products that activate this addiction-like reaction and keep us coming back for more.

As a result of this dietary "pleasure trap," many people are suffering from the diseases of excess, such as diabetes, high blood pressure, cardiovascular disease, cancer, and arthritis. The average American diet is not health-promoting. Fortunately, adopting a health promoting diet is a cost effective and reliable way to achieve optimum weight and avoid, or even reverse, these diseases.

Our brains are wired to crave the most concentrated sources of food available. This ability to distinguish between calorically dense foods, such as bread and avocados, and foods less dense in calories, such as salad and vegetables, was a useful talent in times of scarcity. Yet today we don't think about why we prefer bread or pasta to salad or why gelato tastes "better" to us than non-fat ice cream. In the distant past we never had to think about what to eat — we just ate whatever we could get our hands on. Consequently, we are not well prepared to live in an environment of abundance, not only of natural foods, but of an environment of artificial food-like substances designed to seduce our brains and extract money from our wallets while making us sick. This modern dilemma can be called the "pleasure trap."

We don't live in an environment where we can rely on "instinct." We have to think about the food we put in our mouths if we want optimal health. There just isn't any getting around it. We need to avoid foods that have been processed to the extent that the fiber has been removed and the sugar and fat content has been concentrated or artificially enhanced. There are also many bad vegan choices out there too, and it is entirely possible to consume a totally vegan but terribly unhealthful diet.

Avoiding the "Pleasure Trap"

Two main keys to making wise dietary choices are: (1) Knowing the difference between caloric density and nutritional density, and (2) Understanding the role of food processing. That probably sounds a bit complicated, but it isn't, as we shall see.

First, density: fats and oils contain more calories per gram than any other nutrient, so any food that contains a lot of fat or oil is a high-calorie food. All natural foods contain some fat. Most vegetables and fruits have small amounts, while nuts, avocados, and olives, and, of course, meat and fish contain a lot more. Natural foods also contain carbohydrates and protein, and again, amounts vary. Grains and root vegetables are more concentrated and contain less water, and thus have more calories, while fruits and green vegetables are less calorie-dense. But natural foods, particularly fruits and vegetables, are very high in nutrients other than calories. These include vitamins, minerals, antioxidants and other compounds that are essential for our health. This is what is meant by nutritional density.

The second key to making wise food choices is an understanding of food processing. Processing is anything you do to the food to alter its natural state. You can cut it into smaller pieces or grind it to make it easier to eat or you can cook it, which softens it and makes the nutrients more available. These are fairly minimal forms of processing, and thus do not change the nature of the food too much.

But humans have learned to do a lot more than simple processing. We can squeeze the juice from fruit and get rid of all the fiber, leaving a very sweet, concentrated liquid. We can remove the fibrous coating from grain and grind it finely to make flour and then turn that into bread. We can extract the fat or oil from foods and bottle it to sell separately or add it to other foods. We can extract the sugar from cane, beets, or corn and then use the concentrated sugar to concoct foods that do not exist in nature. Essentially, we've learned to isolate the various components of foods that we find most desirable (mainly sugar, starch and fat) and combine them to form cookies, cakes, ding-dongs — you name it! And it is these artificially concentrated, food-like substances that lead us straight into the "pleasure trap."

The most effective way to get the proper nutrients without overdoing the calories is to include large quantities of high nutritionally dense and low calorically dense vegetables in your diet. This includes salad greens (lettuces, spinach, mescaline, sprouts), root vegetables (carrots, beets, jicama, sweet potatoes, white potatoes), dark greens (kale, chard, collards, purslane), cabbage family (broccoli, cauliflower, bok choy), and green beans and squashes. Most of these can be eaten raw, juiced, blended, steamed, or baked

In addition to vegetables, you will want to include fresh fruit and whole non-glutinous grains like brown rice, quinoa, millet or corn. Also, beans, including lentils and peas, may be included. Limited quantities of high-fat vegetable foods such as nuts and avocado may be included, depending on your goals regarding weight.

As a vegan diet lacks a significant source of vitamin B12, we recommend that all vegans consume 1000 mcg per day of vitamin B12 in the form of methylcobalamin in order to ensure that adequate vitamin B12, an essential nutrient, is present.

The Benefits of Detoxing

In our ancient ancestors' world, fasting occurred primarily by force not by choice when resources became scare. The ability of humans to fast was a biological necessity born from the disproportionate use of glucose by the brain. Were it not for the biological adaptation we call fasting, our species would never have survived. During fasting, the body preferentially utilizes fat for energy and breaks down other tissues in inverse order to their importance to the body.

Today, the environment of scarcity has largely been eliminated in the industrialized countries. Surprisingly, the physiological process of fasting, which once kept us from dying of starvation, can now help us overcome the effects of dietary excess from the consumption of "pleasure trap" chemicals including oil, sugar, and salt as well as highly processed flour products and factory farmed animal foods. Fasting can help counteract the effects of poor diet choices and to help make the transition to a health promoting diet.

In the past 30 years, I have witnessed the effect of medically supervised, water-only fasting in over 10,000 patients. Not every condition will respond to fasting. Genetic disorders and certain types of kidney disease, for example, may not respond but many of the most common causes of premature death and disability respond and often spectacularly.

The following are 6 of the most common conditions that respond and benefit from fasting:

1. Obesity: when fasting is fully implemented, in conjunction with adequate sleep and activity, consistent weight loss will occur that averages 1.5-2 pounds per week for women and 2-3 pounds per week for men.

2. High Blood Pressure: as overstimulation by artificially concentrated calories can confuse normal satiety signals, resulting in persistent overeating, fasting has been shown to be a safe and effective means of normalizing blood pressure

3. Diabetes: fasting, along with a health-promoting diet and exercise program, can dramatically increase insulin sensitivity and bring blood sugar levels under control.

4. Addiction to nicotine, alcohol, caffeine, and other prescription and recreational drugs: fasting can effectively establish healthy habits while eliminating the perceived need for addictive substances.

5. Autoimmune disorders (arthritis, lupus, colitis, Crohn's disease, asthma, eczema, psoriasis): fasting can help to normalize gut permeability and ease the transition to a health promoting, low inflammatory diet.

6. Exhaustion (physical and emotional): fasting can give your body and your mind a complete rest.

If your goal is to "recharge" your system, fasting may help you accomplish your goals and be a powerful tool to help your body do what it does best…heal itself

Alan Goldhamer, DC, DO, *is licensed as a DC in California and a DO in Australia. He served as the Adjunct Faculty in the Department of Naturopathic Medicine at Bastyr University in Kenmore, WA and at the Department of Continuing Education at Western States Chiropractic College in Portland, OR. He is the co-author of "The Pleasure Trap" and author of the "The Health Promoting Cookbook" as well as several published articles. He worked at the TrueNorth Health Clinic*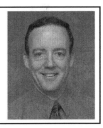

Minimize Toxins with a Plant-Based Diet

David Musnick, MD

One of the major benefits of a plant- based diet is that it greatly minimizes consumption of toxins and free radicals, thereby decreasing inflammation, improving brain function, protecting liver and kidney function and decreasing risk of cancer and heart disease.

Cattle, pigs and chicken are fed diets high in GMO corn and other feed that may have high toxin contents from fertilizers, herbicides, pesticides, metals, among other toxins in the food chain. The fat in these animals concentrate these toxins in their body which we subsequently digest. This is because toxins tend to be fat soluble and deposit in animal fat. In particular, nitrates are found in many processed sliced meat and jerky products and have been linked to colon cancer. Although many people think that ocean and fish products are healthy because they have omega 3 fats (only certain fish are high in omega 3 fats), in reality most farm raised fish are high in toxins such as dioxins, PCBs, and mercury. Ocean fish may be high in mercury and radiation.

In addition to the toxins stored in fat cells, cooking meat releases the toxin polycyclic Aromatic Hydrocarbons (PAHs). When fat drips onto a heat source and smokes, the smoke can transfer carcinogenic PAHs into meat that can contribute to cancer growth. The free radicals in meat and dairy products called AGES or Advanced Glycosylated End Products also cause inflammation throughout the body.[1] These free radicals are produced when proteins are browned which can happen with meats, butter, eggs etc.

Today artificial growth hormones such as Bovine Growth Hormones are widely used to promote growth in beef cattle, dairy cows and sheep. Recombinant bovine somatotropin (rBST), also known as rBGH, causes a significant increase in IGF-1 levels in milk from treated cows. These residues in the meat and dairy products may also increase the risk of cancer in humans. Using hormones this way is banned in most European countries and in Australia, Japan, and New Zealand but it is still common in U.S. beef cattle, dairy cows and sheep.

Vegan diets have many health benefits by avoiding toxins, however it just as important to avoid any deficiencies. Vegans may not get enough of certain nutrients from their diets including vitamin B12, iron, calcium, zinc, omega 3 fatty acids and vitamin D. Did you know that most supplements are put into gelatin capsules? Gelatin capsules are made out of the bone and skin of animals. In general it is better if your supplements are not in gelatin capsules. Having them in liquid, powder or tablet form is preferable. Ensure that your vitamins, minerals and other supplements for B12 are vegan based.

Plant- based eating is fun, tasty, and will contribute to a healthier you!

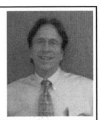

David Musnick, MD, *is a Sports Medicine and Functional Medicine MD physician in Bellevue Washington. He taught sports medicine at Bastyr University for 16 years and is on the teaching faculty of the Institute for Functional Medicine. He has been vegan for most of his adult life and his wife, Subhadra, is also vegan. For more information:* www.peakmedicine.com*.*

sixteen

DITCH THE DIETS!

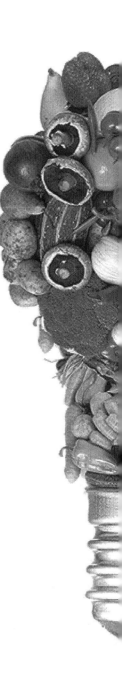

Walk into any bookstore or glance at the covers of grocery store magazines and the shelves are crowded with the new dietary secrets claiming to help us lose our fat fast. The problem with these diets, programs, and surgery options is that they don't last AND they don't properly nourish us. As more and more people are becoming overweight, these fad diets are becoming ever more ubiquitous in the market. Yet, most people today are still left searching for the next secret tip to shed those extra pounds.

As a society, we have become obsessed with counting carbs, gorging on lean meat protein, and frantically exercising away our midnight snacks. Chicken is the most touted "lean" meat. However, the EPIC Panacea study in Europe, one of the largest dietary studies to date, found that eating chicken is most associated with weight gain. In fact, researchers concluded that losing weight was directly associated with *decreasing* meat consumption.[1]

This chapter's weight-loss experts show why a plant-based diet will be your last diet. Unlike caloric dense meat and dairy that are also high in bad fats and contain zero fiber, plant-based foods are not only high in fiber and low in calories, but they also contain the right amount of antioxidants and nutrients to maintain a healthy weight. As obesity is the foundation for the leading non-communicable diseases such as heart disease, cancer and diabetes, it is a key step in combating our global chronic disease epidemic. We don't need to be counting calories, avoiding carbohydrates or working off our dinners at the gym. There is an easier and lasting solution to weight-loss and it starts with a plant-based diet.

Keep the Pounds Off the Right Way

Garth Davis, MD

Although I had practiced weight-loss surgery for a few years, I had never tied disease to nutrition. Nutrition was never even presented as an option for patients that had failed surgery, which is most directly associated to a poor diet. The only guidance was to do another surgery. However, I started seeing patterns among my patients. Everybody had the same diseases, was overweight, and was eating similar foods. Looking at their food logs – breakfast consisted of eggs and bacon and a healthy dinner was considered to be of either steak or chicken. As I was a big meat eater, my diet mirrored my patient's diet and so did my health problems. When I was diagnosed with high cholesterol, fatty liver, and high blood pressure at the young age of 35, I began to investigate the connection between diet and health.

As I researched America's healthcare in comparison to the health in other countries, I found that we are by far one of the sickest countries. We have the most heart disease, the most obese population, and the highest rates of diabetes and cancer. Where are we going wrong? Why are other populations in the world much healthier?

In the 1970s, President Nixon was attuned to the fact that as a population we were getting more overweight and heart disease was on the rise. He organized a commission together to discuss three questions: Why are we getting sick? Why are we getting fatter? Why are we getting heart disease? After reviewing the literature, the McGovern Committee came to the conclusion that eating animals is bad for our health.[1] When they came out with this conclusion the industry lobbied Congress, voted McGovern out of office and food libel laws were passed that you cannot really say that certain foods are bad for health. For instance, you can say eat a low-fat diet but you cannot say a low-meat diet, even though they are synonymous.

As a society we stopped talking about food, and started talking about nutrition in terms of macronutrients. This led to our national obsession with proteins, carbohydrates and fats. The common thought is we need a high intake of protein, and a low intake of carbs. We eat more protein than any other country in the world. The recommended daily allowance for protein for a man is about 57 grams, and for a woman it is about 45 grams. Yet depending on what you read, we eat between 100 and 130 grams of protein a day. This recommendation is two standard deviations above what we need to survive. The World Health Organization, and the FAO, came up with even lower recommendations.[2]

Yet when you look around the world at the healthiest people they eat categorically different to this message of "more protein, less carbs." Studies such as the Blue Zone Project looked at areas of the world where people were the healthiest and lived the longest.[3] This was not a diet program but a study of the culture to find commonalities that could influence healthier lives such as diet, family ties, exercise, etc. A definite theme throughout all of the Blue Zones was a plant-based diet. For instance the Okinawas live longer than anyone else in the world and have the least weight issues and zero cases of heart disease. The majority of the Okinawas diet is carbs. They eat about 80% carbs and it mainly comes from potatoes. Only about 8% of their calories come from protein.

Another Blue Zone is located in Loma Linda, New California, where the Seventh Day Adventists live. As not every Seventh Day Adventist is vegan, studies have been conducted to see how diet influenced disease by comparing those who were vegan to those people that ate meat, people that ate milk and cheese, and people that ate fish. What they found is that those who consumed more animal products were the least healthy.[4]

Beyond these studies, the research on plant-based diets is unbelievable. I have experienced the benefits of a plant-based diet as well as seen its benefits in my patients. While we tend to treat surgery as the answer, it is really just a tool. If we return to the same eating habits after surgery, we still will not be healthy. This is why many weight loss surgeries can fail and people can gain weight back. Instead I use the surgery to preface dietary changes, which are lasting. I instituted a medical weight-loss program at my clinic that teaches how to cook and eat plant-based meals. The benefits for my patients have been life-changing.

The Connection Between Animal Protein and Obesity

Weight gain and loss is all about calorie intake. Animal protein is almost always tied with fat and weigh-gain because it is extremely calorie dense. Dairy, and especially, cheese is very high in saturated fat and calories. The main reason that people eat or drink dairy is because they think calcium is good for our bones. Yet, when you look around the world, cultures that drink the most milk have the most bone disease. The Harvard Nurses Study also found that the nurses that drank the most milk had the most hip fractures.[5] This is because milk is very acidic and to buffer the acid, calcium from our bones is used as a neutralizer to bring our body's pH back to a more alkaline state. So, you are actually creating bone disease by drinking milk.

When we drink dairy-based protein shakes, eat chicken breasts, and steaks, we are consuming excess calories and excess protein. Our body can only process about 15g to 30g of protein at a time. When people digest anything over that such as taking 40g protein shakes, it becomes straight calories because your body cannot utilize that protein.

Extra calories turn into fat. Our high protein diet then is just adding to calorie excess.

Our body is actually designed to thrive on carbohydrates, not protein. Our body needs carbohydrates for energy and when there are no carbs our body panics. The common misunderstanding is that carbohydrates and insulin are the problem. The prevailing thought is that carbs cause an insulin rise and insulin creates fat. The truth is meat causes insulin to rise. Even if it was just insulin contributing to the problem, eating meat would still be a culprit. Meat consumption is intimately tied to not just weight gain but also chronic conditions that are killing us such as diabetes, heart disease, and cancers.

Eating Chicken is Not Eating Clean

Chicken is the most advertised meat for eating clean. Yet chicken is loaded with bacteria, antibiotics, and fat. The Epic PANACEA is the largest study that has ever been done on weight, and what we eat.[6] The study followed 500,000 people for 10 years and looked at a variety of variables from exercise to food logs to see what caused weight gain. They found that the food group most tied to weight gain is animal meat, and specifically chicken. The number one factor causing weight-gain, in Europe, over time is chicken. Since the study held calories equal, this finding is more than just a story about consumption. One possibility is people think chicken is a health food so they consume more of it.

Lose Weight and Reduce Heart Disease Risk

It is well documented that vegetarian diets, and specifically, vegan diets can reverse heart disease. Losing weight is fundamental to lowering heart disease risk because our cholesterol levels improve. When you eat meat, it causes a state of inflammation, causing your blood vessels to constrict. Meat causes a problem with the enzyme that breaks down arginine to nitrous oxide, which dilates your vessels. When we do not get nitrous oxide, the vessels constrict and blood flow is slowed. This can cause any built up plaque to rupture causing a heart attack.

In contrast, plants do not cause our vessels to constrict because they have a lot of arginine. Arginine actually causes vessels to dilate because arginine is broken up into

---

Reverse Diabetes in Days

Obesity lays the foundation for many chronic conditions including type 2 diabetes. Diabetes can be reversed in the first week with a Gastric Bypass and continual weight-loss, as it dramatically changes our hormones. When we bypass the pancreas, and the duodenum, we send food to the intestine quicker. This releases a hormone called GLP1, (used in many new medications) which causes the pancreas to create more insulin. Sugar production is stopped in the liver and the body becomes more sensitive to insulin. The effect is immediate: as your fat gets out of your cells, your cells become more sensitive to insulin.

nitrous oxide. The meat protein do not block the arginine conversion so you have easy conversion into nitrous oxides, which is what our body needs for healthy blood flow and flexible vessels.

We are Made to Eat Plants

Weight-gain can be attributed to the fact that we are not eating the food sources we are designed to consume. Most of our diet consists of processed foods with added sugar and salt and meat and dairy products. Yet our bodies are designed closer to herbivores than carnivores or even omnivores. For example, our teeth and mouth are not made to rip meat like a bear or a dog. Our jaws are made to move side-to-side for the express purpose of chewing plants. Additionally our digestive system is long and contains enzymes to break down starches from plant-type products. By comparison, carnivores have a short digestive tract as meat will putrefy. When we eat meat and dairy, meat sits in our digestive tract and putrefies, causing gastro-intestinal problems.

A high animal protein diet lacks fiber which is instrumental to maintaining a healthy diet and weight as it keeps us full and our blood sugar stable. When we are nutrient deficient it drives hunger. The beauty of a plant-based diet is it is nutrient dense but not calorie dense. A diet plan should look like this: oatmeal with berries, and some flax seed, and a grapefruit in the morning, salad for lunch, an apple and some almonds for snack, and then beans and vegetables for dinner. It is simple, easy, inexpensive, and tastes fantastic. When I switched to a plant-based diet, I felt amazing. Now when I look at my once favorite meal- a double cheeseburger- I see a heart attack.

Garth Davis, MD, *graduated from the University of Texas in Austin and attended medical school at Baylor College of Medicine. Dr. Davis completed his surgical residency at the University of Michigan in Ann Arbor where he was elected as Chief Administrative Resident. He is certified by the American Board of Surgery and is a Fellow of the American College of Surgeons and the American Society for Metabolic and Bariatric Surgery. Dr. Davis is a recognized expert in initial bariatric procedures as well as revisional bariatric surgery, and frequently gives lectures to both patient and physician audiences. As a leader in the field of bariatric medicine, Dr. Davis was again recently recognized as a Texas Monthly Super Doc and stars with his father, Dr. Robert Davis, on the hit docu-reality medical series, BIG MEDICINE. His recently published bestseller, "The Expert's Guide to Weight Loss Surgery" is available in bookstores nationwide.*

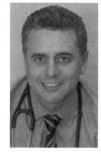

"Get Waisted"

Mary R. (Clifton) Wendt, MD

In the US, everybody was reasonably thin, until increased availability of meats, dairy, and processed foods changed the content of our diets in the 60s and 70s. As we consumed more processed food and our diets became heavily meat and dairy laden, our weight increased. Back then epidemiologists were scratching their heads, thinking that their data must be incorrect. How could people be getting so fat so quickly? Study after study reveals that our metabolic disorders arise from one core problem- our food.

For my first 10 years of practice as an internal medicine doctor, I worked hard to control these chronic diseases. I was an expert at the pharmaceutical options available for disease control. But I started to realize that I wasn't healing anybody. I treated patients with various metabolic disorders, like, high blood pressure, cholesterol, diabetes, as well as chronic rashes, lupus, or rheumatoid arthritis. I would see these patients every three months for check-ups to ensure the prescriptions were not damaging their liver or kidneys. As time passed, I saw my sickest patients grow even sicker, developing cancer and heart disease. Something needed to change, but I didn't know what.

Then about 5 years ago I was diagnosed as a pre-diabetic and had elevated cholesterol. I was only in my late 30s, I exercised almost every day, and I had a normal body weight. I ate a healthy high protein diet, and had about 3 servings of dairy per day. I thought I was on the right track.

When I started to read about how to control diabetes without medicine, I kept finding the same answers in the literature: decrease the consumption of animal protein and dairy in order to decrease inflammation, and metabolic disorders. Within 3 days of going plant-based, my sugar levels were back to normal range. When I visited my doctor 6 months later, my cholesterol had dropped by 70 points.

The change was so dramatic, and the substitutions were relatively simple: eating grains, and beans, instead of meat and chicken and choosing soy instead of dairy milk. I started sharing these simple changes with my patients, with extraordinary outcomes. I started to cure people, instead of just treating the conditions. A plant-based diet is anti-oxidant rich, high fiber, low fat foods, and makes it very, very easy to lose weight, because all of the food is so healthy and very low calorie.

The Question is: HOW do our meat and dairy diets lead to pre-diabetes, metabolic syndrome and undesired weight gain?

It all starts with choosing sources of healthy fats and proteins. When you are eating healthy fat, not in excess, you will not be adding it to your stomach or your backend. Your body uses healthy fats to create cell walls. Healthy fats keep the cell walls supple to transport proteins, and make cell-to-cell communication much easier. All of the fats that line your nervous system and cell walls are comprised of the fat from whole grains, beans, fruits, and vegetables.

The saturated fat from meat, eggs, and dairy greatly damage the health of your cell walls, and the lining of your nerves, throughout your nervous system. When we eat unhealthy fat, the cell walls become more rigid, and inflexible. This makes it very difficult for proteins to cross over the cell wall, for cell-to-cell communication. The cells have to work much harder to work together as a team.

The Lean Meat Myth

There is a common misunderstanding that white meat is significantly better than red meat. Trying to improve your health by converting from red meat to chicken is not enough. Chicken is still 30% calories from fat, and virtually all of those fats are unhealthy saturated fats. If you want to really make a difference, you are going to need to go from a piece of meat to wholesome grains and beans.

Arguably the bigger problem with eating meat and dairy is the form of protein itself. Many people think, "I need a good protein. I have got to make sure I get my protein from meat." But this is the wrong nutrient to focus on. It has been a disaster to our health to keep such a strong focus on that single macronutrient.

Animal proteins induce inflammation in the intestine, which causes the intestinal wall to become leaky. This means that bits of bacteria and protein that should stay inside the intestine are allowed to leak outside of the intestine. These proteins look very much like the proteins in your own body.

The body responds to this "bacterial translocation" using a variety of mechanisms that may contribute to autoimmune diseases. For instance, Type I diabetes, rheumatoid arthritis, and osteoarthritis are the result of the immune system responding to these inflammatory proteins. When you quit eating animal proteins, and choose plant proteins that do not inflame your gut, it stabilizes the gut wall, and prevents this inflammatory response to food.

The Connection Between Diabetes and Obesity

Diabetes is when the cells become resistant to insulin, and resistant to normal metabolism. While it is possible to control type 2 diabetes to a degree simply by restricting calories, more often than not we choose the wrong calories to restrict. For example, we may still eat the hamburger, but not eat the bun. We might eat it with mustard instead of ketchup to cut back on sugar. While we have ultimately cut back on calories in the short run, in the long run we are still eating high fat foods that will clog our arteries with fatty plaques. Eating plant-based foods makes it much easier to be able to eat an appropriate amount of food. Plus, whole healthy plant foods are loaded with fiber, which slows carbohydrate absorption and makes diabetes control a breeze.

"Everything in moderation" is a theme that pervades our approach to diet, diabetes, and losing weight. We have to rethink what moderation means from a world perspective. The whole idea of cutting a chicken breast in half and sharing it with your husband is not going to work in terms of getting healthier and losing weight. That is not moderation. If it is hard to completely change your diet overnight, you can take steps to first change the perspective of what moderation even means. Gradually reducing your meat portion each day is a great first step.

A Better Way

We pride ourselves on our independence. The irony is that we now allow ourselves to follow advice on nutrition driven largely by financial desires, and not by what is best for us at all. We need to seek the truth, and honor the science that supports a healthy diet with the exclusion of meat and dairy in favor of grains and beans. There is a better way.

Mary R. (Clifton) Wendt, MD *has been an Internal Medicine doctor for almost 20 years. Dr. Clifton regularly speaks at health and inspirational seminars, medical and heath conferences, corporate wellness events, Universities, and for private groups. Dr. Mary is the author of the best-selling book, "Waist Away", co-author of the book "Get Waisted: 100 Addictively Delicious Plant-Based Entrees", and CEO of the healthy weight loss program Get Waisted. Mary most enjoys spending time with her daughters, husband, and reveling in the deliciousness of decadent plant-based food!*

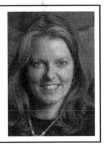

ReThinking Thin and Understanding Obesity

Mark Berman, MD

As a top executive at several Fortune 500 companies throughout her career, Meghan had worked extraordinarily hard, but she could not seem to control her weight. At 60, despite more than 20 major dieting attempts, she weighed 290 lbs. Along with that extra weight came diabetes, high cholesterol, depression, and daily heartburn. One day, Meghan lost consciousness and almost died, suffering a modest size stroke. Forced to rethink her lifestyle, she started exercising daily and changed her diet-eliminating meat, dairy, eggs, and fish. Before, a meal was only a meal if it had large amounts of animal protein. After losing 140 lbs from this new diet, most of her health conditions had fully reversed and she felt the best she had in her life.

Unfortunately, much about obesity and weight-loss is misunderstood and is perpetuated by diet fads and incessant advertisements for miracle weight-loss cures. Let's begin by clarifying and illuminating facts and trends key to rethinking obesity.

Understanding Obesity

Past generations have worked very hard to make food progressively cheaper, more convenient, and more plentiful over the last century. To their credit, phenomenal technological advances in the ability to mass grow, prepare, and market food, have enabled dramatic increases in cheap, readily accessible food.[1]

When it becomes easier and less energy-intensive to consume food, we gain weight. Millions of years of biological evolution are more powerful than our ability to *think thin*. Animal- based foods, like meat and dairy products, are calorically denser than plant foods. As animal foods typically contain lots of fat, which is by far the most energy dense food, whole plant foods are invariably lower in calories than animal foods. Unlike animal products, plants also contain fiber, which is critical to human health and has an added benefit of increasing satiety while providing no direct calories.[2] Today we consume considerably fewer whole grains then we did 100 years ago, when obesity rates were less than a tenth of what they are now.[3] It's not surprising in the least that as our diet has increased in processed foods and animal foods, so has our collective waistline expanded.[4]

We are now beginning to understand how excess food intake leads to the metabolic diseases associated with weight gain and obesity. A key emerging mechanism has been dubbed *meta-inflammation*, a complex set of interactions between our gut bacteria (aka microbiome) and our immune system in response to excess nutrients.[5] Meta-inflammation is a chronic low-grade inflammation that impairs specific cells in the liver, pancreas, blood vessels, brain, and fat cells, ultimately leading to type 2 diabetes, heart disease, and other inflammatory diseases.[6] Meta-inflammation is not only made worse by extra calories in general, but also by diet-induced changes in the gut microbiome. While much about this mechanism is yet to be understood, we do know that over time eating meat alters the gut microbiome in deleterious ways.[7] This can possibly explain why meat eaters have a harder time maintaining a normal weight then vegans and vegetarians.[8]

If more protein intake was helpful in preventing obesity, our obesity rates would be amongst the world's lowest. Average protein consumption far exceeds the amount we need and both per capita and total animal protein intake have increased significantly in the past century.[9] What is shameful about the current protein obsession, often promoted by poorly educated health enthusiasts, is that excess protein is likely very harmful. For instance, higher protein intake increases the rate of thyroid cancer,[10] and animal protein in particular is associated with higher rates of type 2 diabetes,[11] as well as with increased all-cause mortality when paired with a low carb dietary pattern.[12]

Once someone gains excess weight, it leads to conditions that further weight gain—*creating a "snowball" effect.* For example, obesity and weight gain lead to osteoarthritis, obstructive sleep apnea, and insulin resistance. Pain and fatigue from these conditions limit physical activity and increase the desire to eat or an inability to efficiently utilize dietary carbohydrates, which promotes overeating.[13] This snowball effect can explain why so many have difficulty losing weight and why national prevention strategies are critical. On the flip side, there is a positive snowball effect that we see in people who lose weight and experience relief from so many health problems as a result.

The idea of moderation has failed. The notion that we can simply eat everything and anything in moderation and this will solve the obesity epidemic is absurd. What you might consider moderate would be considered great excess by someone just like you living 50 or 100 years ago. We will only solve obesity if we change what we now consider normal.

We have an increased collective awareness of the harm of food marketing, food consumption persuasion, growth in portion sizes, and inadequate safe places to be active and play. Of all American adults, 83% are actively doing something to lose or maintain their weight.[14] Unfortunately diets are by nature short lived, and exercise is not the major determinant of weight. A recent study showed that even though people are exercising more, our collective waistline nonetheless worsened.[15]

It is time to make a massive change. Ultimately, we need to decrease the net amount of calories and to do this requires an immense reduction in the amount of animals we consume.

Mark Berman, MD, *is an internal medicine physician and social entrepreneur whose work focuses on obesity, plant-based diets, and health information technology. Dr. Berman was born in South Africa and grew up in Canada. He studied physical therapy at McGill University, medicine at Yale University, and primary care internal medicine and population medicine at Harvard's Brigham and Women's Hospital. He was a Doris Duke Clinical Research Fellow at UCSF and later served as the Special Assistant to the CEO and President for Childhood Obesity at the Robert Wood Johnson Foundation. At present, Dr. Berman directs and practices lifestyle and obesity medicine at One Medical Group in San Francisco. He is also a director of the American College of Lifestyle Medicine. (San Francisco, CA)*

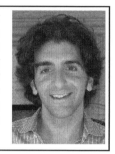

Every Woman's Favorite Weight-Loss, Cancer-Prevention Diet

Racheal L. Whitaker, MD

My gastric reflux was so bad it would wake me at night. I had been having episodes of reflux off and on for years, and accepted it as par for the course. As a doctor specializing in obstetrics and gynecology, I knew the rules—typical foods to avoid (coffee, citrus foods, alcohol) as well as the medications to take. However, despite following these guidelines my discomfort and symptoms only worsened. As I knew the consequences of long-term irritation of my esophagus by gastric acid, such as difficulty swallowing, irreversible changes in my voice, and even cancer of my esophagus, the doctor finally had to see a doctor.

An upper GI scope (light-guided examination of the upper gastrointestinal—GI—tract) revealed that the entire lining of my esophagus and stomach was very irritated and inflamed. I was placed on Nexium (an expensive medication that inhibits stomach acid) twice daily, and given information on foods to avoid (all of which I was well aware).

After listening to the *Forks Over Knives* documentary, about food and health, I cleared my refrigerator of eggs, cheese, and meats, and went shopping for vegetables and fruit to start my vegan journey. Within 7 to 10 days, I was able to decrease my Nexium to once daily and was no longer waking up in the middle of the night searching for my apple cider vinegar. After another week, I was no longer requiring Nexium at all. Quite, honestly, I was in disbelief. For years, I had been speaking to patients about proper diet to control/cure their diabetes, stop obesity, and decrease blood pressure, but dairy and meat had always been okay on my list of options.

The Connection Between Diet and Obesity

Meat and dairy products are leading contributors to obesity as they are calorie-dense foods that are low in nutrients and high in fat. When we fill up on fiber-rich, plant-based foods, we become full and satisfied with a high amount of nutrients and a low amount of calories. We are also satiated longer because the digestion is slower and steady. When we eat, stretch receptors in our stomach tell us when we are full. It takes approximately 20 minutes for these receptors to communicate to our brain that the stomach is full, and our brain then tells us to stop eating.

When we eat calorie-dense foods that are low in nutrients and high in fat, simple carbohydrates and sugar, it takes much more food to become satiated. Simple carbohydrates and sugars also result in the release of insulin. Excess insulin causes resistance in its ability to control blood sugar levels and results in storage of fat around our waistlines. Excess fat anywhere on our bodies is not good for our health, but fat storage at our midsections is the worst. The fat is essentially surrounding our vital organs (heart, lungs, liver, pancreas) and is associated with higher risks of heart disease, fatty liver disease, diabetes, and visceral cancers (e.g. cancers of the stomach and pancreas). By eating plant-based foods, we don't get unhealthy cravings, we maintain healthy insulin levels, reduce our cancer risks, and maintain healthy weights.

The Connection Between Obesity and Cancer in Women

For women, obesity also increases the risk for benign conditions such as uterine fibroids, urinary incontinence, and pelvic organ prolapsed, and the more serious conditions such as breast and uterine cancers.[2] These cancers are often associated with hormones, and excess fat cells increase the amounts of circulating hormones.

Breast Cancer: 1 in 8 women will get breast cancer in her lifetime.[3-4] While there are some contributing factors that we can't control such as genes and the environment we are exposed to, we can control our diet and weight.

One of the main female hormones is estrogen. Estrogen is good for us in moderation and at normal levels. In women who are normal weight, estrogen levels are low. In overweight women, fat cells are a source of higher levels of estrogen. In particular, the breasts have a large number of estrogen receptors. With the combination of higher amounts of circulating estrogen and a dense amount of estrogen receptors in the breast, the risk for breast cancer in obese patients increases.

Endometrial Cancer: Cancer of the lining of the uterus also results from the effects of high amounts of circulating estrogen. It is the fourth most common cancer in women and one of the biggest risk factors is obesity.[2] Endometrial cancer is 2 to 4 times more likely in overweight and obese women, despite menopausal status.[5]

Because overweight women have excess hormones from fat cells, the normal menstrual cycle often becomes disrupted, and these women tend to stop ovulating regularly.

When irregular shedding of the endometrial lining occurs, the lining becomes thick and menstrual periods become erratic and heavy. Eventually the thickened lining becomes disorganized and precancerous changes occur that turn into cancer if not addressed. Since endometrial cancer is almost always seen in women who are overweight, losing and maintaining a healthy weight greatly decreases uterine cancer incidents. Unfortunately, fad diets and pills get more attention than the easy, healthy, and less expensive way.

Although the time that we spend on this earth is increasing, many of us merely exist instead of living, simply due to our diet choices. When we load up on raw vegetables and fruit, we get the nutrition we need and the satisfaction of being satiated without the calorie load.

Racheal L. Whitaker, MD, *is a Board Certified Obstetrician/Gynecologist. She received her Bachelor's degree in Biology from Dillard University in New Orleans, Louisiana, and her MD degree from Meharry Medical College. She completed her internship and residency training at Ochsner Medical Center in New Orleans where she served as Executive Chief Resident. Dr. Whitaker has served as Assistant Professor in the Department of Obstetrics and Gynecology at Louisiana State University Health Sciences Center. She is a member of the prestigious Alpha Omega Alpha Honor Society. Dr. Whitaker is author of Cold Knife Conization of the Cervix, a chapter in: Mayeaux, E.J. Jr. MD The Essential Guide to Primary Care Procedures. Philapelphia: Lippincott Williams & Wilkins. Dr. Whitaker is a women's health lecturer, and believes in empowering the total woman— mind, body and soul.*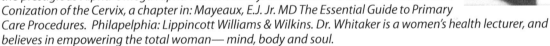

The High Protein- Low Carb Fad

Magda Robinson, BM

High protein/low carbohydrate diets that consist of less than 40% carbohydrates and at least 30% protein (mainly animal protein) are typified by the popular *Atkins Diet, South Beach Diet,* and *Dukan Diet.* These diets are widely promoted for weight loss in the media and in many commercial weight-loss programs. But are they to be recommended? The answer is no.

Overloading the body with protein is unhealthy and detrimental to liver and renal function. Additionally unless the diet is low in saturated fat and animal protein, and high in fiber, high protein diets can lead to a host of medical complications such as high cholesterol, high blood pressure, cardiovascular disease, type 2 diabetes, osteoarthritis, depression, and several different cancers.

The Myth Behind High Protein/Low-Carbohydrate Diets

The theory behind high protein/ low carb diets centers on the principles of blood sugar, insulin, the process of "fat burning," and ketosis. According to this theory, depriving the body of carbohydrates forces it to use up its fat stores to provide energy, as in the process of fasting. Allegedly, this diet causes insulin levels to fall, and because insulin is a "fat-storing hormone, the net result is fat loss. This theory, however, is flawed and the benefits of a high protein/low carb diet are a myth. The problems with this diet are as follows:

Ketosis is not essential for weight loss and has dangerous side effects. The fat oxidation process is incomplete and produces ketones, a toxic by-product. Elimination of the ketones via the kidneys causes loss of both water and sodium, resulting in false weight loss, dehydration, and offensive halitosis. Ketosis also causes an acidotic state in the blood, encouraging the leaching of calcium out of the bones in order to neutralize the acidity.

Low-carbohydrate diets contain excessive amounts of protein and fat. Protein cannot be stored in the body, so excess protein is converted into glucose for fuel and fat for storage. Excessive levels of animal protein are particularly detrimental to kidney function. It is recommended that diabetics consume no more than 16% protein (or 80g a day).[1] However, substituting soy protein for animal protein does not have the same detrimental effect and causes less stress on the kidneys.[2]

Low-carbohydrate diets are seriously deficient in various vitamins, minerals, and

fiber. (The Atkins diet demands that 63 different vitamin, mineral, and fiber supplements should be taken to make up the shortfall.) There have even been cases of people losing their eyesight on low-carbohydrate diets due to the development of optic neuropathy from thiamine (vitamin B1) deficiency.[3] The lack of whole grains is particularly unhealthy, as a diet rich in whole grains is known to reduce the risks of developing diabetes by up to 40%, cardiovascular disease by 26%, and stroke by 43%. Also, colon cancer risk is reduced by 55% in people consuming at least 25g of fiber a day.[4] Current medical recommendations are to include a fiber intake of 25g to 50g a day, of which 7g to 13g should be soluble fiber (found in oats and barley, fruits, and vegetables), which improves glycemic control and lowers total and LDL cholesterol.

It is a myth that only carbohydrates cause insulin release. Certain amino acids and fat are also known to stimulate the insulin response. The more saturated the fatty acid, the greater the insulin release. The accumulation of fat in muscle cells also causes impaired insulin-mediated glucose intake, or insulin resistance. In the long term, saturated fat has a lipotoxic effect on the beta cells of the pancreas, causing impaired insulin synthesis and progression to diabetes.

Without a minimum of 130 g carbohydrate a day, the body eats up its own muscle tissue to provide the essential substrates for the glucose-dependent tissues such as the brain, neurons, red blood cells, testes, and renal cortex cells. Loss of muscle tissue is the exact opposite of any dieter's aims.

Carbohydrate-rich meals induce optimum conditions in the brain for the synthesis of serotonin. This is the neurotransmitter responsible for feelings of elevated mood. Serotonin is made from the amino acid tryptophan. Protein-rich meals reduce the flux of tryptophan into the brain, and carbohydrate-rich meals increase the flux of tryptophan into the brain.[5] This can attest to why low-carbohydrate dieters tend to suffer from lower mood than normal-carbohydrate dieters.[6] (Note that plant proteins such as soy, pumpkin seeds, sesame seeds and sunflower seeds all contain more tryptophan than turkey.)

Low-carbohydrate diets have numerous side effects because they contain too much animal protein, saturated fats, and cholesterol and too little fibrous complex carbohydrates, and not enough fruit, vegetables, or whole grains.

The Link Between Eating High Protein Animal Products and Obesity

There is a direct connection between eating animal protein and weight gain leading to obesity. A review of forty studies associated people who are vegetarian or vegan with having reduced body weight, on average between 3 kg and 13 kg less than meat eaters (up to 20% slimmer).[7] In fact, one study reported that vegetarians have an average BMI of over 2 points lower and vegans over 5 points lower than meat eaters.[8] Conversely, consumption of red meat, sausages, and hamburgers are all significantly associated with a higher risk of weight gain.[9,10]

Meat-based diets are high in fat and protein but contain zero fiber. Protein above normal body requirements (0.8g/kg/day) cannot be stored, and is converted into fat and carbohydrate. As there is protein in all foods, aside from pure oils and pure sugars, eating a diet rich in whole grains, legumes, and vegetables supplies all the protein that the body needs. For example, per calorie, dried soy mince contains 63% protein; broccoli contains 45% protein; lentils contain 36% protein; and even oranges and raspberries contain 10% protein.

Animal products also contain zero fiber, which adds to weight-gain. Fiber decreases the energy density of the food, and leads to reduced energy intake due to increased satiety. Indeed, a higher intake of fiber is linked to a reduced BMI, while a lower intake of fiber is associated with obesity.[11] The only source of fiber is plant foods such as whole grains, legumes, nuts, seeds, fruit, and vegetables.

The connection between obesity and the consumption of animal products is illustrated in the health crisis epidemic occurring in Japan. Since the 1950s, when the Japanese changed their diet, meat consumption rose 10-fold, egg consumption nearly 9-fold and dairy consumption nearly 20-fold, all at the expense of carbohydrate (rice and grain) consumption.[12] As the Japanese gradually incorporated typical Western diets, even while keeping caloric intake consistent, the rates of obesity, type 2 diabetes, bowel, and breast cancer increased dramatically.[13]

Thus the answer to healthy weight loss is not to *reduce* carbohydrates, but to *replace* refined or bad carbohydrates, such as white bread, white rice, biscuits, and desserts with unrefined complex carbohydrate such as brown rice, whole-grain bread, oats, barley, steamed potatoes, and quinoa. I highly recommend a plant-based diet to anyone.

Magda Robinson, BM *was born in Oxford, UK, and studied psychology at university, followed by a degree in medicine. After qualifying as a doctor, she began her career as a GP, and subsequently developed a keen interest in nutrition. She has been practicing as an obesity management consultant in London, UK for 18 years. She specializes in using nutrition to aid weight loss and to combat cardiovascular disease, diabetes, and cancer. She is a member of the Association for the Study of Obesity, and the National ObesityForum. She recently published* **Eat Carbohydrates: Get Thin (And Healthy)** *available online.*

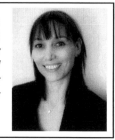

Eat to Lose Weight

Joseph Gonzales, RD, LD

Sick of exercising? It seems we are always pointing to exercise as a staple for weight loss when the truth is it plays little role, if any, with maintaining a healthy weight.

Most people indulge in a bag of chips or burger with the expectation of later "burning" off the dietary calories. But the average person is not going to achieve weight loss by exercising post meals. Physical activity has changed very little in recent decades but calorie intake has greatly increased, accounting for virtually all observed weight gain. What we need to focus on is what we are putting into our mouths, not how many calories we can burn.

The Physicians Committee for Responsible Medicine (PCRM) has conducted randomized research control trials on plant-based nutrition and weight loss for decades. Our latest and largest publication to-date found that a low-fat vegan diet (with no portion control, carbohydrate counting, or changes in exercise) could reduce body weight by roughly a pound per week and lower blood sugar and cholesterol levels as well as, if not better than, typical medications.

The study tracked 291 GEICO employees who were either overweight or diabetic. Over 18 weeks, half of the participants were counseled on how to follow a low-fat vegan diet and choose low glycemic foods (such as oatmeal, barely, beans, berries, and green leafy vegetables). The results were impressive: all intervention participants lost weight, LDL cholesterol lowered by 13 points, and those who were diabetic lowered their A1c (measurement of how much sugar is attached to the blood) by 0.7 points. By comparison, a typical diabetes medication can only lower A1c by 0.5 points. Interestingly, not only were participants on the vegan diet losing weight and lowering their cholesterol, they were commenting on other health benefits such as their arthritis pain was decreasing, or their energy had improved!

When you change to a plant-based diet, you are going to tackle every spectrum of health. The same diet working for a multitude of diseases? This is something every healthcare professional needs to know, and every one of their patients deserves to know.

Joseph Gonzales, RD, LD, *worked the past 4 years as a staff dietitian for the Physicians Committee for Responsible Medicine where he spearheaded the Food for Life program. Mr. Gonzales conducts lectures at hospitals and universities. Currently he assists the Vegetarian Nutrition Dietetic Practice Group - a group of the Academy of Nutrition and Dietetics. Mr. Gonzales earned his Bachelor of Science degree in nutrition at Bastyr University and completed his supervised dietetic internship through the Coordinated Program of Dietetics at Washington State University.*
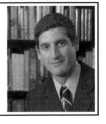

seventeen

THE SKIN SECRET TO ANTI-AGING

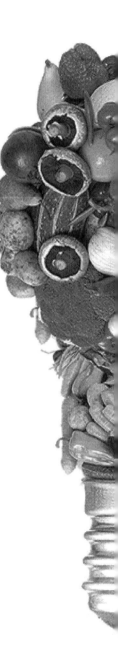

Our skin acts as a mirror- reflecting our true state of wellness from the inside out. Women reportedly spend $426 billion dollars a year on beauty products.[1] We spend hours in front of the mirror and an astronomical amount of money on our appearance, but our best skin care products are plant-based foods. Filled with antioxidants and anti-inflammatory agents, plant-based foods fight off free radicals that damage our skin and accelerate the aging process.

As the following experts attest, from dry to oily skin and acne and eczema to wrinkles, what we eat has a profound effect on our skin. Meat and dairy products flush our cells with toxins, altering and damaging our cells and thus leading to aging. This is because meat consumption is directly associated with inflammation, the building blocks of disease, and it breaks down collagen and elastin in our skin. Vitamin C is vital to collagen- which repairs damaged cells and gives us that smooth, wrinkle-free complexion. Dairy, a known allergen, is a leading contributor to some of our most common skin conditions including acne. We spend close to $2 billion a year alone on trying to rid ourselves of those pesky blemishes.[2] Yet these creams, prescriptions and lotions can be extremely harsh and leave our skin more dry and damaged than before.

We can rekindle and rejuvenate a glowing complexion by choosing antioxidant rich food. It's the simplest secret to looking and feeling younger.

The Effect of Food On Skin- And Everything Else!

Michael Klaper, MD

My colleagues and I in clinical medicine spend the vast majority of our time in operating rooms, emergency departments and outpatient offices largely cleaning up the wreckage of the "Standard American Diet." Whether they choose to recognize it or not, the medical practice of every physician across the medical specialties - from internists to surgeons, from pediatricians to radiologists, from gastroenterologists to dermatologists, rheumatologists to public health and preventive medicine specialists – is largely focused upon repairing the damage resulting from what our patients are eating.

The time has come – for physicians and patients alike - to recognize that our food is chemically "alive." The nutrients – or contaminants – from every meal and snack flow through our cells within minutes of eating, playing our un-coiled DNA like a piano, turning on some genes and turning off others – inducing the production of some enzymes and inhibiting the production of others that determine who we are and how well we function. This means that every bite does matter. Food affects our functioning on the most fundamental levels, moment to moment, year in and year out - from determining our skin's oil production to turning cancer-promoting genes on or off.

Eating a fast-food hamburger predictably sends a witch's brew of denatured muscle proteins, saturated fats, pro-inflammatory arachidonic acid, endotoxin, and sialic acid Neu5Gc, growth-promoting hormones, along with antibiotics and bio-concentrated pesticide residues though the bloodstream. This toxic mixture is bathing every cell in the body within minutes of swallowing the meal and can promote cellular reactions that lead to inflammatory diseases in artery walls, inhibit the function of insulin receptors and promote the growth of several kinds of cancers.

The polluted river of pizzas, chili dogs and their ilk, flowing through one's tissues creates a far different symphony of cellular reactions than an antioxidant-rich meal of a colorful fresh salad, hearty lentil stew, steamed green and yellow vegetables and fresh fruit for dessert. The phytonutrients in these foods generally promote healing and stability of tissues, and, thus, play a key role in the prevention and reversal of most of our common degenerative diseases.

We can look at any organelle in the cell such as the mitochondria, ribosomes, Golgi bodies or endoplasmic reticulum and see how flooding them with arachidonic acid,

Neu5Gc and other substances from animal-based foods might adversely affect its structure and function. The interaction between our food and the genes on our chromosomes that determines the function of our cells is called nutrigenomics. Understanding that relationship gives us tremendous power to stop using foods to create disease states in our body and to start using each meal to foster deep and true healing.

The influence diet has on the cellular level is even more apparent when we look at the telomeres at the ends of our chromosomes, the tightly wound coils of our DNA that contain all our genetic information that let's our cells function normally. Telomeres are special regions on the ends of the chromosomes that keep the chromosomes healthy and protect them from damage. Long, healthy telomeres are directly correlated with long, healthy lives; conversely, the shorter the telomere length, the shorter the lifespan.[1] As we get older and subject ourselves to the chemical barrage of modern life, we can see under the electron microscope how eating a diet filled with free radicals and oxidizing agents damages our telomeres. When we eat food that abuses our chromosomes, the damage is akin to going outside in the snow without a jacket. The telomeres become damaged and shortened, and expose the DNA within the chromosomes to genetic injury that can affect every aspect of cellular function - and echo down the generations through every subsequent cell division. Conversely, we can see evidence under the same electron microscope of injured, shortened telomeres visibly healing and becoming longer as plant-based nutrients exert their restorative effects.[2]

All this has profound implications for all practicing physicians, like dermatologists, most of who apparently still do not believe that their patient's diet affects the health of their skin, especially in cases of acne. There are now numerous studies showing how cow's milk products, with their powerful concoction of growth factors such as estrogens and IGF-1 can launch a cascade of reactions that can play a direct role in acne eruptions.[3]

Of course, our diet alters everything in the skin, from blood flow that determines wound healing, to the lubricating quality of skin oils, to the populations of bacteria living down in the hair follicles. Since most skin conditions have a strong component of inflammation - which can be promoted by many factors in animal-based foods - dramatic improvements in skin conditions such as acne[4], atopic dermatitis[5], and psoriasis[6] are predictably observed when the diet becomes one based upon whole, plant-based foods.

We find ourselves in a seminal time for medicine and public health as we recognize each individual's power to largely determine the course of their health – and, thus, their lives - though their food choices. As physicians, nutritionists, and scientists, we must stop hiding behind the linguistic barrier of "Etiology Unknown" when it comes to most of health challenges in the Western world. As we grow ever more ravenous for a meat-heavy, fast-food diet, waistlines expand, children become obese, and the costs for diabetes and stroke care alone threaten to bankrupt our nation, we must stop overlooking the obvious. "It's the food!" Physicians, government policy makers, food producers - and all of us - need to grasp that the molecules that we choose to flush through our cells on a daily basis hold the key to preventing and overcoming disease and to creating abundant health and optimal function. Such a powerful tool, and it is available to everyone. "Let food be your medicine," indeed. As the title of this book so aptly states, the time has come for scientists and physicians who want to effectively treat the cause of diseases – not just to deal with symptoms - to rethink food.

Michael Klaper, MD, *has over 40 years of experience in general practice and acute care medicine. He practices in California and Hawaii as well as counsels patients through private virtual consultations. He hosted the popular radio program "Sounds of Healing" on WPFW in Washington D.C. and KAOI on Maui, Hawaii for over 10 years. Dr. Klaper contributed to 2 PBS television programs, "Food for Thought," and the award-winning, "Diet for a New America." As a pilot, he served as an advisor to the NASA project on nutrition for long-term space colonists on the moon and Mars. Dr. Klaper practiced acute care medicine in New Zealand for 3 years and currently serves on the staff of the TrueNorth Health Center in Santa Rosa, CA. Visit DoctorKlaper.com*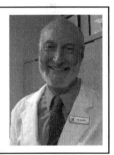

Vitamin C: The Key To Healthy, Younger- Looking Skin

Clayton Moliver, MD, FACS

Our bodies are constantly breaking down and sustaining micro injuries to our cells that can potentially damage our DNA. As a practicing Plastic Surgeon for 23 years, I can see this damage on a cellular level. For example, we can actually feel the elasticity of the vessels. The firmer the artery indicates a less healthy patient. Our body is very good at consistently repairing itself. However, our body cannot repair itself without the proper nutrients. Vitamin C, obtained from plant-based foods, is vital to aiding collagen in healing and repairing daily micro injuries through cell recovery, acceleration, and replenishment. When our body cannot properly repair itself, it weakens the tissue, allowing harmful bacteria into the tissue. Over time this leads to the breakdown of this wonderful machine we call our bodies.

When it comes to recovery, Vitamin C promotes wound healing; as it is absolutely essential to collagen cross-linking. Collagen is part of the connective tissue in the skin that helps keep it firm, supple, and in the constant renewal of skin cells. Collagen is made of amino-acids that comprise about 30% of the protein within the body. Collagen is essentially the protein "cement" within the skin that holds everything together and greatly influences the quality of our hair, skin, and nails.[1]

Many of my patients come to me for filler or collagen to make their skin thicker, a procedure that ultimately makes a person look younger. One type of collagen is called elastin, which is responsible for the elastic nature of young people's skin. Although collagen depletion happens at different rates depending upon our genetic make-up, generally we begin to lose elastin around 50 years of age. Essentially our skin changes from being more like Spandex to that of linen. For example, when you get older and bend your wrist backwards, you can see the skin folding on top of the wrist. This is because your skin has lost the spandex quality or collagen, and becomes more relaxed.

Besides the natural process of aging, the 3 main factors that cause our skin to breakdown are sun damage, smoking, and lack of Vitamin C. Vitamin C is an integral part of a cell that requires a sustained release throughout the day, not just 1 massive dose. The best way to achieve this release is through food, and, in particular, vegetables.

Our heavily meat based diets prove problematic for recovery and healing as they do not contain Vitamin C. There are 3 mammals in the world that do not produce Vitamin C: primates, fruit bats, and guinea pigs. Studies on guinea pigs indicate that if they are deprived of Vitamin C, their life expectancy is halved. By contrast, no other carnivorous animal needs Vitamin C. This is one mechanism that distinguishes humans from being carnivores or even omnivores.

A plant-based diet provides a continuous source of Vitamin C, as well as other vital nutrients. Since Vitamin C is water soluble, it is not enough to take a vitamin or supplement because they wash through our body in a matter of hours. Rather, our body requires a slow release of Vitamin C which can be adequately provided through consumption of plant-based foods throughout the day.

As surgeons concerned with repair and recovery, we finally understand that diet is unbelievably important. Humans are currently the only species that eats differently from the species closest to us, and we are experiencing the backlash in our current spike in chronic, degenerative conditions. We have to protect and maintain our bodies from the environmental toxins, and a first step is looking at our food choices and feeding our bodies the right ingredients.

Clayton Moliver, MD, FACS, *is Board Certified in General Surgery, and Plastic Surgery. Dr. Moliver is a graduated of Texas Tech University School of Medicine. He was a Clinical Professor at The University of Texas Medical Branch, Department of Surgery, Division of Plastic Surgery. Dr. Moliver has been published in the Aesthetic Surgery Journal, Texas Medicine, and Southern Medical Journal. He is a retired major in the United States Army Reserves.*

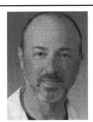

Clean, Clear, Radiant Skin

R. Saravanan, BHMS

As the human body's largest organ, the skin can reflect our state of health and well-being. The skin needs proper nourishment with the right type of foods as it plays a vital role in protecting the body from microorganisms, mechanical damage, ultraviolet radiation, and dehydration as well as excreting toxins such as urea, uric acid, and ammonia. While we tend to overlook the dietary connection, unhealthy eating habits negatively affect our skin condition, and can even increase the rate at which our skin ages. Acne and eczema are common skin diseases which can be directly related to the consumption of animal-based foods.

Acne is mostly caused by the increased level of sebum (oily secretion that lubricates the skin) under the influence of hormones such as androgens and insulin-like growth factor (IGF-1). Animal protein in meat and dairy products naturally contain IGF-1 growth factors that stimulate the body to make even more IGF-1. This in turn raises androgen levels leading to acne.[1] Today it is common practice on dairy farms to inject cows with artificial growth hormones called recombinant bovine growth hormone (rBGH) to increase milk production. This can also increase the IGF-1 levels in milk. This increase in IGF-1 in dairy products due to rBGH contributes to various health issues ranging from acne to cancer.

Studies show an association between dairy consumption and acne. One study looking at the diets of 47,000 adolescent girls and diagnoses of severe acne found a 95% confidence indicating the positive association between intake of total skim milk and acne.[2] The researchers concluded that this association could be due to the hormones present in milk products. A similar study on about 4,000 adolescent boys found the same positive correlation between dairy and the presence of acne.[3]

If you are prone to acne, a great way to prevent and possibly reverse acne is to eliminate animal-based foods (particularly dairy), decrease sugar consumption, and follow a whole food, plant-based diet.

Eczema is a chronic inflammatory skin disease characterized by redness of skin, itchy patches and eruptions that may ooze or bleed, and discolor the skin. Atopic dermatitis is the most common type of eczema in infants and children, and is often associated with food allergies.[4] Food allergies account for at least 20% of the incidences of eczema in children less than 4 years old.[5] Children having a family history of hay fever, asthma, or eczema may be prone to atopic dermatitis. Eczema is often associated with food allergies and can be aggravated by the intake of foods such as eggs, fish, and dairy products. Many people are not aware that this offending skin disease can be reversed by eliminating these animal based foods.

Plant- Based Diet For Healthy, Glowing Skin

To have healthy and glowing skin it is crucial to pay attention to what we eat every day. Foods that are high in trans fatty acids such as meat, dairy products, processed, and fast foods can dehydrate the skin. This is because trans fats in animal based foods increase the free radical load and lead to premature aging of the skin.

Whole plant-based foods such as fruits, vegetables, greens, legumes, nuts, and seeds are storehouses of the vital nutrients needed for healthy skin. Vitamin A, biotin, vitamin C, vitamin E, selenium, zinc, silica, and omega 3 fatty acids are some of the important nutrients required for healthy and glowing skin.[6,7]

Vitamin A helps in maintaining and repairing skin cells. Carotenoids, the precursors of vitamin A, may help prevent ultraviolet induced skin damage and wrinkling. Vitamin A deficiency may result in dry and flaky skin. This vitamin is present in dark greens and yellow colored vegetables such as sweet potatoes, carrots, and pumpkins. Papaya and mango are good fruit sources of Vitamin A.

Biotin is a water soluble B vitamin and is needed for the formation of skin, nail, and hair cells. Biotin is found in whole grain cereals, nuts such as almonds and walnuts, and vegetables like carrots, cucumbers, cauliflowers, and onions.

Vitamin C is a powerful antioxidant that helps protect the skin against free radical damage.[8] Factors such as exposure to environmental pollutants, smoking, and an unhealthy diet could lead to the production of these free radicals. Free radical damage is thought to be the basis of the aging process.[9] Citrus fruits such as oranges, grape fruits, lemons,

---

Morning Shine Fruit Smoothie

Ingredients:

½ cup of apple slices

½ cup of mango slices

½ cup of papaya slices

1 cup of chilled almond milk

3-4 dates (deseeded) as natural sweetener.

1 teaspoon Salba or chia seeds

Blend all these ingredients in a blender to get a nutritious and delicious smoothie.

Super Nutrient Smoothie

Ingredients:

1 cucumber

1 carrot

½ cup of fresh greens (iceberg lettuce / kale or any other greens)

1 tomato

1 cup of tender coconut water

2 tablespoon of coconut meat

Blend all these ingredients thoroughly in a blender and a super nutrient smoothie is ready.

and limes as well as apples, papayas, watermelon, and leafy vegetables such as spinach and cilantro are rich in Vitamin C.

Vitamin E is an antioxidant that is essential for healthy and youthful skin. Vitamin E is found in green leafy vegetables, whole grains, almonds, and sunflower seeds.

Selenium is a trace mineral and a potent antioxidant which also helps protect the skin from the damage caused by free radicals. Selenium has anti-aging effects and is found in whole grains, soya beans, mushroom, apple, tomato, onion, garlic, and walnut, and sun flower seeds.

Zinc, needed for repairing damaged tissues, has role in cellular growth and wound healing. It is beneficial for people who suffer from acne, as it helps control excess oil production in the skin. Peanuts, sesame seeds, watermelon seeds, and pumpkin seeds, as well as whole grains and legumes, are rich in zinc.

Omega-3 fatty acids act like moisturizers for skin and improve suppleness. Flax seeds, salba/chia seeds, sesame seeds, and walnuts are natural sources of omega-3 fatty acids.

Although many people think sun exposure is not good, our skin needs sunshine for Vitamin D. At least 15 – 20 minutes of sunlight exposure is needed for the skin to synthesize Vitamin D. Vitamin D is important for healthy skin and immunity. If you have a Vitamin D deficiency, supplementations are advised.

Whole plant-based foods, adequate water intake, sunlight exposure, and exercise[10] will keep the skin healthy, youthful and attractive!

R. Saravanan, BHMS, *is a qualified Homeopath from the Tamil Nadu Dr. M.G.R. Medical University in India. Dr. Saravanan has received special training in Nutritional disease reversal from SHARAN, the pioneer organization in India offering Nutritional disease reversal programs. Currently he is serving as a Health advisor with SHARAN (www.sharan-india.org). He can be contacted at saravanan@sharan-india.org.*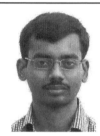

eighteen

FORGET ABOUT ALZHEIMER'S

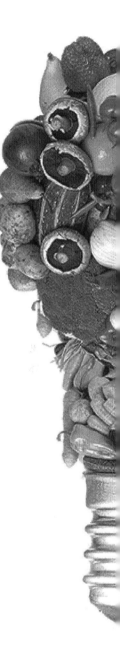

We can think of our genes as committees. They give recommendations and suggestions but they do not solely determine our fate. The same is true in many cases for most cognitive disorders. For years, Alzheimer's has been understood as a genetic condition. Rather, new research is suggesting that dietary factors such as metal intake (copper, iron, zinc, and aluminum), saturated fat, and excess cholesterol intake are significantly associated with increased Alzheimer's incidence.

The Rush University Medical Center study found that those with excess copper in their body combined with diets high in "bad" fats found in animal products and processed snack foods- showed a loss of mental functions equivalent to 19 years of aging![1] High cholesterol level in midlife can predict Alzheimer's risk 20 to 30 years later. This connection between saturated fat intake and Alzheimer's is eye-opening-demonstrating the strong connection between nutrition and disease and our potential to take charge of our health.

The following doctors discuss exciting new research showing how a whole food plant- based diet can shield our brain from destructive toxins, provide us with healthy fats and omega- 3 fatty acids, and necessary sources of Vitamins E, B, and folate nutrients that along with continual mental and physical activity reduces cognitive decline. With no cure, prevention is paramount to preserve our memories.

Power Foods For The Brain

Neal Barnard, MD

Five million Americans have Alzheimer's disease. Many more fear that it could be in their future. However, the good news is that research studies at major research centers have shown that foods may help protect your memory and dramatically reduce your risk of Alzheimer's disease.

First, diets high in "bad fats" (saturated fats and trans fats) are linked with increased risk of developing Alzheimer's disease. Saturated fat is found primarily in dairy products, meat, and eggs. Trans fats are found in snack foods. Evidence suggests that avoiding these "bad fats" can dramatically reduce your risk.

Second, studies have shown that iron and copper, when ingested in excess, may increase the risk of memory problems, presumably because they promote the production of free radicals in the brain. Iron is found in meat, cookware, and supplements. Copper is found in copper pipes, shellfish, and some supplements, as well. Some evidence also suggests that aluminum may play a role. It comes to us in cookware, some antacids, and certain food additives.

Additional benefit comes from exercise. Physical exercise helps protect the brain and reduces the risk of memory problems. Mental activities help too; reading newspapers, working crossword puzzles, listening to documentaries, or learning a language. And sleep allows your brain to rest and recover.

If you would like to try a healthful diet, it pays to break the process into 2 phases. First, take a week or two to find meals that you like that skip meat and other animal products. Then, once you have found good choices, stick to an entirely plant-based diet for 3 weeks. (Be sure to include a daily source of vitamin B-12, such as a B-12 supplement or fortified foods.) Then see how you feel. Chances are you'll want to stick with it for life.

For more Information: The Physicians Committee for Responsible Medicine offers books, DVDs, and an online 21-Day Vegan Kickstart program. Please visit www.PCRM.org.

Power Foods for the Brain, by Neal Barnard, MD, shows findings of scientific studies and builds them into simple steps for improving the health of your body and mind.

Neal Barnard, MD, *is an Adjunct Associate Professor of Medicine at the George Washington University School of Medicine in Washington, DC. Dr. Barnard has authored dozens of scientific publications as well as 15 books including Power Foods for the Brain, Neal Barnard's Program for Reversing Diabetes, and Breaking the Food Seduction. As president of the Physicians Committee for Responsible Medicine, Dr. Barnard leads programs advocating for preventive medicine, good nutrition, and higher ethical standards in research. He has hosted 3 PBS television programs on nutrition and health and is frequently called on by news programs to discuss issues related to nutrition and research. Originally from Fargo, North Dakota, Dr. Barnard received his MD degree at the George Washington University School of Medicine and completed his residency at the same institution. He practiced at St. Vincent's Hospital in New York before returning to Washington to found PCRM.*

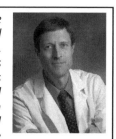

Dietary Guidelines For Reducing Alzheimer's Risk[1]

Physicians Committee for Responsible Medicine (PCRM)

1. Minimize your intake of saturated fats and trans fats. Saturated fat is found primarily in dairy products, meats, and certain oils (coconut and palm oils). Trans fats are found in many snack pastries and fried foods and are listed on labels as "partially hydrogenated oils."

2. Vegetables, legumes (beans, peas, and lentils), fruits, and whole grains should be the primary staples of the diet.

3. One ounce of nuts or seeds (one small handful) daily provides a healthful source of vitamin E.

4. A reliable source of vitamin B12, such as fortified foods or a supplement providing at least the recommended daily allowance (2.4 mcg per day for adults) should be part of your daily diet.

5. When selecting multiple vitamins, choose those without iron and copper, and consume iron supplements only when directed by your physician.

6. While aluminum's role in Alzheimer's disease remains a matter of investigation, it is prudent to avoid the use of cookware, antacids, baking powder, or other products that contribute dietary aluminum.

7. Include aerobic exercise in your routine, equivalent to 40 minutes of brisk walking three times per week.

*The 7 dietary principles to reduce the risk of Alzheimer's disease were prepared for presentation at the International Conference on Nutrition and the Brain in Washington on July 19 and 20, 2013.

The Diet For A Healthy Brain, Happy Mind

Carol A Tavani, MD, MS, DLFAPA

A carnivorous diet can be seen as deviant to our anatomy and physiology, and therefore associated with a host of diseases evident by consuming a Western diet. Nowhere are the dangers of a carnivorous diet more evident - and disastrous - than in the brain and central nervous system. When we eat a diet high in animal protein we consume an excess of minerals such as iron, copper, aluminum, and zinc as well as toxic additives such as arsenic, dioxins and cholesterol that seem to contribute to cognitive disorders. Some of these contributors and cognitive disorders are discussed below, but please note that this list is not comprehensive.

Excess Consumption of Minerals is Linked to Dementia

Copper: Excess dietary copper can damage neurons. In a study in Southern California, 1,451 subjects were mentally sharper and displayed better long and short term memory than those with high copper levels. There is a synergistic effect that occurs when copper is combined with excess dietary fat. This can result in a loss of mental function equivalent to *19 years* of aging. In plant based foods, substances called phytates limit the absorption of this metal. We only need about 0.9 mg a day.

Iron: Excess iron is associated with decline in cognitive function including an increased risk of developing dementia. It is interesting that a plant- based diet can contain at least as much iron as in meat, but our bodies are better able to regulate how much iron is absorbed and utilized. Our bodies have a way of regulating iron from plant-based sources. We absorb more non-heme iron (iron not derived from the blood of another animal) when needed, but we absorb less when not needed.

> ### How Much Iron Do You Need?
>
> In adults ages 18 to 50, about 8 mg daily is sufficient, unless one suffers from iron deficiency anemia or a chronic illness such as kidney disease. Unless a woman is pregnant, still menstruating, or there is a known deficiency, ordinarily it is best to choose a vitamin preparation without iron.

With age, iron accumulates in the gray matter of the brain, and can contribute to the risk of developing age-related diseases, such as Alzheimer's disease. In a small study, which examined iron level and tissue damage in the hippocampus and the thalamus, 31 Alzheimer's patients and 68 healthy participants were imaged with MRI, to quantify the ferritin iron content. Compared with healthy controls, the dementia patients had increased ferritin iron in the hippocampus but not the thalamus. Although this study is small, the data reveals that in Alzheimer's disease at least in these subjects, hippocampus damage is correlated with ferritin iron accumulation. We still need good prospective studies over time to evaluate just how increasing iron levels may influence the trajectory of tissue damage and cognitive and pathological manifestations of Alzheimer's disease and possibly other types of dementia.

Can We Trust Food Additives As Safe?

It is important and revealing to know that about 22% of additive notices were written by employees and consultants of the additive manufacturers. The manufacturers are allowed to use them on their own, without notifying the Food and Drug Administration (FDA), if the additive has gained the status of Generally Recognized as Safe (GRA). GRAs account for 43% of the 10,000 or so additives in use. Thomas Neitner, states "rules governing the chemicals that go into a tennis racket are more stringent than (those for) the chemicals that go into our food." For example, N-nitroso compounds, used as a preservative in red meat, increase the risk of childhood primary tumors of the brain if mothers ate them in pregnancy, by way of these cured meats. Colon Cancer risk increases by 10% with meat consumption.

In particular, excess iron is detrimental to the hippocampus, an area of the brain critical to forming new memories and also in recall. It can damage free radical reactions throughout the body, not just in the brain. Abnormally high stores of iron in the body lead to deposits known as hemochromatosis.

Where does excess iron come from? Aside from meat, excess iron can come from cast iron pots and pans, especially if acidic foods are cooked in them. Similarly, many cereals are fortified with iron; thus care in reading labels is wise so as to avoid excess or unnecessary supplementation.

Zinc: A vital nutrient for the immune system and healing, zinc is essential in the diet. Excess, however, is thought to promote the formation of amyloid, the dreaded substance found in the plaques seen microscopically in the brains of individuals with Alzheimer's disease. Men need about 11 and women 8 mg a day of dietary zinc. In most diets, zinc actually is derived from supplements.

Additives and Substances in Animal Products Can Alter Cognitive Functioning

Arsenic: This toxin can be found in some unlikely places including meat. Chickens have been known to have been fed antibiotics containing arsenic, as have other animals. Roxarsone, an especially carcinogenic form of arsenic, is used as an antibiotic on factory farms. According to the USDA, about 1/3 of a chicken breast (or 2 ounces) exposes its consumer to 3-5 micrograms of inorganic arsenic. Exposure to low doses such as these can dramatically increase the risk of cancer, dementia, and other neurological problems as well as other human ailments.

Cholesterol: The brain contains about 25% of all the cholesterol found in the body, which is an essential substance in the production of hormones and in the formation and composition of cell membranes. It is utilized in the synthesis of neurotransmitters, and is an integral part of the composition of the blood brain barrier. The brain must produce its own supply of cholesterol; it cannot utilize circulating amounts of this substance. Cholesterol is only found in animal-based products.

In a typical Western diet, atherosclerotic changes, or clogging of the arteries, can be seen in the coronary arteries of children, adolescents and young adults. This finding is observed over and over in autopsies of those who have met untimely deaths, as in wartime, accidents or other tragedies.

Atherosclerotic vascular disease affects the entire body, not just the coronary arteries. In the brain, incidence of ischemic strokes (caused by accumulation of atherosclerotic plaque in the vessels within it), is significantly increased in men with high blood LDL and tends to cause vasoconstriction as well. Fat soluble statin drugs, such as atorvastatin, which decrease synthesis of cholesterol by the liver and lower LDL, also decrease brain cholesterol production. Some preliminary work has associated these agents as having a favorable or protective effect on the development of dementia. More work must be done on this important relationship.

Dioxins: Dioxins are carcinogenic, affect the immune system, can cause birth deformities and miscarriages, and neurologic disorders. Environmental chemicals absorbed by an animal into its flesh become concentrated in the animal tissues, making meat highly toxic. According to the Environmental Protection Agency (EPA), nearly 95% of dioxin exposure occurs not by inhalation or contact, but by ingesting meat, fish and dairy products. Thus even "organically" raised animals do not escape conveying to the humans who eat them these concentrated toxins.

Homocysteine: This compound is linked to inflammation and related to various diseases wherein inflammation is an important part of pathology. Built from the amino acid methionine, 2 to 3 times the amount of homocysteine is contained in animal protein as in plants. A study at Harvard Medical School showed that subjects who adopted a vegan diet showed serum levels to drop by 13-20% in just one week.

Plant-Based Diet Can Possibly Prevent and Slow Progression of Cognitive Diseases

Consuming the above discussed substances is a contributor to cognitive disorders such as dementia, Multiple Sclerosis, and stroke. By contrast, a plant-based diet has been shown to be protective and even helpful in slowing the progression of some of these conditions.

Cognitive Disorders: A Dutch study on cognition showed that men aged 69 to 89 who have high omega 6 intake (found in red meat) have an increased incidence of cognitive impairment. Another study found that those who ate meat, including poultry and fish, were more than twice as likely to develop dementia as their vegetarian counterparts. Individuals who eat meat more than 4 times a week over time have a 3 fold incidence of developing dementia than do vegetarians. Even in young adults, a diet rich in omega 3 fatty acids has been shown to improve working memory even in young adults. In one University Study, vegetarian students scored higher on exams than meat eaters, showed less frustration and scored lower on irascibility scales than did their meat eating counterparts. A diet rich in polyphenols (found in darkly pigmented fruits and vegetables) may slow cognitive decline by helping cells clean up debris linked to memory loss and decrease cardiovascular disease by decreasing oxidative stress and inflammation.

Deadly Prions: The infectious prions producing this disease and its equally devastating counterpart or variant in humans, Creutzfeld-Jacob Disease (CJD), could account for substantial increases in "Alzheimer's Disease over the years. It is increasingly thought that prion disease, the transmission of tiny, difficult-to-kill particles, is more common than formerly believed due to a long incubation period. Consumption of not just cows, but deer, sheep, and pigs could also transmit these prions. Dementias attributed to the plaques and neurofibrillary tangles of Alzheimer's, if properly diagnosed, would be found to be more properly ascribed to this prion disease. At least 12% of dementias diagnosed as Alzheimer's are actually CJD, an under diagnosed entity. Confirmation is difficult since this can only be accomplished by brain biopsy.

Multiple Sclerosis (MS): Multiple sclerosis is the most common degenerative inflammatory neurological disease in the United States, affecting approximately half a million people. Yet its etiology has remained elusive. Interestingly, when people from countries where multiple sclerosis is rare, immigrate to the United States, Canada and Northern Europe, the risk of developing this disease increases. The brains of individuals with MS have been found to contain higher saturated fat content than normal subjects. During World War II, when people could not afford a steady diet of meat, there were 2.5 times fewer hospitalizations for this diagnosis. MS patients at the University of Oregon's Neurology Department who tried a diet low in saturated fat had improved motor functioning by as much as 95%.

Parkinson's Disease: Metals contained in meat affect the basal ganglia, which plays an important role in movement disorders. Interestingly, elimination of red meat from the diet of patients already diagnosed with Parkinson's disease has been shown to improve their symptoms.

Stroke: Carnivores are 10 times more likely to develop coronary artery disease, and that number rises for men between the ages of 45-55. Consumption of processed red meat is positively associated with risk of stroke. The largest meta-analysis to date on atherogenic effects of meat shows that the risk for a fatal stroke increased by a staggering 13% for each increase in a single serving of fresh or processed meat and total amount of red meat consumed a day. Conversely, a diet rich in flavonoids, found in grapefruit and oranges, lowers risk of ischemic stroke in women by 19%. In a Finnish study published in Neurology, a diet high in lycopene found in tomatoes may decrease the risk of stroke in men as well.

Mood and Behavior Disorders: A diet rich in monounsaturated fatty acids, (think Mediterranean Diet) decreased levels of depression in men over time, and is associated with a 30% decreased risk of developing depression, compared with meat and dairy rich diets with trans fatty acids. Similar statistics exist for risk of postpartum depression. For ADHD, a diet rich in unsaturated fatty acids has been used to treat ADHD as well as improve working memory in young adults. Deficiencies in omega-3 fatty acids is associated with increased symptoms.

Little exists to suggest a benefit of a meat- based diet. Food pyramids have been lagging behind the literature for years, but the evidence for adoption of a plant- based diet is undeniable and the evidence continues to accumulate. Are we capable of accepting this evidence and having the flexibility to heal ourselves and our own maladies simply by re-adopting that for which we were designed? The choice is up to us.

Carol A. Tavani, MD, M.S., D.L.F.A.P.A., *is a board certified Neuropsychiatrist practicing in the state of Delaware. A graduate of Jefferson Medical College, she practices neuropsychiatry as Executive Director of Christiana Psychiatric Services. She is the director of a large consultation service, and her outpatient private practice, she is a respected forensic expert in both criminal and civil arenas. Dr. Tavani is the first woman to be the President of the Medical Staff of Christiana Care, and former President of the Medical Society of Delaware. She is a Diplomate of the American Board of Psychiatry & Neurology, a Distinguished Fellow of the American Psychiatric Association, and current President of the Delaware Psychiatric Society. Dr. Tavani serves on the Board of Directors of Faithful Friends, and is a member of the Steering Committee of Physicians Committee for Responsible Medicine.*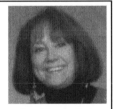

Protein Deposits, Inflammation, and Neurodegenerative Disease

Luca Vannetiello, MD, DC

Brain activity especially in humans, is the ultimate expression of living beings. Our nervous system is both a receiver and transmitter of all stimuli and response. When you have a system that is engineered to be efficient at super fast speed, it is very sensitive to disruption, and signs of it are quickly observed. However, when we experience decay of brain functions, our motor responses generally decrease which can cause a cascade of consequences.

Neurodegenerative chronic diseases are highly linked to protein deposits and a chronic inflammatory state. Proteins are continuously degraded and replaced, to renew biological substrates. Deposits of alpha-synuclein and Tau protein in Lewy body are found in neurodegenerative conditions such as Parkinson disease or Multiple System Atrophy, dementia, Alzheimer's disease. Recent therapeutic strategy in these conditions is to promote autophagy through fasting, pushing the body to eat its own protein deposits.

Nerve transmission of an impulse is highly dependent on cellular membrane integrity and is influenced by our food choices. Cellular membranes are formed by a double layer of fatty acids with embedded proteins that allow communication between intra and extracellular environments. This communication or action potential is ultimately an electronic pulse that translates into daily functioning from moving an arm to planning a holiday.

Optimal brain function is dependent upon neuron cell membrane health. Omega 3-fatty acids (DHA and EPA) are critical to neuron electric impulse transmission and for the membrane fluidity. They are needed in high concentrations in the synaptic membranes of the brain. Research fields are merging in exploring nutrition and child development, cognitive aging, psychiatric disorders etc. and results will surely be of great interest.

Health and optimal brain functioning needs to include the food that we eat, with a conscious awareness of where it comes from and its impact on our land, water and air resources.

Luca Vannetiello, MD, DC, *graduated medical school from "Federico II" University of Naples Italy and graduated Doctor of Chiropractic from "Life Chiropractic College West" Hayward CA. (USA). Dr. Vannetiello is trained in Functional Neurology and received the Geriatric Faculty Fellowship at John Hopkins Medical Institutions. He is certified in Geriatrics.*
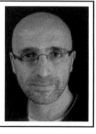

What a Headache

Adina W. Mercer, MD
Graduated from Loma Linda University School of Medicine
Currently works at an Urgent Care Clinic in Riverside, CA.

Jennifer's migraines were so severe that for years she would show up at the Urgent Care as often as once or twice a week for an injection of Dilaudid. I had several CT scans over the years to verify that she didn't have a brain tumor or internal bleeding.

As I learned about the how a whole food, plant based diet could improve headaches, it made sense that processed foods and animal based foods were the likely culprits. Rather, foods like fruits and vegetables provide the needed nutrients for our nervous system. I recommended that Jennifer follow the meal plans outlined in Dr. Joel Fuhrman's book *"Eat to Live".*

As Jennifer changed her diet, her headaches became less frequent and severe. Her skin even had a different glow. She started to buy her produce from the weekly farmer's market and exercising. She replaced drinking sodas with water which greatly improved her sleep. Now, I rarely see Jennifer. She's empowered.

Although headaches are difficult to manage, adopting dietary changes can help control headaches and pain can be used to notify patients of an imbalance. By providing my patients with resources such as lectures, books and audio tapes, I am empowering them to play a role in their own healthcare.

Alzheimer's Disease: Decreasing Risk Through Lifestyle Changes

William M. Simpson Jr., MD

Losing a loved one to Alzheimer's disease is one of the most painful experiences and most dreaded diagnoses I make as a geriatrician. While some cases of Alzheimer's disease are heavily affected by a person's genetic make-up, fortunately the majority of cases are not genetically pre-determined, making Alzheimer's risk reduction possible.

There are 2 main forms of Alzheimer's disease (AD), early- and late-onset. While early-onset of AD is genetically related, this only accounts for 15% of cases. The APOE e4 gene is present in 40% of people who develop late-onset disease.[1] This gene is also present in 25-30% of the general population, indicating that genetics is not the whole story. The remaining 85% or more cases of AD are late-onset and more related to diet and lifestyle factors.

While there are several contributing factors to the development of Alzheimer's disease, neurologic and vascular research is beginning to unravel some of the lifestyle behaviors and environmental mechanisms which either increase or lower our chances of developing this disease. For example, diet is related to risk of Alzheimer's. Foods high in fat, meat and dairy products, foods high in saturated fat such as fried and processed foods as well as fish high in mercury, refined sugars and sugary beverages are all associated with increased AD risk.

Foods such as fruits and vegetables, whole grains, legumes, sweet potatoes, broccoli (all high in Vitamin E and folate), beans, brown rice, corn (high in Vitamin B6), almond milk, and fortified cereals (high in Vitamin B12) all decrease risk of Alzheimer's.[2]

The significant differences in the reported rates of Alzheimer's disease around the world give credence to the influence of lifestyle factors. In general, Western-lifestyle countries have higher reported rates of AD than those of the East and Africa Differences in animal fat consumption seem to play a role in lower rates of AD in countries with more plant-based diets. The same behaviors that increase the risk of cardiovascular disease appear to increase the risk of late onset AD. These include: lack of exercise, smoking, hypertension, hypercholesterolemia, poorly-controlled diabetes mellitus, the metabolic syndrome and poor diet (lacking in fruits and vegetables, coupled with excess calories, resulting in excess weight).[3] Essentially all of above illnesses are associated with increased levels of inflammation in the body. These same inflammatory changes seem to also influence the risk of Alzheimer's.

So, how can we decrease our risk of developing AD? Here are 5 key lifestyle changes[4]:

1. Get moving and lose weight. Inactivity is linked to greater weight gain which is associated with increased levels of inflammation. Walking on a regular basis is associated with decreased brain shrinkage and exercising outside lowers the rate of depression, associated with increased risk of AD.

2. Don't smoke. Smoking is inflammatory and damages our respiratory and cardio-vascular system.

3. Eat more fruits and vegetables. The more fruits and vegetables consumed, the higher the intake of anti-oxidants, potassium and other micronutrients and the lower the average blood pressure, all of which tend to lower AD risk.

4. Get enough sleep. Recent research points to poor sleep patterns as increasing risk for type 2 diabetes, which can increase chances of developing AD.

5. Increase mentally stimulating activities such as social engagement, work, or mentally challenging leisure activities exercising the brain is important to prevent cognitive decline.

Although this only scratches the surface of Alzheimer's, a healthy lifestyle is currently our best point of attack in the battle against AD.

William M. Simpson Jr., MD *is the Emeritus Professor of Family Medicine at the Medical University of South Carolina.*

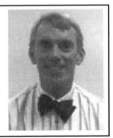

Preventing and Treating Parkinson's Disease with a Plant-Based Diet

Michael Greger, MD

All 9 prospective studies so far published have found dairy products or milk consumption associated with greater Parkinson's disease risk.[1,2] Researchers suspect that it may be because dairy products have been found to be contaminated with neurotoxic chemicals. Autopsies have found higher levels of pollutants and pesticides in the brains of Parkinson's disease patients, and some of these toxins are present at low levels in dairy products, such as tetrahydroisoquinoline, a parkinsonism-related compound found predominantly in cheese. Although the amount of this neurotoxin in cheese is not very high, the concern is that the chemical may accumulate in the brain over long periods of consumption.[3]

A plant-based diet may help treat the disease as well. At its root, Parkinson's is a dopamine deficiency disease, because of the die-off of dopamine-generating cells in the brain. These cells in the brain make dopamine from levadopa derived from an amino acid in our diet. However, the amino acid profile of animal proteins blocks the transport of levadopa into the brain. At first researchers tried what's called a "protein redistribution diet," in which patients were instructed to eat most of their protein in the evening meal, so that they would only suffer the effects while they sleep, but when it was discovered that fiber consumption appears to naturally boosts levodopa levels researchers suggested patients would benefit by cutting animal products out altogether.[4] The researchers conclude: "[A] plant-based diet, particularly in its vegan variant, is expected to raise levodopa bioavailability and bring some advantages in the management of the disease through two mechanisms: a reduced protein intake and an increased fiber."[5] That's why plant protein is the best, because it comes packaged with fiber. A strictly plant-based diet was found to significantly improve Parkinson's disease symptoms.

Michael Greger, MD, *is an author, and internationally recognized speaker on nutrition, food safety, and public health issues. A founding member of the American College of Lifestyle Medicine, Dr. Greger is licensed as a general practitioner specializing in clinical nutrition. Currently he serves as the Director of Public Health and Animal Agriculture at the Humane Society of the United States. Dr. Greger is a graduate of the Cornell University School of Agriculture and Tufts University School of Medicine. Stay up to date with the most recent nutritional science at NutritionFacts.org.*
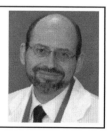

nineteen

DON'T THINK, JUST EAT

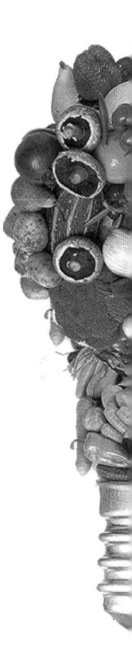

"If we could give every individual the right amount of nourishment and exercise, not too little and not too much, we would have found the safest way to health."

—Hippocrates

We tend to think of breakthroughs in science as new drugs, surgery, or technology. As our knowledge of science advances in relation to the role of diet and disease, it is becoming ever more evident that well balanced, plant-based food choices are some of the most effective disease preventative tools we have. Plant foods contain about a 100,000 different antioxidants or phytonutrients that are disease-preventing nutrients.[1] These phytonutrients are ONLY found in plant-based foods.

One of the most comprehensive studies to date on anti-oxidants in food found that plant foods have 64 times the number of antioxidants than animal based foods including meat, fish, dairy, and eggs.[2] This study which surveyed over 3,000 different types of foods from beverages, to cereals, vegetables, baked goods, fruits, and meats found that when we eat animal-based foods, we are missing out on essential nutrients that are only contained in plant-based foods. Given our daily caloric limit, this means every meal or snack can either promote or hinder disease.

The experts in this chapter can help you plan your next meal and trip to the grocery store as they showcase how and why certain plant-based foods can provide us with the best form of preventative medicine, highlighting why nutrition should be at the forefront of everyone's mind.

Choose Live Foods For ChemoPrevention

Pamela Wible, MD

What's all the confusion about food? Daily, patients come into clinic to ask me what they should be eating. Have we *really* forgotten what to eat?

This week, a woman told me that she's allergic to carbohydrates. Really? That's impossible. Then I saw my vegan raw-foodist family. The parents just divorced with split custody and Dad adopted the paleo diet. Now the kids enjoy kale smoothies and cashew-carob-coconut desserts by week and eat loads of meat like cavemen on the weekends.

Some of my patients claim to be eating right for their blood type; others don't eat anything with a face—or anything that had a mother. Many still follow the good old Standard America Diet (SAD), just meat and potatoes, please. The latest fad is the Paleolithic plan—a Stone-Age diet of wild plants and animals. I see a wide gamut from opportunivores—omnivores who eat whatever is around to pescatarians—who eat no meat except fish, and vegans—who eat no animal products whatsoever.

Today, people study self-help cookbooks and organize meal plans, they track ingredients and count calories. But it should not be such a chore just to figure out what to eat for breakfast.

All of these patients seem to be searching for the same thing: What's the best diet?

I try to make things simple, but I find people are more confused than ever. At the grocery store, I understand why. Currently, everything is gluten-free and twice as expensive. There are gluten-free chips and salsa, gluten-free ice cream, gluten-free cupcakes and cookies. From a patient's perspective it would be easy to fall for each new diet fad seen in the grocery stores.

Unplug Your Refrigerator

Are you a midnight muncher? Do you sneak to the fridge when nobody is looking to get your ice cream fix? Overeating is an American pastime. Unfortunately, so have diseases of excess consumption—and diets of confusion.

In medical school, I witnessed first- hand the devastation of diets of excess: diabetes, heart disease, stroke, and cancer. After completing my medical training, I opened my refrigerator one day and had a big epiphany. I discovered a few jars of condiments and a bottle of beer. My fridge was basically empty. As someone who enjoys a plant-based diet, I was getting most of my food right out of my garden. Whole grains, nuts, seeds, produce, and even most plant-derived condiments remain stable at room temperature. I didn't need to own a refrigerator. So I unplugged. Then I got rid of my fridge. And I felt great.

Think about what you have in your refrigerator. Refrigeration decreases the rate of bacterial growth and slows the spoilage of food. In effect, it allows us to keep unstable foods from rotting. Essentially it means our fridge is often just a graveyard for dead food.

What happens when people eat so much dead food? Could we be killing ourselves with this food? The short answer is yes.

Here's an experiment: Empty your cabinets and refrigerator. Put everything on the kitchen counter that doesn't have artificial preservatives. Then walk away for 2 days. What happens? Upon your return, you would smell rotting flesh. Milk, meat, and cheese will be in varying states of decay. But the apples and oranges, mangos and bananas would still look and smell appetizing.

Plant foods are whole foods. They haven't been processed and broken down into smaller components. Plant foods have an array of natural antioxidants and phytochemicals that animal foods just don't have. In other words: plants preserve themselves.

Antioxidants and Phytochemicals

An antioxidant is a substance that inhibits oxidation by removing damaging oxidizing agents from a living organism thereby protecting the organism from damage and cell death. Oxidative stress is linked to many human diseases. Plants give us the protection we need from our own oxidative stress because they contain such a variety of antioxidants.

There are 2 types of antioxidants in foods: endogenous antioxidants and exogenous antioxidants. It's important to know the difference.

Endogenous antioxidants are antioxidants that are native to foods. Plants are full of antioxidants such as vitamin A, vitamin C, and vitamin E. Plants also have antioxidant enzymes and pigments. Without enough native antioxidants, the plant begins to rot because it is unable to protect itself from oxidative damage and cell death.

Exogenous antioxidants are antioxidants added to preserve packaged food. Read the ingredients on boxes and cans of processed food and you will notice that antioxidants such as vitamin C are added as preservatives to extend shelf life.

Phytochemicals

Phytochemicals are non-nutritive chemical compounds that are naturally occurring in plants. Some phytochemicals are responsible for the deep red and purple colors of foods such as in raspberries and blueberries. Others are responsible for the odor of plants such as in onions and garlic. Phytochemicals have biological benefits for human health. Antioxidants are also classified as phytochemicals. Tens of thousands of phytochemicals have been discovered, but it's likely that even more have yet to be identified. Bottom line: you can never have enough plant chemicals fighting for your health.

What about antioxidant and phytochemical supplements. Many people choose to use supplements. But remember: supplements are supplemental to a healthy diet. Several studies have even suggested that antioxidant supplements offer no benefit or have even caused damage at excess levels.[1]

Dietary Chemoprevention

It's never too late to begin ingesting a low level of "chemotherapy" through medicinal foods as a preventive strategy against cancer. These foods may also have some action against established cancers and can improve your overall immunity. A dietary chemoprevention lifestyle can be used as an adjunct to your current medical treatments. As always, consult with you health care professional for specific advice.

Dietary Chemoprevention: Top 10 Foods

1. Burdock root has been used to treat cancers for centuries and is the active ingredient in many natural cancer remedies such as Essiac tea.[2] It is a popular vegetable in Asian countries that is actually a weed found growing throughout North America, Asia, and Europe. Burdock root tastes like a crisp, sweet carrot and has a plethora of phytochemicals and antioxidants that are mostly stored in the root. Chop fresh burdock root and add to your salads or eat as a snack. Be sure to ask your doctors about the use of burdock as adjunctive therapy for cancer.

2. Flax seeds have been used medicinally for centuries and recent studies reveal that flax can lower cholesterol and stabilize blood sugar.[3] Flax contains the highest plant source of lignans (a plant estrogen) and alpha-linolenic acid, an omega-3 fatty acid. The high lignan content may be beneficial in prevention of breast and prostate cancers. Store flax seeds whole and grind the seeds when needed to prevent rancidity and deterioration of nutritional content. Therapeutic intake is 2 to 4 tablespoons ground flax daily which can be sprinkled on salads and oatmeal.

3. Cruciferous vegetables such as broccoli, kale, and collard greens are loaded with phytochemicals. Indole-3-carbinal (I3C) is one of the most studied and has been found to help the body detoxify and de-activate carcinogens once exposed. Be sure to have multiple servings of crucifers daily for maximum benefit. Plant sterols and organosulfur compounds in crucifers have been found to decrease cholesterol levels.

4. Leafy green vegetables such as parsley, lettuces, and beet greens have the highest nutrient density of any food. Flavonoids and polyphenolic acids help inhibit blood clots and coronary artery disease and are helpful in cancer prevention.

5. Blueberries are high in antioxidants which protect humans from oxidative stress and can prevent cancer as well as a myriad of degenerative diseases such as heart disease and cataracts.[4] Blueberries also decrease the ability of bacteria to cling to the mucous membrane of the urinary tract, thus preventing and sometimes treating urinary tract infections.

6. Turmeric root is a bright yellow spice that comes from the root of *Curcuma longa*, a plant from the ginger family. Curcuminoids (primarily curcumin) which give turmeric its color, act as an anti-inflammatory agent as well as an antioxidant. Turmeric can also help prevent cancers through a variety of pathways including killing cancer cells directly and preventing blood flow to cancerous tissue.[5]

7. Cumin seeds contain a cocktail of phytochemicals with antioxidant effects found to be beneficial to human health. One such phytochemical, cuminaldehyde has strong anti-inflammatory and anticancer activity. Sprinkle on salads, cereals, and even desserts to add a rich and earthy flavor to meals.

8. Green tea is made from the dried leaves of *Camellia sinesis* plant and is popular in Asian culture. Drinking green tea can help prevent cancer, heart disease. Green tea contains polyphenols that are responsible for the antioxidation and anticarcinogenic effects of the plant. Drink green tea after meals or as midday treat to maximize health benefits.

9. Mushrooms are known for their healing potential in Asian culture. With a plethora of phytochemicals, mushrooms such as shiitake and maitakes have been shown to reverse tumors in humans through multiple pathways.[6] Ensure mushrooms are a part of your next stir fry or salad.

10. Citrus fruits Contain a host of phytochemicals with bioprotective effects. For example, citrus peel is one of the most underutilized and accessible sources of phytochemicals in the diet. Two phytochemicals most studied in citrus peel is limonene and perillyl alcohol, both of which have been found to deactivate cancer cells in the human body.[7] Use liberal amounts of citrus peel in your meals.

Choose Life

To help prevent cancer, choose living foods that are full of phytochemicals and antioxidants over dead foods like milk, chicken, and fish that require refrigeration. Plants know how to protect and preserve themselves and when we eat them they pass their protection on to us.

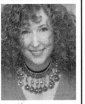

Pamela Wible, MD, *is a family physician born into a family of physicians. While her parents warned her not to pursue medicine, she followed her heart only to discover that to heal her patients she had to first heal her profession. She invited her community to design their own ideal clinic. In 2005, patients created the first community-designed ideal medical clinic in America. An expert in patient-centered care, Dr. Wible helps citizens design cutting-edge clinics and hospitals nationwide. She has been interviewed by CNN, ABC, CBS, and is a frequent guest on NPR. Pamela Wible is the coauthor of 2 award-winning anthologies and the bestselling author of, "Pet Goats & Pap Smears: 101 Medical Adventures to Open Your Heart & Mind". Contact her at* www.IdealMedicalCare.org.

The Nutritional Value of Food

David J.A. Jenkins, MD, PhD, D.Sc.
Professor, Canada Research Chair in Nutrition and Metabolism
Director of Risk Factor Modification Centre, St. Michael's Hospital

A plant-based diet can help us lower our cholesterol, control our blood glucose levels, and aid in weight-loss. In particular, legumes, beans, lentils, chickpeas, seeds and nuts have shown to be especially effective for improving both the risk factors for heart disease and preventing type 2 diabetes. These foods not only lower blood pressure but also are low on the glycemic index, which is important for diabetics and they are a wonderful source of plant protein.

I recommend consuming about 200g of nuts, seeds, and beans per day. Consuming nuts along with temperate fruits such as apples and oranges, are a wonderful mini meal that can prevent a large breakfast and lunch. Nuts, seeds, and pulses are a triple threat: they can not only help prevent disease, but also serve to help reverse disease while aiding in weight loss.

Foods For A Healthy, Happy Life

Jill Nussinow, MS, RD

As a Registered Dietitian who has taught the McDougall Program (a no-fat added vegan diet) for more than 11 years, the key to a great diet is including a high percentage of antioxidant-rich and fiber-rich foods with a focus on the following: cruciferous vegetables, herbs and spices, alliums, mushrooms, peas, beans and lentils (legumes), seeds and nuts. Here is what eating these foods can do for you and your health:

Cruciferous Vegetables

This category includes: arugula, bok choy (and other Asian leafy greens), broccoli, Brussel sprouts, cabbage, cauliflower, collard greens, horseradish, kale, kohlrabi, mustard greens, radish, rutabaga, turnips and turnip greens and watercress.

These vegetables have some of the highest levels of antioxidants and phytochemicals, especially those that are protective against various types of cancer. They are easily fermented foods that introduce beneficial bacteria (probiotics) into your body. Many contain important minerals and vitamins such as folic acid, magnesium and Vitamins C, E and K. All of these vegetables are good sources of fiber and the darker colored ones are also good sources of Vitamin A.

Cruciferous vegetables are best eaten either raw or lightly cooked, because their biologically active components, isothiocyanates, enhance your body's defenses against DNA damage. They can also fuel your body's ability to block cancer growth, rendering them highly effective against human cancers. Since there are so many of these vegetables, you can find one or more them of them in-season throughout the year and they are low in calories. (Note: if you have thyroid issues, be sure to check with your doctor before you eat too many of these cruciferous vegetables.)

Herbs and Spices

Some people mistakenly believe that plant-based food is bland and boring. Herbs and spices taste delicious on vegetables and are amazing sources of antioxidants and phytochemicals that offer a variety of health-promoting properties.

First, let's make a distinction between herbs and spices: herbs are usually shrubby plants of which you use their leaves and flowers, while spices are the bark, seeds, roots, berries and twigs or anything that is not a leaf. It is best to buy organic because they have the most concentrated sources of antioxidants.

Leafy greens such as Italian parsley, basil, oregano, thyme, mint and cilantro are more than just garnishes. For example, pesto is a great way to use more herbs by blending them to make a paste or sauce. Aside from tasting great, most of these herbs are antibacterial and antiviral.

Some common spices with wonderful health benefits include:

- Cinnamon, a favorite, can help regulate blood sugar.

- Ginger has been shown to help reduce nausea, settle your stomach, and aid digestion. You can use it fresh, grated, minced, blended, or powdered. Candied ginger can even help with car sickness. Eat it on a medium-full stomach, 20 minutes before you travel. It works wonders!

- Turmeric, the major component of curry powder, is one of the most potent spices for taming inflammation. In some countries, they make a paste with turmeric and put it on areas that need healing from the outside in, such as burns, bruises and joint pain. Eating turmeric daily can help your health dramatically by possibly keeping cancer at bay, especially with colon and pancreatic cancers. The taste is strong so start with just a little bit of this spice.

Alliums

These vegetables such as onions, garlic, leeks, chives, shallots and scallions- are often the underlying foundation to many cooked dishes. Alliums are flavor enhancers that add depth and nutrition. High in antioxidants they help with inflammation. In particular, they affect cardiovascular disease by lowering blood pressure and cholesterol and possibly preventing plaque buildup.

In particular, garlic is antibacterial, antiviral, and antifungal, which boosts the immune system. Crushing or cutting garlic creates allicin which is the sulfurous compound that offers beneficial anti-inflammatory effects including cancer prevention and treatment. To increase and protect the allicin, when you do use garlic, chop or cut it and let it sit for 10 minutes before using. Garlic is also high in a variety of nutrients, including Vitamin C, vitamin B6, selenium, and manganese. Eat it daily raw or add it toward the end of cooking to add flavor, and preserve the nutrients and potent compounds. For maximum nutrition, buy heads of garlic and peel your own cloves, rather than buying large jars of peeled or already chopped garlic.

Mushrooms

Mushrooms are fungi, not vegetables, and contain an indigestible fiber called chitin which is also found in the exoskeletons of shellfish. This substance helps reduce cholesterol and can help regulate blood sugar. Additionally the soluble fiber, Beta- glucan (β-glucan), found in all mushrooms, from the common white button mushroom to the large portabella mushroom helps lower cholesterol, regulates blood pressure, and aides in weight loss.

Mushrooms are known for their immune-boosting properties. For example, shiitake mushrooms are known to help fight cancer cells. The Japanese synthesize lentinan, a component from the shiitake mushroom, and use it for cancer treatment because it stimulates monocytes which work in conjunction with T cells that boost immune function.

Additionally, if you put your shiitake mushrooms gill-side up in the sunlight, the mushrooms manufacture Vitamin D, which among other benefits aids in calcium absorption. Other mushrooms do the same when exposed to light and some producers are selling Vitamin D mushrooms, which you will find labeled on the bag.

Possibly the best part about mushrooms is their flavor, often called umami- a Japanese word loosely translated as deliciousness. For maximum health benefits, mushrooms should always be cooked as cooking deactivates the mild mycotoxin found in cultivated mushrooms. *Never* pick and eat wild mushrooms without an experienced guide.

Legumes: Peas, Beans, and Lentils

These are the true powerhouses and superstars of the plant-based palette. Not only are there so many varieties that one could probably eat a different one each day of the year, but there is also such a variety in the ways they can be eaten. Beans are the vegan chameleon and can be used in dishes from morning smoothies and salad dressings to even dessert brownies.

Most beans, except for soybeans, are low in fat. They are all high in fiber, especially insoluble fiber which can help lower cholesterol and improve heart health. The darker the color of the bean (as with all other foods, too), the more antioxidants they contain. Beans can help diabetics even their blood sugar as they slow down absorption in your GI tract. They also can help trim waistlines as they are filling and satisfying.

While whole soybeans are preferable, tempeh and tofu are great soy alternatives. Be sure to choose organic and non-GMO sources and avoid isolated soy protein and other highly processed soy foods.

Seeds and Nuts

Nuts and seeds are a wonderful way to add healthy fat, crunch, and flavor to your diet. Flax, chia and hemp are three seeds that are important sources of omega-3 fatty acids, the "essential" fatty acids which are good for your immune system and can only be obtained through food. Since this fatty acid is extremely sensitive to heat and light, it is best to use them raw or cooked into foods, rather than cooking them directly. Flax must be ground to get the most benefit. Chia is good soaked and hemp is a wonderful addition to salads. All other seeds contain beneficial vitamins and minerals such as sesame (a good source of calcium), sunflower and pumpkin (a good source of zinc which is important for your immune system).

Seeds and especially nuts are good sources of plant protein. Walnuts also contain omega 3 (essential) fatty acids and Brazil nuts provide generous amounts of selenium. Selenium is a heart-healthy mineral, and is an important cofactor for antioxidant enzymes within the body. Although nuts contain mostly unsaturated and monounsaturated fat, it is best to eat up to 2 ounces a day, as they are concentrated sources of calories.

Tips for Optimum Health

Below are helpful reminders for planning your meals:

- A large green leafy salad daily is an important addition to your diet. A good rule is pair a cooked dish with something raw, even as a garnish.

- More brightly colored vegetables contain more phytochemicals.

- The vegetables in season provide the lowest cost, best taste and most nutrition. If possible grow your own or shop at a farmer's market or store with high produce turnover.

- Fruit is also a great source of fiber. Careful of overeating in-season fruit and dried fruit. If someone has cancer, avoiding all sugars might be the smartest move.

- Add healthier fats such as olives and avocados in moderation.

- If you eat grains, choose whole grains instead of whole grain bread. In general, the less processed the food, the better.

Eating well for health does not have to be difficult, expensive or boring. Food should and can taste great!

366

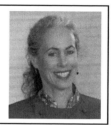

Jill Nussinow, MS, RD, *aka The Veggie Queen™ has been teaching the benefits of a plant-based diet for more than 25 years. She is the author of 2 cookbooks, "The Veggie Queen: Vegetables Get the Royal Treatment" and "The New Fast Food: The Veggie Queen Pressure Cooks Whole Food Meals in Less than 30 Minutes". Her latest book is Nutrition CHAMPS: The Veggie Queen's Guide to Eating and Cooking for Health, Happiness, Energy and Vitality published October 2013. Her website is* http://www.theveggiequeen.com.

Everyone Can Eat Plant-Based

William Harris, MD

All of the carbon-based nutrients required in the human diet are photo-synthesized by green plants, so there is really no reason why any human could not become a successful vegan. Humans have been adaptive omnivores for around the past 4 million years but they never lost the vegetarian genes of the large arboreal vegan apes from which they sprang. This is evidenced by the diets of large contemporary primates and the observation that there are several million healthy human vegans.

Nutritional Guidelines For Foods To Avoid

Michela De Petris, MD

Nutrition is one of the most powerful tools able to influence our current trend of diseases.[1] A diet rich in vegetarian anti-inflammatory foods decreases severity and symptoms, decreases remission periods, and the occurrence of exacerbations. On the other hand, a high-calorie intake of refined foods and proteins and animal fats, produces free radicals, perpetuates inflammation, and favors progression of tissue damage.

All animal foods, not only meat and fish but also animal-derived foods such as milk, cheese, butter, cream, eggs, are a source of acidic proteins that damage tissues (by producing hydrogen sulfide), saturated fats and arachidonic acid (precursor to inflammatory prostaglandins). Furthermore, these foods completely lack antioxidant protection.[2]

Animal based foods abnormally stimulate the immune system which causes a chronic inflammatory state presenting as a variety of different symptoms depending on the organs involved: fatigue, joint pain and swelling, cutaneous lesions, intestinal bleeding, metabolic abnormalities, neurologic deficits, and tissue damage that can even lead to irreversible loss of function.

The only way to naturally decrease inflammation, and cease production of free radicals, favor tissue regeneration and ameliorate this disease trend (particularly autoimmune diseases) is by introducing greater quantities of anti-inflammatory fatty acids (omega 3), vitamins, minerals and antioxidant trace elements particularly abundant in fruit and vegetables.

Here are some of most effective nutritional guidelines for your next trip to grocery store:

AVOID:
- Animal saturated fats and milk, cheese, butter, eggs, meat, salami, fish which contain arachidonic

Animal Products Can Cause Your Body to Mistakenly Kill Itself

High intakes of animal based foods contribute to chronic inflammation which can lead to auto-immune diseases. An **autoimmune disease** is a condition caused by an immune reaction where constituents of the organism (cells, proteins, peptide fragments) are mistakenly identified as exogenous dangerous agents and therefore targeted to be "killed." The most frequent autoimmune diseases are: rheumatoid arthritis, type 1 diabetes, Crohn's Disease, ulcerative colitis, multiple sclerosis, systemic lupus, Sjogren syndrome, psoriasis, scleroderma, polymyositis, autoimmune connectivitis and Hashimoto thyroiditis.

acid-precursors of inflammatory prostaglandins and tissue damage enhancers

- Omega 6 fatty acids (they promote the synthesis of arachidonic acid) found in soy oil, sunflower oil, corn oil, sesame oil, seed oil, margarine, mayonnaise

- Industrial products containing simple sugars (cookies, cakes, sugared drinks, honey, ice cream, all sweets in general). Instead prepare desserts with dehydrated fruit, apple juice, and agave syrup. Replace milk, eggs and butter with rice, soy, oats, almond milk to make cakes, cookies and vegetable muffins

CHOOSE:

- Foods rich in omega 3 fatty acids (they inhibit the production of inflammatory molecules, reduce platelet aggregation, ameliorate tissue response to insulin, lower cholesterol and plasma triglyceride levels, have a powerful anti-inflammatory activity) found in flax oil, flax seeds, hemp seeds, chia and pumpkin seeds, nuts, rosemary, oregano, soy beans, almonds, hazelnuts and seaweed

- Daily foods rich in antioxidant vitamins A, C, E and in anti-inflammatory polyphenols found in green tea, cocoa and raw chocolate, tumeric and curry, wild berries, dried fruit and oil seeds

- Seasonings such as ginger (active ingredient gingerol) and chilli (active ingredient capsaicin) fresh or in powder

- Whole grain cereals for their higher content in antioxidant minerals (magnesium, zinc, selenium)

- Moderate and regular physical activity. Excess caloric intake stimulates the production of free radicals and promotes tissue inflammation

A plant-based diet is the only one able to inactivate free radicals, decrease cellular aging and preserve tissue function in a natural and benign way.[3]

Do You Know Your Vitamin Sources?

<u>Vitamin A:</u> parsley (fresh or dried), carrots, red pepper, basil, yellow pumpkin, green radicchio, peppers, cantaloupe, apricots

<u>Vitamin C:</u> hot peppers, blackberries, nettle, parsley, peppers, oranges, leons, kiwi, Goji berries, acerola. *Note: cooking significantly reduces vitamin C content.*

<u>Vitamin E:</u> hazelnuts, almonds, sunflower seeds, wheat germ, extra virgin olive oil, pine nuts, sage, rosemary

---

Michela De Petris, MD, *graduated with honors in Medicine and Surgery, specializing in Food Science in Milan. She was the medical researcher at the National Cancer Institute and is currently the specialist at the San Raffaele Hospital in Milan. She is a dietitian at the Center for Anthroposophical Medicine Artemedica and Professor of Nutrition in Clinical Nutrition and Wellness courses organized by the Lombardy Region and the Province. Dr. De Petris is the author of "Choice and Vegetarian Life by Bike" Il Pensiero Scientifico Editore (April 2012)*

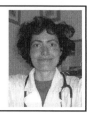

Our Food Sources: Plants, Animals, and Factories

Ana M. Negrón, MD

People in the U.S. have consumed exaggerated amounts of meat, dairy, and unnatural factory foods for over half a century. This has resulted in unprecedented rates of obesity and disease, even in children. It is common for immigrants to gain weight and develop diabetes after just a few years of living on the mainland.

There is ample scientific evidence that we can correct this trend by switching to a diet of whole plants. However, we desperately need food literacy. The current generations of children and their parents are unfamiliar with whole foods like quinoa, collards, kale, daikon, and kohlrabi.

I have been plant-based for 25 years. After introducing oats, quinoa, and steamed kale to one of my patients in 2003, I started a bilingual cooking workshop and gathering that today is an essential part of my medical practice. The patients' rewards are a life with less arthritis medication, cholesterol lowering drugs, medicines to reduce acid reflux, asthma inhalers, diabetic medications, or insulin and a return to wellness.

Food is non prescription medicine. Our bodies' dynamic turnover is so remarkable that within 2 weeks of eliminating dairy and meat and nourishing ourselves well, I see blood pressure, blood sugar, and triglycerides return to normal just as joint aches, acid reflux, bloating, and constipation disappear.

Why Phytonutrients?

Richard A. Oppenlander, D.D.S.

An optimal state of health and wellness is achieved when adopting a purely plant-based diet because of two significant reasons:

1. The elimination of animal products eliminates numerous inflammation stressors, contaminants, and cancer and disease-causing substances.

2. Consumption of plants provides healing and preventive agents, primarily through phytonutrients. Not ONE animal product will give you fiber or phytonutrients.

Phytonutrients play a vital role in preventing and controlling disease, as well as improving longevity by increasing immunity and providing antioxidants and anti-inflammatory properties. Phytonutrients have 5 main categories of actions: 1. Apoptosis (programmed cell death), 2. Repair DNA, 3. Increase immune response, 4. Anti-inflammatory, and 5. Antioxidant.

Antioxidants scavenge free radicals (chemically active atoms with an unpaired electron that contain charged oxygen). Free radicals bombard your other cells and can be formed from stress, either endogenous (respiration, inflammation, disease) or exogenous (pollution, stress factors, chemicals, meat and animal products, and even sunlight). Free radicals can damage DNA and cause acceleration of the aging process and cancer. Plants contain hundreds of these antioxidant-scavenging phytonutrients that help them survive sunlight, chemicals, insects, and stress.

When you consume plant-based foods, these phytonutrients will protect you in similar ways that they protect plants. Most plants have a number of different phytonutrients. Polyphenols, such as flavonoids (quercetin and kaempferol), are powerful antioxidants and can be found in many fruits and vegetables. Catechins are found predominantly in tea, with the highest concentrations in green and white tea. Beans contain lignans, and anthocyanidins can be found in brightly colored berries. Carotenoids (b-carotene, lutein, lycopene) are found in high amounts in orange- and red-colored vegetables, and green leafy vegetables contain isothiocyanates.

Although eating raw plant foods provides many benefits, lightly steaming most vegetables actually increases phytonutrient availability. In an *American Journal of Clinical*

Nutrition article, researchers found that by lightly steaming (without overcooking), the antioxidants in many foods were raised substantially—broccoli by 640%, spinach and asparagus by 100-200%, tomatoes by 150%, carrots by 291%[1]

Read Dr. Oppenlander's "Food Choice And Our Future" in Our Future chapter

Maximizing Nutrition in the Vegan Diet

Jana Bogs, PhD

Author of the recently published "Beyond Organic...Growing for Maximum Nutrition".
www.BeyondOrganicConsulting.com

A major argument against the vegan diet is that it does not supply adequate nutrition. A plant-based diet can provide optimal nutrition but the foods need to be grown properly so they contain the full, balanced array of amino acids and other phytonutrients.

By "grown properly" I mean more than just grown organically. Soils lacking a balanced array of minerals result in plants which do not contain an excellent amino acid profile. Consequently these plants do not fully supply the minerals and other phytonutrients needed by humans. Although I have personally experienced the amazing benefits of a raw, plant-based diet (my weight dropped, and after just 2 months my eye sight dramatically improved), it is important to know that our foods are not what they could or should be from a nutritional standpoint. Food nutrient density has dropped as much as 70% in a 50 year time span. We need to create health from the soil up.

Nine Important Facts About B12

Eric Slywitch, MD

Vitamin B12 is one of most important nutrients for the nervous system. When Vitamin B12 is deficient it affects memory, concentration, and attention. Vitamin B12 is produced by bacterium and is only naturally found in meat, milk, cheese, eggs, and supplements. However, this is not a reason to consume animal products as we can adequately get B12 on a plant-based diet through supplements.

B12 absorption is more about metabolism than frequency as our body can store B12 for a long time, (although the time frame is different from person to person.) Interestingly, B12 deficiency is almost equal across vegetarians and meat-eaters: 50% of vegetarians and about 40% of non-vegetarians have vitamin B12 deficiency. The Institute of Medicine of the United States recommends that everyone over 50 years old use B12 supplements as at least 30% of this population is deficient.

Let's discuss some common questions about B12 and how to address any deficiencies.

1) What are the first symptoms of deficiency and how is it diagnosed? B12 deficiency can have nonspecific symptoms, but the earliest symptom I have seen in patients is tingling in the legs after a few minutes sitting cross-legged. Similarly, complaints of reduced cognitive activity (concentration, memory, and attention) are common. Additionally B12 deficiency can manifest with altered sensitivity of the feet and legs, reduced proprioception (the person has difficulty properly perceive their own body), and psychiatric symptoms.

As B12 is transported in the blood, diagnosis is made primarily by a blood test with or without symptoms of deficiency. Note: there is discrepancy about what physicians deem to be the 'normal range' since B12 levels vary per person.

2) What is the optimal value that B12 should be maintained? Simple rule: always keep the B12 above 490 pcg / mL. Published studies show that when B12 is below 490 pg / mL (the reference being from 200 to 900 pg / ml), it is potentially deficient.

3) How do you maintain proper levels of B12 in your body on a plant-based diet? In a plant-based diet, B12 comes from fortified foods or supplements. Theoretically, to replace the daily loss of B12 in the body, we have to absorb about 1 mcg of B12 per day. (Note: dietitians have a more conservative advisement of 2,4 mcg/day intake per day).

There are 3 ways we can get B12: 1) taken daily orally, 2) taking a weekly oral supplement or 3) via an injection.

- *Daily Orally:* The doses to maintain levels above 490 pg/mL may vary from 5 mcg to

2,000 mcg/day depending upon the person and the way the body metabolizes B12.

- *Weekly Orally:* recommended dose is 2,000 mcg per week. Our body can only absorb 1 to 1.5 mcg every 4 or 6 hours however, but when a big amount of B12 is ingested at the same time, B12 can reach the blood in larger quantities and the body maintains it as stores. For many people, this amount per week might not be sufficient.

- *Injection:* recommended does is 5,000 IU every 6 months or a year. However, quickly raising and reducing the levels of B12 in blood, may not be the optimal way to maintain normal levels in the body.

4) How do you fix B12 deficiency? To correct deficiency, the frequency and dose of B12 should be in accordance with the characteristics of the person treated and its evolution front applications (injections) or pills intake. The oral route (provided in adequate dose and for an adequate period), is much more efficient to correct deficiencies. However, the injection form is the most utilized.

5) How can you explain why some long time vegetarians have no B12 deficiency symptoms? People who are vegetarian for a long time may not have deficiency symptoms, but often have low levels of it. Our body can store B12 for many years. Although you need to absorb B12 daily, when B12 is released daily into our intestine it can return to the blood plasma after being absorbed. Essentially, we can "recycle" our B12 internally preventing loss through this cycle called enterohepatic (the intestine to the liver). However, even with this cycle, we do lose some B12 through our waste and blood levels are reduced.

6) Can algae, fermented foods and brewer's yeast be used for B12? None of these foods can be considered reliable sources of B12. Although algae and fermented foods such as miso can provide small amounts of vitamin B12, it is considered an inactive form of the vitamin is not suitable for humans.

7) Do you have to worry about B12 if you eat eggs, dairy products and fortified foods? Simply put, yes. I have seen countless ovo-lacto-vegetarians patients with low levels of B12. Eating meat and dairy products does not mean you adequately absorb B12.

8) What precautions should you take during pregnancy and infancy in relation to B12? Vitamin B12 has the same importance as folic acid for the formation of the baby. Pregnant women and children should closely maintain their B12 levels.

9) Why do we eat good amount of B12 and still be deficient?
B12 levels depend more on your metabolism than your diet. There are 2 main ways to lose the B12 that is in our body. The first is the internal recycling process. Our gallbladder can launch up to 10 mcg per day of vitamin B12 into the intestine. The amount

released to the gut and the body's ability to absorb each vitamin varies from person to person. And a diet rich in meat, cheese and eggs (sources of B12) can barely reach 7 mcg. This means that there may be greater losses of B12 in the waste than in what a person intakes, which is why a meat and dairy diet does not guarantee adequate B12 levels.

Eric Slywitch, MD, *has a Masters in Nutrition and Graduate Degree in Clinical nutrition. Dr. Slywitch earned his medical degree at the Faculty of Medicine of Jundiai in Brazil. He attended the University of Sao Paulo. He specializes in nutrology and is the head of the Department of Medicine and Nutrition at the Brazilian Vegetarian Society. Dr. Slywitch is author of "Meat Free Meal" (Alimentação sem carne) and "I Turned Vegetarian." And now? (Virei Vegetariano. E agora?). Dr. Slywitch is a professor at GANAP and resides in Sao Paulo.*

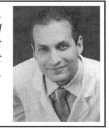

twenty

OUR FUTURE

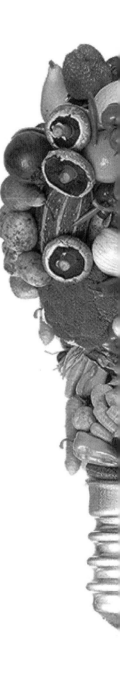

Meat and dairy products have long been associated with the status symbol of wealth and prosperity. Worldwide as populations come into financial security meat and milk becomes part of their meals. This view of social progress is promoting our global health epidemic as Eastern nations aim to follow the Western diet and lifestyle.

Contrary to our stigma of "poor" foods consisting of fruits, vegetables and grains, studies around the world reveal that the societies who live the longest and healthiest are those who primarily eat a whole foods plant-based diet filled with vegetables, fruits, grains, legumes and nuts. The Okinawas, on average, live well into their 90s on a staple diet of potatoes and yams. Meat, fish and dairy are almost non-existent. In fact, as western diets heavy in meat and dairy become more prominent in Asian societies, a dramatic rise in diseases occurs-mirroring the rates in the US and Europe. This correlation is a direct effect from changes in diet.

More than the health epidemic, our global demand for meat and dairy is ravaging our finite and precious resources. Think about this: to produce one hamburger from start to finish, (land for crops needed to feed the animals, fertilizers, insecticides, machinery, transportation, drugs, manure spills etc.) it requires 55 acres of rainforest, about 5,000 gallons of water and 284 gallons of oil.[1] Although hard to believe, it is true. Our desire to produce these unhealthy foods as cheaply as possible is creating virulent strains of bacteria that are predicted to lead to the next pandemics to wipe out populations. We are simultaneously approaching the end of the antibiotic era and the age of large scale water wars. We have one Earth and we cannot afford to decimate our only resources. We desperately need to re-evaluate how to produce food, drastically reduce our meat and dairy consumption, and restore the health of our Earth as we restore our own.

Can Plants Save The World?

Hope Ferdowsian, MD, MPH, FACP, FACPM

For the first time in history, poor nutrition is becoming at least as important a problem to address as tobacco.[1] The World Health Organization and the Food and Agriculture Organization emphasize that chronic diseases, often associated with animal fat and protein consumption, are now responsible for the majority of deaths worldwide. It is not just products from factory-farmed animals either – all sources of animal products contribute to chronic diseases.

Despite the relatively recent Western transition to a diet high in meat and dairy products, much of the rest of the world has traditionally followed a primarily or entirely, plant-based diet. Worldwide meat production has increased more than 10 times faster than the population growth rate over the past several decades,[2] and dairy consumption has followed a similar trend. The world's population is projected to top 9 billion by the middle of the 21st century; if the rest of the world consumes anywhere near the amount of meat the average American eats each year, we will face a health and economic disaster from increased rates of heart disease, diabetes, stroke and cancer – diseases for which industrialized, middle and low income countries do not have adequate resources to fully address.

The Leading Global Killers

Approximately 60% of global deaths occur because of chronic diseases.[3] Today, more than 1.5 billion people are overweight (1 in every 5 people).[4] Heart disease is the leading cause of death, claiming about 17 million lives per year.[5] Diabetes is expected to affect 300 million people by 2025.[6] Close to 2/3 of the 3 million deaths attributable to diabetes

Case Study: Micronesia

Before World War II, there were zero cases of diabetes in Micronesia, according to the United States Navy.[15] People ate diets rich in breadfruit, yams, citrus fruits, bananas, coconuts, and other plant-based foods. Now only half a century later, about one-third of people in Micronesia are affected by diabetes.[16]

So what changed? After World War II, imports from the United States and other countries began to change the ways in which Micronesians eat, consuming more of a "Western diet," full of animal products and processed foods. Genetic factors that could have once protected people from starvation now set Micronesians up for obesity, diabetes, heart disease, and certain forms of cancer. Since Micronesians do not have access to the same levels of medical care many Americans do, complications like blindness, limb amputations, kidney failure, and heart attacks, are more difficult to treat.

The Global Costs of Rising Disease

Worldwide, obesity accounts for at least 2-7% of total health care costs.[17] Diabetes, heart disease, and stroke will contribute dramatically to lost national income in the next 10 years. Projected losses over the next decade include more than $550 billion in China, $330 billion in India, $300 billion in the Russian Federation, $49 billion in Brazil, and $2.5 billion in Tanzania.[18] These projected losses are a significant portion of each country's gross domestic product (GDP).

Current trends indicate that the overall chronic disease prevalence will continue to rise. Projections suggest that non-communicable diseases will account for 57% of all disability in developing countries within 25 years.[19] Although chronic degenerative diseases are typically associated with elderly persons, about 80% of productivity is lost by the working age population in developing countries.[6] These trends will result in a dwindling workforce, and severely impact children who depend on the support of disabled parents.

each year occur in developing countries.[7] By 2030, more than 80% of individuals with diabetes will be in developing countries. India has the largest population of individuals with diabetes, with China closely approaching. China's urban population has increased its animal protein and fat consumption leading to dramatic increases in heart disease mortality compared with rural inhabitants who follow more plant-based diets.[8]

Chronic diseases are even becoming more prevalent in areas such as Sub-Saharan Africa, where historically infectious diseases has most influenced health.[9] In 2009, 5 in every 120 Kenyan children had type 2 diabetes.[10] Death rates from chronic diseases as a whole are higher in Africa than in practically any other region in the world,[11] and over the next decade, the African continent is expected to experience the largest increases in death rates for heart disease, cancer, and diabetes.

The solution is quite simple. Large studies have shown that populations consuming low-fat, plant-based diets are less likely to be overweight and obese, or have heart disease or diabetes.[12,13,14] These diseases are actually reversible when people switch from eating meats and dairy products to strict vegetarian or vegan diets.

What YOU Can Do

Sometimes health problems seem overwhelming, but it is never too late to make changes.

One of my patients, a 73 year old woman, discovered she had diabetes, elevated blood pressure, and dangerously high cholesterol when she was admitted to the hospital for an orthopedic emergency. Less than 2 years after adopting a low fat, plant-based diet, she lost more than 70 lbs, completely reversed her diabetes, lowered her cholesterol, and her blood pressure returned to normal. She feels empowered and is ecstatic that her lifestyle choices also have positive "side effects" for animals, the environment, and people living on the other side of the world. My younger patients equally experience health benefits including weight loss, improved blood pressure, diabetes and cholesterol, as well as positive changes in their skin, menstrual cycles, and energy levels.

We need a radical shift in our diets if we are going to reverse the out-of-control growth rate of chronic diseases. Choose fruits, vegetables, beans, and whole grains. Keep meat, cheese, and eggs off your plate and dairy milk out of your glass – we don't need these products. As adults, let's set a better example and help kids choose healthier options. Spread the word and speak up for people living in your own community and abroad by lobbying for healthier options at school, work, and religious institutions. We are at a time in history desperate for revolution, and the revolution begins within each of us.

Hope Ferdowsian, MD, MPH, FACP, FACPM, *is an Assistant Professor of Medicine at The George Washington University and Adjunct Associate Professor at the Georgetown University Medical Center Department of Microbiology and Immunology. She is double-board certified in General Internal Medicine and General Preventive Medicine and Public Health. Dr. Ferdowsian is a volunteer physician for Health Right International and Physicians for Human Rights (PHR), and she serves as a consultant for the PHR Program on Sexual Violence in Conflict Zones. Internationally, she has worked in Malawi, South Africa, Kenya, Uganda, Ethiopia, and the Federated States of Micronesia.*

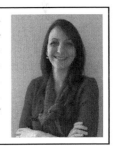

The New Laboratories For Deadly Viruses

Aysha Akhtar, MD, MPH

Suppose we learned that a rogue scientist was producing deadly influenza viruses around the clock in a laboratory and that the scientist planned to release these viruses into the general population. How would we react? What if we learned that these deadly viruses are already being produced, not in scientific laboratories, but in animal factory farms?

New and dangerous pathogens are emerging and spreading rapidly throughout the world at an increasing pace. Novel influenza A viruses (such as bird flu variants H5N1 and H7N9 and swine flu variants H1N1 and H3N2) have already caused a significant number of human illnesses and deaths as the virus has spread through China, Pakistan, Southeast Asia, and the Middle East.

So far, we have been lucky that, though many of the viruses are extremely lethal, they have not yet been very contagious among humans. However, as long as we continue to confine billions of animals on factory farms, we are unwittingly creating a global laboratory of dangerous pathogens. In spite of our current low risk, it is just a matter of time before H5N1, H7N9, or another influenza strain evolves from a factory farm into a contagious form that leads to a pandemic.

The Rise of Factory Farms

Factory farming is a leading contributor to the rise in infectious diseases and antibiotic resistance.[1] Once viewed as a luxury, meat is now becoming a dietary staple due to a worldwide growth in urbanized populations and affluence. Annually, over 64 billion land animals are raised and killed for food worldwide.[2] In the United States alone, over 9 billion land animals are slaughtered for food each year—that is about 1 million per hour.[3]

With this increasing demand for animal products come the intensification of animal agriculture and the suffering of more animals than ever before seen in human history. Farmed animals are treated as "production units" and are denied their most basic needs in the name of efficiency. The overwhelming majority of animals raised for food are housed in extremely filthy, overcrowded conditions without access to fresh air, sunlight, or space to move around normally. This demand-driven transformation of animal agriculture is so dramatic that it has been dubbed the "Livestock Revolution."[4]

The conditions in these farms greatly contribute to the creation of deadly influenza viruses. For example, let's look at wild aquatic birds, the primordial source of all influenza A viruses--the ones that have the potential to cause pandemics. People rarely become infected directly from wild aquatic birds. Usually an intermediate host is involved—providing the right biological setting for the virus to transform into something that can easily infect humans. This is where chickens and other farmed animals play a role.

Viruses pass readily from animal to animal in factory farms, not only because they are tightly crowded together, but also because their ability to fight off infections is severely reduced by the distressful situations in which they are forced to live. Once these viruses enter poultry operations they can rapidly mutate into highly pathogenic (very lethal) viruses within very short periods of time.

Since 1990, outbreaks of highly pathogenic virus subtypes have increased substantially among farmed birds, and the intensive confinement of birds has been found to facilitate both the increasing frequency and scale of these outbreaks.[5,6,7] Every transmission of the virus from one animal to another brings us closer to a pandemic. H5N1 demonstrates how a virus emerged from wildlife, adapted to domestic poultry, and, after circulating in these populations, acquired the ability to infect humans.[8]

As pigs are highly susceptible to both avian and human influenza viruses, they could be the means by which H5N1 and other viruses gain the ability to widely infect humans. Among the scientific community, pigs are commonly referred to as "mixing vessels" in whom viruses from birds, humans, and other pigs co-mingle. In pigs, influenza viruses swap genes, accelerating their mutation into forms that can widely infect humans. A 2010 study not only confirmed widespread H5N1 infection in pigs, but also the lack of symptoms in pigs carrying H5N1. This means that the virus can easily evolve and evade detection in pig populations transported throughout the world.[9] Even more concerning is the fact that one viral isolate from pigs acquired the ability to recognize a cell receptor in both pig and human noses, a change that could allow it to spread more easily among humans.

If we really want to prevent H5N1and other deadly viruses from causing a pandemic, we need to turn our attention to how we are producing meat, eggs, and dairy products. By densely confining animals, by the billions to feed our global appetite for animal products, we are unwittingly accelerating the mutation of the influenza A virus into a form more deadly than we have yet seen. While governments have tried vaccination, surveillance, and "culling" animals who are infected, the only lasting solution is to prevent the viruses from emerging in the first place.[10]

Traditionally we have viewed our health in an evolutionary vacuum, ignoring its connection to our relationship with other animals. However, our health is inextricably tied with how we treat animals.[10] By significantly reducing our consumption of animals, or better yet going vegan, we can make lasting changes that benefit all of us. By simply choosing one plate of food over another, we can each single-handedly help thwart a pandemic, reduce climate change, keep ourselves slimmer and healthier, and reduce animal suffering.[11] I challenge anyone to name a drug that can accomplish all of that!

   The opinions expressed here are those of the author and do not represent the official position of the U.S. Food and Drug Administration or the U.S. government."

Aysha Akhtar, MD, MPH *is a neurologist and public health specialist with the Office of Counterterrorism and Emerging Threats of the Food and Drug Administration and a Fellow of The Oxford Centre for Animal Ethics. She also serves as LCDR in the US Public Health Services Commissioned Corps. She is the author of Animals and Public Health. Why treating animals better is critical to human welfare.* www.ayshaakhtar.com

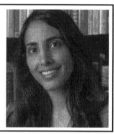

Food Choice and Our Future

Richard A. Oppenlander, D.D.S.

While health is important, it will not matter how healthy we are as individuals if our planet is not healthy.

'Sustainability' vs. Global Depletion

Estimates from the Global Footprint Network show that we are and have been, in an "overshoot" mode-- using our planet's resources at a rate of 1.6 times over what it can provide. It is predicted that by 2030 we will need 2 full Earths to sustain our current rate of consumption.

Perhaps the most appropriate manner in which to view sustainability issues is with an understanding of what we are *losing*. I call this global depletion: the loss of our primary resources, as well as our own health. As we deplete our natural resources, we add 230,000 new human mouths to feed each day. It is predicted that in just 18 years, there will be a 40% global water shortage (already over 1 billion people are without adequate drinking water; 2 billion are without running water for cleaning and hygiene). Nearly 6 million children will starve to death in 2013. Contrary to common belief, global depletion is not as much a matter of overpopulation as it is what we are all doing to our planet.

What Is The Extent Of The Problem? [1]

The largest contributing factor to all areas of global depletion is the raising and eating of more than 70 billion animals each year and the annual extraction of 1 to 2 trillion fish from our oceans. This consumption is most responsible for the following set of problems:

- Increased risk of the most common degenerative diseases and cancers found in the Western world

- Increased health care costs and loss of productivity

- Prevalence of world hunger (77% of all coarse grain produced globally per year is given to livestock, impacting food prices, resource use and availability)

- Depletion of our oceans (commercial fishing has caused the collapse and near extinction of numerous species, loss of coral reefs, and destruction of ecosystems)

- Depletion of freshwater supplies (nearly 30% of all freshwater used in the world goes to livestock)

- Climate change (30-50% of all human-induced greenhouse gas emissions are due to the raising and eating of animals)

- Inefficient agricultural land use (45% of all land on Earth is now being used by livestock)

- Pollution (our atmosphere, land, freshwater, and oceans are all adversely affected by raising and harvesting animals to eat)

- Loss of biodiversity (plants, animals, and insects are becoming extinct at a rate up to 10,000 times what has been seen for the past few millions of years)

Comparing Agricultural Systems

Agricultural systems use massive quantities of land, water, and energy inefficiently to produce meat and dairy products. Each year the U.S. plants approximately 56 million acres of alfalfa and over 120 million acres for feed crops—all going to livestock and poultry— but only 50,000 acres in buckwheat, an exceptional plant that provides numerous human health benefits. Over the years, 75% of all buckwheat harvested has been fed to livestock.

More than 260 million acres of U.S. forest have been cleared just to create cropland to grow grain to feed farmed animals. This is the equivalent of 7 football fields of land bulldozed worldwide *every minute.*[2] For every acre of land in the U.S. that is used for raising a fraction of a cow (as each grass-fed cow requires more than one acre to graze), as well as the acre next to it used to grow grains to supplement feed for that cow, we could grow ancient grains, beans, green leafy vegetables, fruit, nuts, and herbs and spices, providing us with literally thousands more pounds of resource efficient and healthier food per acre.

Freshwater Crisis

One of the most pressing concerns we face today is our supply of fresh water. Fresh water constitutes just 2.5% of all water on earth and is not fully renewable in our lifetime, nor infinite in quantity. From 1941 to 2011 the world's freshwater consumption has quadrupled. This is predicted to leave 40% of the world's population facing severe water stress by the year 2020. By 2050 one third of all counties in the lower United States spanning 14 states will face water shortages.

While many scientists and organizations are researching new technologies, the matter is really one of water management. Rather than focusing on individual acts of everyday water consumption (flushing toilets, taking showers, doing laundry, etc.), we need to manage the more water-intensive practices involved in production of our food choices and particularly animal products. Nearly half of U.S. annual water consumption goes toward raising livestock, while less than 1% is used for human drinking purposes. The meat and dairy industries combine to account for 29% of all the fresh water used in the world today.

Think about this: producing a pound of meat requires approximately 50 times more water than producing a pound of vegetables, fruits, or grain for us to eat directly. Between 1,700 and 4,000 gallons of water are needed to produce 1 pound of beef (depending on location), 880 gallons to produce 1 gallon of milk, and over 100 gallons to produce a single egg! Additionally some animals use 40 or more gallons per day—that's over 100 times what we as individuals need to consume daily.[3]

The average American consumes 206 pounds of meat each year (broken down: 46 pounds of pig, 58 pounds of cow, and 102 pounds of chicken and turkey), as well as 248 eggs and 616 pounds of dairy products. This equates to 405,000 gallons of water per person per year, consumed just to support that animal-based diet.[4] A more accurate account of the water consumption for the average U.S. household of 3 people is over a million gallons of water each year. Ninety-six percent of that water use results directly from the choice to eat animals.

To appease this consumption, aquifers are being drawn down at rates as high as 250 times their ability to recharge. As much as 75% of the water withdrawals from groundwater aquifers such as the North China Plain, the Ogallala, the Columbia River Basin, and California's San Joaquin Valley are given to livestock. The 12 million-year-old Ogallala Aquifer, which has supported 50% of our cattle industry since the mid-1940s, is predicted to run completely dry within the next 20 years.

A new era of water scarcity has arrived, and it will require an enormous paradigm shift regarding how we view and manage water sources. This will be critical in the developing world. The most effective water-management changes relative to the time lines we are on is the *eradication* of meat and dairy from our diet, not simply "*limiting*" it as the United Nations Environment Programme (UNEP) advised, for true progress.

World Water Wars

Freshwater scarcity coexists with hunger, poverty, and inefficient use of marginal natural resources. Soon countries downstream will be battling those upstream for freshwater supplies. Pakistan, Afghanistan, and Saudi Arabia are raising livestock and crops to feed these animals while running their water supplies dry. Sixty percent of Ethiopia's population suffers from hunger and thirst, and yet their parched land is being used to support a growing herd of over 50 million cattle.

Taking Action

How can our land and freshwater be used most efficiently with the least amount of greenhouse gas emissions, and have the least impact on sea life and our oceans? Which foods will best solve world hunger, most likely to reduce overall food prices and health care costs, and which will be most beneficial to our own human health?

As a civilization, we are just now beginning to recognize the food choice-planetary-human health connection. Many of our planet's concerns can be eliminated or, at least significantly minimized by a simple, collective change to a healthier, more peaceful, plant-based food choice and thereby more efficient, more compassionate food-production systems. We all have the ability to make the change and inspire others to do the same—for our sake and for that of future generations.

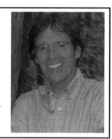

Richard A. Oppenlander, D.D.S., *is the author of the newly released "Food Choice and Sustainability" and the award-winning book "Comfortably Unaware", endorsed by Ellen DeGeneres, Dr. Jane Goodall, and Dr. Neal Barnard, among others. Dr. Oppenlander is a sought after lecturer and keynote speaker for several conferences and events. Dr. Oppenlander also serves as an advisor to municipalities in the U.S. and to world hunger projects that are designing programs from his model of multidimensional sustainability. He is president and founder of an organic vegan food production and education business, as well as the founder of the non-profit organization, Inspire Awareness Now.* http://comfortablyunaware.com/

Taking the Next Step

Sometimes it can seem overwhelmingly making dietary changes. Below are some of our favorite plant-based resources from cookbooks to health and fitness books that will get you on track to a delicious and invigorating plant-based lifestyle.

If you need or would like medical care, we highly recommend reading the doctors' bios which can direct you to their helpful and informative websites as well as their plant-based clinics and programs.

Health, Fitness, and Cookbooks:

1. *Artisan Vegan Cheese* by Miyoko Schinner
2. *Betty Goes Vegan* by Annie and Dan Shannon
3. *Chloe's Kitchen* and *Chloe's Vegan Desserts* by Chloe Coscarelli
4. *Crazy, Sexy, Diet* by Kris Carr author of Crazy, Sexy Cancer
5. *Comfortably Unaware* by Dr. Richard Oppenlander
6. *Eat to Live* and *Disease-Proof your Child* by Dr. Joel Fuhrman
7. *Eat Carbohydrates, Get Thin (And Healthy)* by Dr. Magda Robinson
8. *Eat Vegan on $4 a Day* by Ellen Jaffe Jones
9. *Fast Food Nation* by Eric Schlosser
10. *Food Prescription for Better Health* by Dr. Baxter Montgomery
11. *Health Power* by Dr. Hans Diehl
12. *Holistic Heart* by Dr. Joel Kahn
13. *Isa Does It* by Isa Chandra Moskowitz
14. *Just be Well* by Dr. Thomas Sult
15. *Mad Cowboy* and *No More Bull* by Howard Lyman
16. *Mayim's Vegan Table* by Mayim Bialik with Jay Gordon
17. *No Meat Athlete* by Matthew Ruscigno
18. *Pet Goats and Pap Smears* by Dr. Pamela Wible
19. *Pillars of Health* by Jean Pierre
20. *Power Foods for the Brain* and *The 21 Day Weight-Loss Kickstart Dr. Neal Barnard's Program to Reversing Diabetes* by Dr. Neal Barnard
21. *Prevent and Reverse Heart Disease* by Dr. Caldwell B. Esselstyn, Jr.
22. *Skinny Bitch Cookbook* by Kim Barnouin
23. *The Candle Café Cookbook* Joy Pierson, Bart Potenza Barbara Scott-Goodman
24. *The Cheesy Vegan* by John Schlimm
25. *The China Study* by Drs. T. Colin Campbell and Thomas M. Campbell
26. *The Conscious Cook* by Tal Ronnen
27. *The Engine 2 Diet* and *My Beef with Meat* by Rip Esselstyn
28. *The Expert's Guide to Weight Loss Surgery* by Dr. Garth Davis

29. *The Food Revolution* and *Diet for a New America* by John Robbins
30. *The Happy Herbivore* by Lindsay S. Nixon
31. *The Joy of Vegan Baking* and *The Vegan Table* by Colleen Patrick-Goudreau
32. *The Kind Diet* by Alicia Silverstone
33. *The Meaty Truth* by Shushana Castle & Amy-Lee Goodman, fall 2014
34. *The Starch Solution* by Dr. John McDougall
35. *The Pleasure Trap* by Dr. Alan Goldhamer
36. *The Thrive Diet* by Brendan Brazier
37. *The Vegan Diner* by Julie Hasson
38. *Unprocessed* by Chef AJ
39. *Veganist* by Kathy Freston
40. *Veganomicon* by Isa Chandra Moskowitz and Terry Hope Romero
41. *Vegan A La Mode* by Hannah Kaminsky
42. *Vegan Chocolate* by Fran Costigan
43. *Vegan Cooking for Carnivores* by Roberto Martin
44. *Vegan Cupcakes Take Over the World* and *Vegan Cookies Take Over Your Cookie Jar* by Isa Chandra Moskowitz, Terry Hope Romero
45. *Vegan for Life* by Jack Norris and Virginia Messina
46. *Vegan Holiday Kitchen* by Nava Atlas and Susan Voisin
47. *Vegan Soul Kitchen* by Terry Bryant
48. *Waist Away* by Dr. Clifton and Dr. Clinton
49. *Whitewash* by Dr. Joseph Keon
50. *Whole* by Dr. T. Colin Campbell with Howard Jacobson

DVD's:

1. Eating
2. Fat, Sick and Nearly Dead
3. Food, Inc
4. Forks Over Knifes
5. Vegucated

Notes

Chapter 1

Hans A. Diehl

1. N Temple, DP Burkitt, *Western Diseases: Their dietary prevention and reversibility*, (Totowa, NJ:Humana Press, 1994). Personal communication with DP Burkitt, 1992.
2. FF Marvasti, RS Stafford, "From sick care to health care- re-engineering prevention into the US system," *N Engl J Med* 367(2012):889-91.
3. G Danaei et al., "The preventable causes of death in the US: comparative risk assessment of dietary, lifestyle, and metabolic risk factors," *PLOS Med* 6(4)(2009):e1000058.
4. HA Diehl, A Ludington, *Health Power*, (Hagerstown, MD: Review and Herald Publishing Association:2011).
5. CC Cowie et al., "Full accounting of diabetes and pre-diabetes in the US population from 1988 to 2006," *Diabetes Care* 32(3)(2011):287-94.
6. Centers for Disease Control and Prevention, *National diabetes fact sheet 2011*, (Atlanta, GA:CDCP, USDHHS, 2012).
7. KM Narayam et al., "Diabetes: a common, growing, serious, costly and potentially preventable public health problem," *Diabetes Res Clin Pract* 50(Suppl 2)(2000):577-84.
8. Centers for Disease Control and Prevention, "Overweight and obesity," 2012, accessed Nov. 30th, 2013, www.cdc.gov/obesity/data/adult.html.
9. AV Finn et al., "History of Discovery: concepts of atherscrlotic plaques," *Atheroscerlosis, Thrombosis, and Vascular Biology*, 30(2010):1282-92.
10. JP Strong et al., "Prevalence and extent of atherosclerosis in adolescents and young adults," *JAMA* 281(1999): 727-35.
11. D Ornish et al., "Can lifestyle changes reverse coronary heart disease? The Lifestyle Heart Trial," *Lancet* 336(8708)(1990): 129-33. D. Ornish et al., "Intensive lifestyle changes for reversal of coronary heart disease," *JAMA* 280 (23)(1998): 2001-7.
12. CB Esselstyn et al., "A strategy to arrest and reverse coronary artery disease: a 5-year longitudinal study of a single physician's practice," *J Family Pract* 4(6)(1995): 560-8. CB Esselstyn, "Updating a 12-year experience with arrest and reversal therapy for coronary heart disease (an overdue requiem for palliative cardiology)," *Am J Cardiol* 84(3)(1999): 339-41.
13. CJ O'Donnell, R Elosua, "Cardiovascular risk factors: Insights from the Framingham Heart Study," *Rev Esp Cardiol* 61(3) (2008): 299-310. J Stamler, "George Lyman Duff Memorial Lecture: Lifestyles, major risk factors, proof and public policy," *Circulation* 58(1978):3-19.
14. D Ornish et al., "Intensive lifestyle changes may affect the progression of prostate cancer," *J Urology* 174(2005): 1065-70. D Ornish et al., "Changes in prostate gene expression in men undergoing intensive diet and lifestyle intervention," *Proc Nat Acad Sciences* 102(24)(2008): 8369-75. WJ Aronson et al., "Growth inhibitory effects of a low-fat diet on prostate cancer cells: results of a prospective randomized dietary intervention trial in men with prostate cancer," *J Urology* 183(2010): 345-50.
15. CB Esselstyn, *Prevent and Reverse Heart Disease*, (New York: Penguin Group, 2007).
16. ND Barnard et al., "A low-fat vegan diet improves glycemic control and cardiovascular risk factors in a randomized clinical trial in individuals with type 2 diabetes," Diabetes Care 29(8)(2006): 1777-83.
17. Pritikin Program clinical results bibliography, accessed Nov 30, 2013, www.pritikin.com/you-health/pritikin-research/research-foundation.html.
18. CHIP Program clinical results bibliography, accessed Dec. 1st, 2013, www.CHIPhealth.com/About-CHIP/Scientific-Publications/.
19. Gordon Wardlaw, Anne Smith, *Contemporary Nutrition*, McGraw-Hill: 192. http://highered.mcgraw-hill.com/sites/dl/free/007501855/191973/war01855_ch06.pdf

Juliet Gellatley

1. J. V. Ferraro, et al., "Earliest Archaeological Evidence of Persistent Hominin Carnivory," *PLoS ONE* 8 (2013), e62174.
2. J. Wilkins, et al., "Evidence for Early Hafted Hunting Technology," *Science* 338 (2012): 942-46.
3. K. Milton, "A Hypothesis to Explain the Role of Meat-Eating in Human Evolution," *Evolutionary Anthropology* 8(1) (1999): 11-21.
4. The National Health Service, "Lactose Intolerance," in the *NHS Direct Online Health Encyclopaedia*, from the NHS Direct website (2005), http://www.nhsdirect.wales.nhs.uk/encyclopaedia/l/article/lactoseintolerance
5. H. Pringle, "Neolithic Agriculture: Reading the Signs of Ancient Animal Domestication," *Science* 282 (1998): 1448.

Zarin Azar

1. Heather J. Baer, Robert J. Glynn, Frank B,Hu, Susan E. Hankinson, Walter. C. Wilett et al, "Risk Factors for Mortality in the Nurses' Health Study, A Competing risk," *American J. of Epidemiology* 73(2012). Michael Greger, "Eggs, Cigarettes, and Atherosclerosis," NutritionFacts.org, September 2013, http://nutritionfacts.org/2013/09/10/eggs-vs-cigarettes-in-atherosclerosis/.
2. W.H. Wilson Tang, Zeneng Wang, Bruce S. Levison, Robert A. Koeth, B.S., Earl B. Britt, et al., "Intestinal Microbial Metabolism of Phosphatidylcholine and Cardiovascular Risk," *New England Journal of Medicine* 368(17)(April 25,2013):1575-1584.
3. MC Morris, EA Evans, JL Bienias, et al., "Dietary fats and the risk of incident Alzheimer disease," *Arch Neurol* 60(2003):194-200.

4.   MH Laitinen, T Ngandu, S Rovio, et al., "Fat intake at mid life and risk of dementia and Alzheimer's disease: A population-based study," *Dement Geriatr Cogn Disorder* 22(2006):99-107.

5.   Tulika Arora, Rajkumar Sharma, Gary Frost, "Propionate, Anti-Obesity and Satiety Enhancing Factor?" *Appetite* 56(2011)511-515. www.elsewier.com/local/appetite

6.   Jacob Exler, Linda lemar and Julie Smith, "Fat and Fatty Acid Content of Selected Foods Containing Tarns-Fatty Acids: Special purpose table #1," *US Department of Agriculture Research Service*, www.usda.gov. Ida Laake, Jan I.Pedersen, Rundi Sclmer, Bente Kirkhus, Anja S. Lindman, Aage Tverdal, and Marit B. Veienrod, "A Prospective Study of Intake of Trans-Fatty Acids from Ruminant Fat, Partially Hydrogenated Vegetable Oils and Marine oils and Mortality from CVD," *British.J.of Nutrition* (2011):1-12.

Chapter 2

James Loomis

1.   SM Grundy, JI Cleeman, SR Daniels, *et al,* "Diagnosis and management of the metabolic syndrome: an American Heart Association/National Heart, Lung, and Blood Institute Scientific Statement". *Circulation* 112 (17) (2005): 2735–52.

Chapter 3

Sahara Adams

1.   Iain L C Chapple, Michael R Milward, Nicola Ling-Mounford, et al, "Adjunctive Daily Supplementation with Encapsulated Fruit, Vegetable and Berry Juice Powder Concentrates and Clinical Periodontal Outcomes: a Double- Blind RCT". *Journal of Clinical Periodontol* 39 (1)(2012): 62-72

2.   Cyril O. Enwonwu, Reshma S. Phillips and Christine D. Ibrahim et al., "Nutrition and oral health in Africa," *International Dental Journal* 54(2004):344-351.

3.   Iain L C Chapple, Michael R Milward, Nicola Ling-Mounford, et al, "Adjunctive Daily Supplementation with Encapsulated Fruit, Vegetable and Berry Juice Powder Concentrates and Clinical Periodontal Outcomes: a Double- Blind RCT". *Journal of Clinical Periodontol* 39 (1)(2012): 62-72

Ashmit Gupta

1.   Adarsh K Gupta and Ashmit Gupta, "Rhinitis and Acute Rhinosinusitis" in *Treatment Strategies- Respiratory*, ed. Cambridge Research Centre, 2011.

2.   C Lill et al., "Milk allergy is frequent in patients with chronic rhinitis and nasal polyposis," *American Journal Rhinology and Allergy* 25(6): 221-4.

3.   "Foods that Cause Mucus Build-Up" last modified 2013, http://www.healthguidance.org/entry/14588/1/Foods-That-Cause-Mucus-Build-Up.html.

4.   AK Gupta and A Gupta, "Management of Chronic Rhinosinusitis", *Osteopathic Family Physician* 2:4-9.

5.   H Juntti et al., "Cow's milk allergy is associated with recurrent otitis media during childhood," *Acta Otolaryngologica* 119(8): 867-73.

6.   Farahmand et al., "Cow's mildk allergy among children with gastroesophageal reflux disease," *Gut Liver* 5(3): 298-301.

7.   Bradshaw et al., "Associations between dietary patterns and head and neck cancer," *American Journal of Epidemiology* 175(12): 1225-1233.

Martin Root & Ellen Lawrence

1.   RA Silva, JJ West, Y Zhang, SC Anenberg, JF Lamareque, et al., "Global premature mortality due to anthropogenic outdoor air pollution and the contributor of past climate change", *Environment Research Letters,* 2013.

2.   TM McKeever, SA Lewis, PA Cassano, M Ocke, P Burney, J Britton, HA Smit, "Patterns of dietary intake and relation to respiratory disease, forced expiratory volume of 1s, and decline in 5-y forced expiratory volume." *American Journal of Clinical Nutrition,* (2010): 408-15.

3.   F Hirayama, A Lee, C Binns, N Hiramatsu, M Mitsuru, and K Nishumura, "Dietary intake of isoflavones and polysaturated fatty acids associated with lung function, breathlessness and the prevalence of chronic obstructive pulmonary disease: Possible protective effect of traditional Japanese diet", Molecular Nutrition and Food Research, (2010): 909-17.

4.   CS Tabak, D Heederik, MC Ocke, D Kromhout, "Diet and chronic obstructive pulmonary disease: independent beneficial effects of fruit, whole grains, and alcohol (The MORGEN study)", *Clinical and Experimental Allergy*, (2001): 747:55.

5.   BK Butland, AM Fehily, PC Elwood, "Diet, lung function, and lung function decline in a cohort of 2512 middle aged men", *Thoraz.* (2000): 102-8.

6.   Y Cui, H Morgenstern, S. Greenland, D, Tashkin, J. Mao, L Cai, W. Cozen, T Mack, Q. Lu, and Z. Zhang, "Dietary Flavoniod Intake and Lung Cancer- A Population-based Case-Control Study", *Cancer.* (2008): 2241-8.

7.   H Kan, Stevens J, Heiss G, KM Rose, SJ London, "Dietary Fiber, Lung Function, and Chronic Obstructive Pulminary Disease in the Atherosclerosis Risk in Communities Study", *American Journal of Epidemiology.* (2008).

8.   R Varraso, WC Willet, CA Camargo Jr., "Prospective study of dietary fiber and risk of chronic obstructive pulmonary disease among US women and men", American Journal of Epidemiology. 171 (1) (2010): 776-84.

Alireza Falahati- Nini

1.   S. Mishra, J XU, U Agarwal, J. Gonzales, S Levin, and ND Barnard, "A multicenter randomized controlled trial of a plant-based nutrition program to reduce body weight and cardiovascular risk in the corporate setting: the GEICO study." *European Journal of Clinical Nutrition.* 67(7) (2013): 718–724.

2.   Serena Tonstad, MD, PHD, Terry Butler, DRPH, Ru Yan, MSC, and Gary E. Fraser, MD, PHD, "Type of Vegetarian Diet, Body Weight, and Prevalence of Type 2 Diabetes", *Diabetes Care.* 32(5) (2009): 791–796.

3.   JM Berardi, AC Logan, AV Rao, "Plant based dietary supplement increases urinary pH", *Journal of the International Society Sports Nutrition*, 6(2008): 5-20.

4. K Arnberg, C Molgaard, KF Michaelson, SM Jenson et al., "Skim milk, whey, and casein increase body weight and whey and casein increase the plasma C-peptide concentration in overweight adolescents", Journal of Nutrition, 142(12) (2012): 2083-90.

5. Zhifang Yang, Zhumin Zhang, Kristina L. Penniston, Neil Binkley, and Sherry A. Tanumihardjo, "Serum carotenoid concentrations in postmenopausal women from the United States with and without osteoporosis", International Journal of Vitamin Nutrition Research, 78(3)(2008):105-11.
Ambroszkiewicz J, Klemarczyk W, Gajewska J, Chełchowska M, Rowicka G, Ołtarzewski M, Laskowska-Klita T, "Serum concentration of adipocytokines in prepubertal vegetarian and omnivorous children", Med *Wieku Rozwoj* 15(3) (2011):326-34.

6. BL Beezhold, "Restriction of meat, fish, and poultry in omnivores improves mood: a pilot randomized controlled trial." *Nutrition Journal* 11(2012):9.

7. H Kahleova, M Matoulek, H Malinska, O Oliyarnik et al., "Vegetarian diet improves insulin resistance and oxidative stress markers more than conventional diet in subjects with Type 2 diabetes." *Diabet Med* 28(5)(2011): 549–559.

8. U Vij, and A Kumar, "Phyto-oestrogens and prostatic growth." *National Medicine Journal of India* 17(1)(2004):22-6.

Jimmy Conway

1. AR Halabi, JH Alexander, LK Shaw, et al, "Relation of Early saphenous vein graft failure, to outcomes following coronary artery bypass surgery." *American Journal of Cardiology* 96(9) (2005):1254-9.

2. Rothmom RH, Parke WW, "The Vascular Anathomy of the Rotator Cuff." *Clinical Orthopedics* 41 (1965):176-186

3. S Homma, DA Troxclair, AW Zieske, et al., "Histological topographical comparisons of atherosclerosis progression in juveniles and young adults." *Atherosclerosis* 197(2)(2008):791-798.

4. K Yameguchi, AM Tetro, O Blam, et al., "Natural history of asymptomatic rotator cuff tears: a longitudinal analysis of asymptomatic tears detected sonographically." *Journal of Shoulder Elbow Surgery* 10(3)(2001):199-203.

5. SS Anand, S Islan, A Rosengren, et al., "Risk factors for myocardial infarction in women and men: insights from the INTERHEART study." *European Heart Journal* 29 (2008): 932-940. doi:10.1093/eurheartj/ehn018

6. FJ Larsen, TA Schiffer, S Borniquel, et al., "Dietary inorganic nitrate improves mitochondrial efficiency in humans." *Cell Metabolism* 13(2)(2011):149-59. doi:10.1016/j.cmet.2011.01.004.

7. DP Wilkerson, J Tarr, N Benjamin, et al, "Dietary nitrate supplementation reduces the O2 cost of low-intensity exercise and enhances tolerance to high-intensity exercise in humans." *Journal of Applied Physiology* 107(2009):1144-1155. First published August 6 2009. doi: 10.1152/japplphysiol.00722.2009

8. RA Vogel, MC Corretti, GD Plotnick, "Effects of a single high-fat meal on endothelial function in health subjects." *American Journal of Cardiology* 79(1997):350-354.

9. LL Smith, "Acute inflammation: the underlying mechanism in delayed onset muscle soreness?" *Med Sci sports Exerc.* 23(5)(1991):542-551

10. C Erridge, "The capacity of foodstuffs to induce innate immune activation of human monocytes in vitro is dependent on food content of stimulants of Toll-like receptors 2 and 4." *British Journal of Nutrition* 105(1)(2011):15-23. doi: 10.1017/S0007114510003004.

11. RA Koeth, Z Wang, BS Levison, "Intestinal microbiota metabolism of L-carnitine a nutrient in red meat, promotes atherosclerosis." *Nature Medicine* 19(5)(2013):576-85.

12. DE Sellmeyer, KL Stone, A Sebastion, et al., "A high dietary animal to vegetable protein increases the role of bone loss and risk of fracture in post-menopausal women." *American Journal of Clinical Nutrition* 73(2001):118-122.

13. LI Kauppila, "Can low-back pain be due to lumbar artery disease?" *Lancet* 346(1995):888-89.

Daniel Chartrand

1. W.C. Rose, and R.L. Wixom, "The amino acid requirements of man. XIII The sparing effect of cystine on methionine requirement." Journal Biological Chemistry 216(1955): 763-773.

2. E. Knight. "The Impact of Protein Intake on Renal Function Decline in Women with Normal Renal Function or Mild Renal Insufficiency." *Annals of Internal Medicine* 138(6)(2003):460-467.

Roger Greenlaw

1. Stig Bengmark. "Colonic Food: Pre- and Probiotics." *American J. Gastroenterology* 95(1)(2000): S5.

2. Anderson at al. "Health benefits of dietary fiber." *Nutrition Reviews* 67(2009):4, 188–205.

3. L Galland "Gastrointestinal Dysregulation: Connections to Chronic Disease." Institute3 for Functional Medicine, 2008. www.functionalmedicine.org

4. Dean Ornish, Spectrum: A Scientifically Proven Program to Feel Better, Live Longer, Lose Weight, and Gain Health." (New York: Random House, 2008).

Chapter 4

Scott Stoll

1. Graeme L. Close, et al. "The emerging role of free radicals in delayed onset muscle soreness and contraction-induced muscle injury."*Comparative Biochemistry and Physiology Part A: Molecular & Integrative Physiology* 142.3 (2005): 257-266.

2. Scott K Powers, and Malcolm J. Jackson. "Exercise-induced oxidative stress: cellular mechanisms and impact on muscle force production." *Physiological reviews* 88.4 (2008): 1243-1276.

3. Konstantinos Margonis, et al. "Oxidative stress biomarkers responses to physical overtraining: implications for diagnosis." *Free Radical Biology and Medicine* 43.6 (2007): 901-910.

4. Oliver Neubauer, et al. "Exercise-induced DNA damage: is there a relationship with inflammatory responses." *Exerc Immunol Rev* 14.1 (2008): 51-72.

5. A Mastaloudis, T. W. Yu, R. P. O'Donnell, B. Frei, R. H. Dashwood, and M. G. Traber. "Endurance exercise results in DNA

damage as detected by the comet assay." *Free Radic Biol Med.* 36(2004):966-975.

6. SD Balakrishnan, and C. V. Anuradha."Exercise, depletion of antioxidants and antioxidant manipulation."*Cell biochemistry and function* 16.4 (1998): 269-275.

7. V Pialoux, JV Brugniaux et al. "Antioxidant status of elite athletes remains impaired 2 weeks after a simulated altitude training camp." *European Journal of Nutrition* 49(201): 285-292.

8. A. N. N. E McARDLE, and Malcolm J. Jackson. "Exercise, oxidative stress and ageing." *Journal of anatomy* 197.4 (2000): 539-541. Ji, Li Li. "Antioxidants and oxidative stress in exercise." *Experimental Biology and medicine* 222.3 (1999): 283-292.

9. B Halliwell, "The antioxidant paradox." *Lancet* 355(2000):1179–1180.

10. Lucja Pilaczynska-Szczesniak, et al. "The influence of chokeberry juice supplementation on the reduction of oxidative stress resulting from an incremental rowing ergometer exercise." *International journal of sport nutrition and exercise metabolism* 15.1 (2005): 48.

11. DA Connolly, M. P. McHugh, and O. I. Padilla-Zakour. "Efficacy of a tart cherry juice blend in preventing the symptoms of muscle damage." *British journal of sports medicine* 40.8 (2006): 679-683.

12. Normand G Ducharme et al. "Effect of a tart cherry juice blend on exercise-induced muscle damage in horses." *American journal of veterinary research* 70.6 (2009): 758-763.

13. Justin R Trombold et al. "The effect of pomegranate juice supplementation on strength and soreness after eccentric exercise." *The Journal of Strength & Conditioning Research* 25.7 (2011): 1782-1788.

14. E Jokl, "The immunological status of athletes." *J Sports Med Phys Fitness* 14(3)(1974):165–167.

15. M Gleeson, DC Nieman, BK Pedersen, "Exercise, nutrition and immune function." *J. Sports Sci* 22(2004):115–125.

16. D Nieman, "Risk of Upper Respiratory Tract infection in Athletes: An Epidemiologic and Immunologic Perspective." *J Athl Train* 32(4)(1997): 344–349.

17. H Schmitz et al. "Defining the role of dietary phytochemicals in modulating human immune function." *Nutrition and immunology: principles and practice* (2000): 107-119.

18. E Pihl and T. Jürimäe. "Relationships between body weight change and cardiovascular disease risk factors in male former athletes." *International journal of obesity and related metabolic disorders: journal of the International Association for the Study of Obesity* 25.7 (2001): 1057-1062.

19. Roberd M Bostick, et al. "Sugar, meat, and fat intake, and non-dietary risk factors for colon cancer incidence in Iowa women (United States)." *Cancer Causes & Control* 5.1 (1994): 38-52.

20. Geoffrey Rose, "Incubation period of coronary heart disease." *British medical journal (Clinical research ed.)* 284.6329 (1982): 1600.

21. P.J Campbell, *Nature* 467(2010):1109-1113.

22. Fulvia Zanichelli, Stefania Capasso, Marilena Cipollaro, Eleonora Pagnotta, Maria Cartenì, Fiorina Casale, Renato Iori, Umberto Galderisi. "Dose-dependent effects of R-sulforaphane isothiocyanate on the biology of human mesenchymal stem cells, at dietary amounts, it promotes cell proliferation and reduces senescence and apoptosis, while at anti-cancer drug doses, it has cytotoxic effect.

Ellen Cutler

1. Food and Nutrition Board, Institute of Medicine. "Dietary Reference Intakes for Energy, Carbohydrate, Fiber, Fat, Fatty Acids, Cholesterol, Protein, and Amino Acids." Washington, DC: National Academy Press, 2002.

Chapter 5

1. C Erridge, T Attina, CM Spickett, DJ Webb, "A high fat meal induces low-grade endotoxemia: evidence of a novel mechanism of postprandial inflammation," *Am J Clin Nutr* 86(5)(2007):1286-92. RA Vogel, MC Corretti, GD Plotnick, "Effect of a single high-fat meal on endothelial function in healthy subjects," *Am J Cardiol* 79(3)(1997):350-4. SK Rosenkranz, DK Townsend, SE Steffens, CA Harms, "Effects of a high-fat meal on pulmonary function in healthy subjects," *Eur J Appl Physiol* 109(3)(2010):499-506.

Jay Sutliffe

1. P. M. Ridker, "Cardiology Patient Page. C-Reactive Protein: A Simple Test to Help Predict Risk of Heart Attack and Stroke," *Circulation* 108 (2003)**:** e81-85.

2. J. C. Pickup, "Inflammation and Activated Innate Immunity in the Pathogenesis of Type 2 Diabetes," *Diabetes Care* 27 (2004): 813-823.

3. V. Pasceri, J. T. Willerson, and E. T. Yeh, "Direct Proinflammatory Effect of C-Reactive Protein on Human Endothelial Cells," *Circulation* 102 (2000): 2165-2168.

4. C. Julia, N. Meunier, M. Touvier, et al, Dietary Patterns and Risk of Elevated C-Reactive Protein Concentrations 12 Years Later," *British Journal of Nutrition* 110 (2013): 747-754.

5. Y. T. Szeto, T. C. Kwok, and I. F. Benzie, "Effects of a Long-Term Vegetarian Diet on Biomarkers of Antioxidant Status and Cardiovascular Disease Risk," *Nutrition* 20 (2004): 863-866.

6. C. J. North, C. S. Venter, and J. C. Jerling, "The Effects of Dietary Fibre on C-Reactive Protein, an Inflammation Marker Predicting Cardiovascular Disease," *European Journal of Clinical Nutrition* 63 (2009): 921-933.

7. D. E. King, B. M. Egan, and M. E. Geesey, "Relation of Dietary Fat and Fiber to Elevation of C-Reactive Protein," *American Journal of Cardiology* 92 (2003): 1335-1339.

Juliett Gellatley

1. U Alexy, T Remer, F Manz, CM Neu, E Schoenau, "Long-term protein intake and dietary potential renal acid load are associated with bone modeling and remodeling at the proximal radius in healthy children." *American Journal of Clinical Nutrition.* 82 (5)(2005): 1107–1114.

8.   M Ashwell, E Stone, J Mathers, J Barnes, J Compston, RM Francis, T Key, et al. "Nutrition and bone health projects funded by the UK Food Standards Agency: have they helped to inform public health policy?" British Journal of Nutrition. 99 (1)(2008): 198-205.

9.   RS Chan, J Woo, DC Chan, CS Cheung, DH Lo, "Estimated net endogenous acid production and intake of bone health-related nutrients in Hong Kong Chinese adolescents." European Journal of Clinical Nutrition 63(4)(2009): 505-512.

10. JA Kanis, A. Odén, EV McCloskey, H Johansson, DA Wahl, C Cooper, "A systematic review of hip fracture incidence and probability of fracture worldwide." Osteoporos Internationa 2012.

11. SA New, HM MacDonald, M.K. Campbell, JC Martin, MJ. Garton, et al, "Lower estimates of net endogenous noncarbonic acid production are positively associated with indexes of bone health in premenopausal and perimenopausal women." American Journal of Clinical Nutrition 79(2004): 131–138.

12. V. Powell, "Break Free: How to build healthy bones and what really matters in the prevention of osteoporosis." Viva!Health 2012: 10-12, 25-28.

13. WHO/FAO." Diet, nutrition and the prevention of chronic diseases" 2003.

David Bullock

1.   Russel J. Reiter, Dun-Xian Tan, Lucien C. Manchester, Ahmet Korkmaz et al. "A Walnut-Enriched Diet Reduces the Growth of LNCaP Human Prostate Cancer Xenografts in Nude Mice." Cancer Investigation Vol. 31(6)(2013): 365-373. doi:10.3109/07357907.2013.800095

2.   Yun Wang, Chen-Fu Chang, Jenny Chou, Hui-Ling Chen, Xiaolin Deng et al. "Dietary Supplementation with blueberries, spinach, or spirulina reduces ischemic brain damage." Experimental Neurology 193 (1)(2005): 75-84.

Chapter 6

1.   P Pekka, P Pirjo, U Ulla, "Influencing public nutrition for non-communicable disease prevention: from community intervention to national programme- experiences from Finland." Public Health Nutr. (1A)(2002):245-51.

Robert Ostfeld

1.   "Heart disease and stroke statistics-2004 update," American Heart Association, Dallas Texas, (2003).

2.   D Lloyd- Jones, RJ Adams, TM Brown, M Carnethon et al., "Heart disease and stroke statistics- 2010 update: a report from the American Heart Association," Circulation 121(2010):46-215. doi: 10.1161/CIRCULATIONAHA.109.192667.

3.   RJ Ostfeld, Yw Cheung, I Saal, et al., "A brief office intervention is associated with increased days per week of exercise," Int J Cardiol 125(3)(2008):413-5.

4.   RJ Ostfeld, YW Cheung, I Saal, et al., "A brief office intervention is associated with improved health measures," Int J Cardiol 119(2)(2007):239-41.

5.   TC Campbell, TM Campbell II. The China Study. (Texas: Benbella Books, 2006).

6.   CB Esselstyn Jr. Prevent and Reverse Heart Disease. (New York, NY: Penguin Group, 2007).

7.   Campbell TC, Parpia B, Chen J, "Diet, lifestyle, and the etiology of coronary artery disease: the Cornell China study," Am J Cardiol 82(1998):18T–21T.

8.   CB Esselstyn, Jr. "Is the present therapy for coronary artery disease the radical mastectomy of the twenty-first century?" Am J Cardiol, 106(6)(Sept.15, 2010) :902-4.

9.   HC Stary, "Evolution and progression of atherosclerotic lesions in coronary arteries of children and young adults. *Arteriosclerosis,*" 9(1)(Jan-Feb 1989):I19-32.

10. Heart and Vascular Institute. The George Washington University. Heart Facts. http://www.gwheartandvascular.org/index.php/media-center/heart-facts (October 27th, 2013).

11. CG Smith, JP Pell, "Parachute use to prevent death and major trauma related to gravitational challenge: systematic review of randomised controlled trials," *BMJ* 327, no.7429 (Dec 20 2003):1459-61.

12. MW Freeman, C June, "Understanding Cholesterol: The Good, the Bad, and the Necessary," *The Harvard Medical School Guide to Lowering Your Cholesterol,* (New York, NY, McGraw-Hill 2005).

13. JH O'Keefe Jr, L Cordain, WH Harris, et al, "Optimal low-density lipoprotein is 50 to 70 mg/dl: lower is better and physiologically normal," J Am Coll Cardiol 43, no.11 (Jun 2 2004):2142-6.

14. MD Carroll, BK Kit, DA Lacher et al, "Trends in lipids and lipoproteins in US adults1988-2010," JAMA 308, no.15 (Oct. 17th 2012):1545-54.

15. PM Ridker, "Cardiology Patient Page. C-reactive protein: a simple test to help predict risk of heart attack and stroke," *Circulation* 108, (2003): e81-85.

16. P Libby, "The Vascular Biology of Atherosclerosis," In: Bonow RO, Man DL, Zipes DP, Libby P, eds. *Braunwald's Heart Disease: A Textbook of Cardiovascular Medicine,* 9th (Philadelphia, Pa: Saunders Elsevier; 2011): chap 43.

17. CB Esselstyn, "Moderation kills. In: CB Esselstyn Jr.,"*Prevent and Reverse Heart Disease,(* New York, NY: Penguin Group, 2007):chap 5.

18. R Vogel, "Brachial artery ultrasound: a noninvasive tool in the assessment of triglyceride-rich lipoproteins," *Clin Cardiol Suppl* 6, (Jun 1999):II34-9.

19. JM Canty, "Coronary Blood Flow and Myocardial Ischemia," In: Bonow RO, Man DL, Zipes DP, Libby P, eds. *Braunwald's Heart Disease: A Textbook of Cardiovascular Medicine,* 9th ed. (Philadelphia, Pa: Saunders Elsevier; 2011):chap 52.

20. RA Vogel, MC Corretti, GD Plotnick, "Effect of a single high-fat meal on endothelial function in healthy subjects," Am J Cardiol 79, no.3 (Feb 1st, 1997):350-4.

21. J Davignon and P Ganz, "Role of endothelial dysfunction in atherosclerosis," *Circulation* 109, (2004): III-27-32.

22. AG Herman and S Moncada, "Therapeutic potential of nitric oxide donors in the prevention and treatment of atherosclerosis," *Eur Heart J* 26, no.19 (Oct. 2005):1945-55.

23. GS Sainani, and VG Maru, "Role of endothelial cell dysfunction in essential hypertension," *J Assoc Physicians India* 52, (2004):966-9.

24. RG Victor, "Systemic Hypertension: Mechanism and Diagnosis," In: Bonow RO, Man DL, Zipes DP, Libby P, eds. *Braunwald's Heart Disease: A Textbook of Cardiovascular Medicine*, 9th ed, (Philadelphia, Pa: Saunders Elsevier; 2011):chap 45.

25. RS Vasan, A Beiser, S Seshadri, et al, "Residual lifetime risk for developing hypertension in middle-aged women and men: The Framingham Heart Study," JAMA 287, no. 8 (Feb. 27th 2002):1003-10.

26. DJ Millward, "The nutritional value of plant-based diets in relation to human amino acid and protein requirements," Proc Nutr Soc 58, (1999):249-260.

27. Position of the American Dietetic Association, "Vegetarian Diets," *J Am Diet Assoc* 109, (2009): 1266-1282.

28. "Agricultural Research Service," United States Department of Agriculture. Accessed November 2nd, 2013, http://ndb.nal. usda.gov/ndb/foods/show/2920?fg=Vegetables+and+Vegetable+Products&man=&lfacet=&format=&count=&max=25&of fset=&sort=&qlookup=broccoli.

29. A Wachsman, and DS Bernstein, "Diet and osteoporosis," Lancet (1968):958-959.

30. M Hegsted, SA Schuette, MB Zemel, HM Linkswiler, "Urinary Calcium and calcium balance in young men as affected by level of protein and phosphorus intake," *J Nutr* 111, (1981): 553-562.

31. D Feskanich, WC Willett, MJ Stampfer, *et al,* "Protein consumption and bone fractures in women," *Am J Epidemiol* 143,(1996):472–79.

32. BJ Abelow, TR Holford, KL Insogna, "Cross-cultural association between dietary animal protein and hip fracture: A hypothesis," *Calcif Tissue Int.* 50, (1992):14-18.

33. D Ganmaa, XM Li, J Wang, *et al*, "Incidence and mortality of testicular and prostatic cancers in relation to world dietary practices," *Int J Cancer* 98, (2002):262-267.

34. F Bravi, C Bosetti, M Filomeno *et al*, "Foods, nutrients and the risk of oral and pharyngeal cancer," *Br J Cancer*, (Oct. 22nd, 2013).

35. D Armstrong, and R Doll, "Environmental factors and cancer incidence and mortality in different countries, with special reference to dietary practices," Int. J. Cancer 15, (1975): 617-631.

36. J C von der Pols, C Bain, D Gunnell, et al, "Childhood diary intake and adult cancer risk: 65-y follow-up of the Boyd Orr cohort," Am J Clin Nutr 86,(2007): 1722-1729.

37. KM Fairfield, DJ Hunter, Colditz et al, "A prospective study of dietary lactose and ovarian cancer,"Int J Cancer 110, (2004): 271-277.

38. Chan JM, Stampfer JM, Ma J, et al., "Dairy products, calcium and prostate cancer risk in the Physicians' Health Study," Am J Clin Nutr 74, (2001):549-554.

39. K Dahl-Jorgenson, G Joner, KF Hanssen, et al., "Relationship between cow's milk consumption and incidence of IDDM in childhood," Diabetes Care 14, (1991):1081-1083.

40. D Malosse, Perron, A Susco, et al., "Correlation between milk and dairy product consumption and multiple sclerosis prevalence: a worldwide study," Neuroepidemiology 11, (1992):304-312.

41. WG Robertson, Peacock M, Hodgkinson A, "Dietary changes and the incidence of urinary calculi in the U.K. between 1958 and 1976," J Chronic Dis 32, no. 6 (1979):469-76.

42. WG Robertson, "Diet and Calcium stones,"Miner Electrolyte Metab 13 (1987): 228-234.

43. HA Feldman, I Goldstein, DG Hatzichristou et al., "Impotence and its medical and psychosocial correlates: results of the Massachusetts Male Aging Study," J Urol 151, (1994):54–61.

44. Mayo Clinic, "Erectile Dysfunction," 2012, Accessed October 27th 2013. http://www.mayoclinic.com/health/erectile-dysfunction/DS00162/DSECTION=causes

45. K Esposito, F Giugliano, C Di Palo, et al., "Effect of lifestyle changes on erectile dysfunction in obese men: a randomized controlled trial," JAMA 291, no. 24 (2004):2978-84.

46. EJ Behrman and V Gopalan, "Cholesterol and Plants," J. Chem. Educ. 82, no.12 (2005): 1791.

47. Agricultural Research Service, United States Department of Agriculture, Accessed Nov. 2nd, 2013 http://fnic.nal.usda. gov/.

48. AY Chong, AD Blann, GY Lip, "Assessment of endothelial damage and dysfunction: observations in relation to heart failure," QJM 96, no. 4 (2003):253-67.

49. WH Tang, Z Wang, BS Levison et al., "Intestinal microbial metabolism of phosphatidylcholine and cardiovascular risk," N Engl J Med 381, no.17 (Apr 25 2013):1575-84.

50. RA Koeth, Z Wang, BS Levison et al., "Intestinal microbiota metabolism of L-carnitine, a nutrient in red meat, promotes atherosclerosis," Nat Med 19, no. 5 (May 2013):576-85.

Caldwell B. Esselstyn Jr.

1. Caldwell B. Esselstyn Jr., M.D., *Prevent and Reverse Heart Disease: The Revolutionary, Scientifically Prove, Nutrition-Based Cure*, (New York: Penguin, 2007).

Carl Turissini

1. DP Watts, KB Potts, JS Lwanga, and JC Mitani, "Diet of chimpanzees (*Pan troglodytes schweinfurthii*) at Ngogo, Kibale National Park, Uganda, 1. diet composition and diversity," *Am. J. Primatol* 74, (2012):114–129. doi: 10.1002/ajp.21016

2. R Dunn, "Human Ancestors Were Nearly All Vegetarians," *Scientific American* (July 2012). http://blogs.scientificamerican. com/guest-blog/2012/07/23/human-ancestors-were-nearly-all-vegetarians/

3. MT Cerqueira, Am. J. Nutrition 32, (1979): 905-11.

4. ND Barnard, Cohen, J, Jenkins, D, Turner-McGrievy G, et. al., "A low-fat vegan diet and a conventional diabetes diet in the treatment of type 2 diabetes: a randomized, controlled, 74-wk clinical trial," *Am. J. Clin. Nutrition* 89, no. 5 (2009): 1588S-1596S. doi: 10.3945/ajcn.2009.26736H

5. Caldwell Jr Esselstyn, personal communication, and personal experience

6. DE Koshland Jr, "The Molecule of the Year," *Science* 258, no.5090 (Dec. 18th, 1992): 1861. DOI: 10.1126/science.1470903
7. RA Vogel, MC Corretti, GD Plotnick, "Effect of a single high-fat meal on endothelial function in healthy subjects," *American Journal of Cardiology* 79, no.3 (1997):350–354. doi: 10.1016/S0002-9149(96)00760-6
8. RA Koeth, et. al., "Intestinal microbiota metabolism of L-carnitine, a nutrient in red meat, promotes atherosclerosis," *Nature Medicine* 19, no. 5(2013): 576-585.
9. WP Castelli, JT Doyle, T Gordon, et al., "HDL cholesterol and other lipids in coronary heart disease: The Cooperative Lipoprotein Phenotyping Study," *Circulation* 55 (1977): 767-772.
10. D Ornish, L Scherwitz, J Billings, Gould L, et al., "Intensive Lifestyle Changes for Reversal of Coronary Heart Disease," *JAMA* 280, no. 23(1998): 2001-2007. doi:10.1001/jama.280.23.2001.
11. Esselstyn CB Jr, "Updating a 12-Year Experience with Arrest and Reversal Therapy for Coronary Heart Disease: An Overdue Requiem for Palliative Cardiology," *The Am J of Cardiology* 84, (Aug. 1st, 1999):339-341
12. De Longeril, et. al. *Circulation* 99(1999): 117-85.
13. WE Boden, RA O'Rourke, KK Teo, PM Hartigan et al., "Optimal medical therapy with or without PCI for stable coronary disease," New England Journal of Medicine 356, no. 15 (Apr 12th 2007): 1503-1516. DOI: 10.1056/NEJMoa070829

Joaquin Carral

1. K. Bloch, "The Biological Synthesis of Cholesterol," (Nobel Lecture, Dec. 11, 1964), 78–100.
2. M. S. Kim, S. S. Hwang, E. J. Park, and J. W. Bae, "Strict Vegetarian Diet Improves the Risk Factors Associated with Metabolic Diseases by Modulating Gut Microbiota and Reducing Intestinal Inflammation," *Environ Microbiol Rep* 5 (2013): 765-775.
3. K. Sezer, R. Emral, D. Corapcioglu, R. Gen, and E. Akbay, "Effect of Very Low LDL-Cholesterol on Cortisol Synthesis," *J Endocrinol Invest* 31(12) (Dec. 2008): 1075-8.
4. M. S. Brown and J. L. Goldstein, "A Receptor Mediated Pathway for Cholesterol Homeostatis," (Nobel Lecture, Dec. 9, 1985), 284–324.
5. L. M. Morrison, "Reduction of Mortality Rate in Coronary Atherosclerosis by a Low Cholesterol-Low Fat Diet," *Am Heart J* 42(4) (Oct. 1951): 538-45.
6. B. G. Nordestgaard, M. J. Chapman and S. E. Humphries, "Familial Hypercholesterolaemia Is Underdiagnosed and Undertreated in the General Population: Guidance for Clinicians to Prevent Coronary Heart Disease: Consensus Statement of the European Atherosclerosis Society," *Eur Heart J* (Sept. 12, 2013).
7. Liz Szabo, "In Battle of Cholesterol Drugs, Lipitor as Good as Crestor," *USA TODAY* (November 15, 2011, 1:22 pm).
8. R. W. Wissler, "Update on the Pathogenesis of Atherosclerosis," *Am J Med* 91(1B) (July 31, 1991): 3S-9S.
9. D. Ornish, L. W. Scherwitz, J. H. Billings, et al., "Intensive Lifestyle Changes for Reversal of Coronary Heart Disease," *JAMA* 280(23) (1998): 2001-2007.
10. D. Ryglewicz, M. Rodo, and M. Roszczynko, "Dynamics of LDL Oxidation in Ischemic Stroke Patients," *Acta Neurol Scand* 105(3) (Mar. 2002): 185-8.
11. M. Uno, M. Harada, and O. Takimoto, "Elevation of Plasma Oxidized LDL in Acute Stroke Patients Is Associated with Ischemic Lesions Depicted by DWI and Predictive of Infarct Enlargement," *Neurol Res* 27(1) (Jan. 2005): 94-102.
12. T. Imamura, Y. Doi, and H. Arima, "LDL Cholesterol and the Development of Stroke Subtypes and Coronary Heart Disease in a General Japanese Population: The Hisayama Study," *Stroke* 40(2) (Feb. 2009): 382-8.
13. J. K. Ryu, H. R. Jin, G. N. Yin, et al., "Erectile Dysfunction Precedes Other Systemic Vascular Diseases Due to Incompetent Cavernous Endothelial Cell-Cell Junctions," *J Urol* 190(2) (Aug. 2013): 779-89.
14. D. R. Meldrum, J. C. Gambone, M. A. Morris, et al, "The Link between Erectile and Cardiovascular Health: The Canary in the Coal Mine," *Am J Cardiol* 108(4) (Aug. 15, 2011): 599-606.
15. J. C. Vinagre, C. G. Vinagre, F. S. Pozzi, E. Slywitch, and R. C. Maranhão, "Metabolism of Triglyceride-Rich Lipoproteins and Transfer of Lipids to High-Density Lipoproteins (HDL) in Vegan and Omnivore Subjects," *Nutr Metab Cardiovasc Dis* 23(1) (Jan. 2013): 61-7.
16. M. K. Kim, S. W. Cho, and Y. K. Park, "Long-Term Vegetarians Have Low Oxidative Stress, Body Fat, and Cholesterol Levels," *Nutr Res Pract* 6(2) (Apr. 2012): 155-61, doi:10.4162/nrp.2012.6.2.155.
17. F. L. Crowe, P. N. Appleby, R. C. Travis, and T. J. Key, "Risk of Hospitalization or Death from Ischemic Heart Disease among British Vegetarians and Nonvegetarians: Results from the EPIC-Oxford Cohort Study," *Am J Clin Nutr* 97(3) (Mar. 2013): 597-603, doi:10.3945/ajcn.112.044073.
18. H. R. Ferdowsian and N. D. Barnard, "Effects of Plant-Based Diets on Plasma Lipids," *Am J Cardiol* 104(7) (Oct. 1, 2009): 947-56.

Rick Koch

1. R McClelland, K Nasir, M Budoff, R Blumenthal et al., "Arterial Age as a Function of Coronary Artery Calcium (From the Multi-Ethnic Study of Atherosclerosis [MESA])," Am J Cardiol 103, (1)(Jan. 1st 2009): 59–63. doi:10.1016/j.amjcard.2008.08.031. The Multi-Ethnic Study of Atherosclerosis (MESA) is a medical research study involving more than 6,000 men and women from six communities in the United States. MESA is sponsored by the National Heart Lung and Blood Institute of the National Institutes of Health.
2. Centers for Disease Control, 9/26/2013, www.cdc.gov
3. KD Kochanek, JQ Xu, SL Murphy, AM Miniño, and HC Kung, "Deaths: final data for 2009," *National vital statistics reports*, 60(3), 2011.
4. F Lowry. "Coronary atherosclerosis begins at a young age," Medscape, Jun. 5th, 2001, http://www.medscape.com/viewarticle/783668
5. NJ Ward, "A strategy to reduce cardiovascular disease by more than 80%," BMJ 326 (2003): 1419. doi: http://dx.doi.org/10.1136/bmj.326.7404.1419

6. S Okazaki, T Yokoyama, K Miyauchi, "Early statin treatment in patients with acute coronary syndrome. Demonstration of the beneficial effect on atherosclerotic lesions by serial volumetric intravascular ultrasound analysis during half a year after coronary event: the ESTABLISH study," *Circulation* 110, (2004):1061-1068.
7. P Appleby, G Davey, and T Key, "Hypertension and blood pressure among meat eaters, fish eaters, vegetarians and vegans in in EPIC- Oxford," *Public Health Nutr* 5, no.5 (2002): 645-54.
8. R Virmani et al., "Lessons from sudden coronary death: a comprehensive morphologic classification scheme for atherosclerotic lesions," *Arterioscler Thromb Vasc Biol* 20, no. 5 (2000): 1262-75.
9. S Shea, et al., "Family history as an independent risk factor for coronary artery disease," *J Am Coll Cardiol* 4, no.4(1984):793-801.
10. Society for Heart Attack Prevention and Eradication (SHAPE), http://www.shapesociety.org/.
11. PA Heidenreich, JG Trogdon, OA Khavjou, et al., "Forecasting the future of cardiovascular disease in the United States: a policy statement from the American Heart Association," *Circulation* 123, (2011):933-44.

Kristofer Charlton-Ouw & Scott Aronin

1. D. J. Margolis, O. Hoffstad, J. Nafash, et al., "Location, Location, Location: Geographic Clustering of Lower-Extremity Amputation among Medicare Beneficiaries with Diabetes," *Diabetes Care* 34(11) (2011): 2363-7.
2. T. C. Campbell, B. Parpia, and J. Chen, "Diet, Lifestyle, and the Etiology of Coronary Artery Disease: The Cornell China Study," *Am J Cardiol* 82(10B) (1998): 18T-21T.
3. J. J. Koopman, D. van Bodegom, J. W. Jukema, and R. G. Westendorp, "Risk of Cardiovascular Disease in a Traditional African Population with a High Infectious Load: A Population-Based Study," *PLoS One* 7(10) (2012): e46855.
4. P. J. Tuso, M. H. Ismail, B. P. Ha, and C. Bartolotto, "Nutritional Update for Physicians: Plant-Based Diets," *Perm J* 17(2) (2013): 61-6.
5. S. Mishra, J. Xu, U. Aragwal, et al., "A Multicenter Randomized Controlled Trial of a Plant-Based Nutrition Program to Reduce Body Weight and Cardiovascular Risk in the Corporate Setting: The GEICO Study," *Eur J Clin Nutr* 67(7) (2013): 718-24.
6. T. C. Campbell, "Diet, Lifestyle," 18T-21T (see n. 2).
7. M. J. Orlich, P.N. Singh, J.Sabati, et, "Vegetarian Dietary Patterns and Mortality in Adventist Health Study 2," *JAMA Intern Med* 173(13) (2013): 1230-8.
8. R. K. Johnson, L. J. Appel, M. Brands, et al., "Dietary Sugars Intake and Cardiovascular Health: A Scientific Statement from the American Heart Association," *Circulation* 120(11) (2009): 1011-20.
9. L.Mucci, F. Santilli, C. Cuccurullo and G. Davi, "Cardiovascular Risk and Dietary Sugar Intake: Is the Link So Sweet?" *Intern Emerg Med* 7(4) (2012): 313-22.
10. S. Thornley, R. Tayler, and K. Sikaris, "Sugar Restriction: The Evidence for a Drug-Free Intervention to Reduce Cardiovascular Disease Risk," *Intern Med J* 42 (suppl 5) 2012: 46-58.
11. J. J. Carlson, J. C. Eisenmann, G. J. Norman, et al., "Dietary Fiber and Nutrient Density are Inversely Associated with the Metabolic Syndrome in US Adolescents," *J Am Diet Assoc* 111(11) 2011: 1688-95.
12. V. S. Retelny, A. Neuendorf and J.L. Roth, "Nutrition Protocols for the Prevention of Cardiovascular Disease," *Nutr Clin Prac* 23(5) (2008): 468-76.
13. J. A. Nettleton, L. M. Steffen, L. R. Loehr, et al., "Incident Heart Failure is Associated with Lower Whole Grain Intake and Greater High Fat Dairy and Egg Intake in the Atherosclerosis Risk in Communities (ARIC) Study," *J AM Diet Assoc* 108(11) (2008): 1881-7.
14. I. Mehmetoglu, F.H Yerlikaya et al, "Plasma Ω-3 Fatty Acid Levels Negatively and Ω-6 Fatty Acid Levels Positively Associated with other Cardiovascular Risk Factors Including Homocysteine in Severe Obese Subjects," *Asia Pac J Clin Nutr* 21(4) (2012): 519-25.
15. R. C. Masters, A. D. Liese, S.M. Haffner, et al., "Whole and Refined Grain Intakes Are Related to Inflammatory Protein Concentrations in Human Plasma," *J Nutr* 140(3) (2010): 587-94.
16. G.Ruel, Z Shi, S. Zhen et al., "Association between Nutrition and the Evolution of Multimorbidity: The Importance of Fruits and Vegetables and Whole Grain Products," *Clin Nutr* (Jul 22, 2013), doi: 10.1016/j.clnu.2013.07.009, (Epub ahead of print).
17. Gould 1995.
18. D Ornish, , L Scherwitz, J Billings, Gould L, et al., "Intensive Lifestyle Changes for Reversal of Coronary Heart Disease," *JAMA* 280, no. 23(1998): 2001-2007. doi:10.1001/jama.280.23.2001.
19. L Patrick and M. Uzick, "Cardiovascular Disease: C-Reactive Protein and the Inflammatory Disease Paradigm: HMG-Coa Reductase Inhibitors, Alpha-Tocopherol, Red Yeast Rice, and Olive Oil Polyphenols. A Review of the Literature," *Altern Med Rev* 6(3) 2001.
20. P. Lagiou, S. Sandin, M. Lof et al., "Low Carbohydrate-High Protein Diet and Incidence of Cardiovascular Diseases in Swedish Women: Prospective Cohort Study," *BMJ* 344 (2012): e4026.
21. M. J. Orlich, "Vegetarian Dietary Patterns," (see no. 7).
22. T. C. Campbell, "Diet, Lifestyle," 18T-21T (see n. 2).
23. S. Thornley, "Sugar Restriction," (see no. 10).
24. P. Lagiou "Low Carbohydrate-High Protein Diet," (see no. 20).

Jennifer Rooke

1. Centers for Disease Control (CDC) and World Health Organization (WHO), "High Blood Pressure Fact Sheet," 2013.
2. "The Seventh Report of the Joint National Committee on Prevention, Detection, Evaluation, and Treatment of High Blood Pressure," U.S. Department of Health and Human Services, National Institutes of Health, National Heart, Lung, and Blood Institute, National High Blood Pressure Education Program (NIH Publication No. 04-5230, Aug. 2004).

3.   P. M. Kearney, M. Whelton, K. Reynolds, P. K. Whelton, and J. He, "Worldwide Prevalence of Hypertension: A Systematic Review," *J Hypertens* 22(1) (Jan. 2004): 11-9.

4.   R. C. Thompson, et al., "Atherosclerosis Across 4000 Years of Human History: The Horus Study of Four Ancient Populations," *The Lancet* 381(9873) (Apr. 6, 2013): 1211-1222.

5.   G. Finking and H. Hanke, "Nikolaj Nikolajewitsch Anitschkow (1885-1964) Established the Cholesterol-Fed Rabbit as a Model for Atherosclerosis Research," *Atherosclerosis* 135(1) (Nov. 1997): 1-7.

6.   D. Ornish, "Can Lifestyle Changes Reverse Coronary Heart Disease? The Lifestyle Heart Trial," *Lancet* 336(8708) (Jul. 21, 1990): 129-33.

7.   C. B. Esselstyn, et al., "A Strategy to Arrest and Reverse Coronary Artery Disease: A 5 -Year Longitudinal Study of a Single Physician's Practice," *The Journal of Family Practice* 41(6) (Dec. 1995): 560-68.

8.   A. Sachdeva, et al., "Lipid levels in patients hospitalized with coronary artery disease: An analysis of 136,905 hospitalizations in Get With The Guidelines," *American Heart Journal* 157 (1)(January 2009): 111-117.

9.   FDA, "Consumer Updates: FDA Expands Advice on Statin Risks, Apr 12, 2013", DHHS, www.fda.gov/ForConsumers/ConsumerUpdates/ucm293330.htm

10. J. Stamler, "The INTERSALT Study: background, methods, findings, and implications," *Am J Clin Nutr.*, 65(Suppl 2)(Feb. 1997):626S-642S.

James Craner

1.   J Stamler, JD Neaton, DN Wentworth, "Blood pressure (systolic and diastolic) and risk of fatal coronary heart disease," *Hypertension* 13 (Suppl 5)(1989)l):I2-12

2.   J Stamler, R Stamler, JD Neaton, "Blood pressure, systolic and diastolic, and cardiovascular risks, US population data," *Arch Intern Med* 153(5)(1993):598-615.

3.   S MacMahon, R Peto, J Cutler, R Collins, P Sorlie, J Neaton, et al., "Blood pressure, stroke, and coronary heart disease. Part 1, Prolonged differences in blood pressure: prospective observational studies corrected for the regression dilution bias," *Lancet* 335, (8692)(1990):765-774.

4.   J Stokes 3rd, WB Kannel, PA Wolf, LA Cupples, RB D'Agostino, "The relative importance of selected risk factors for various manifestations of cardiovascular disease among men and women from 35 to 64 years old: 30 years of follow-up in the Framingham Study," *Circulation* 75(6 PT 2)(1987):V65-73.

5.   FM Sacks, EH Kass EH, "Low blood pressure in vegetarians: effects of specific foods and nutrients," *Am J Clin Nutr.* 48(Suppl 3)(1988):795-800.

6.   Z Huang, WC Willett, JE Manson, B Rosner, MJ Stampfer, FE Speizer, et al., "Body weight, weight change, and risk for hypertension in women," Ann Intern Med 128, (2)(1998):81-88.

7.   DA McCarron, ME Reusser, "Nonpharmacologic therapy in hypertension: from single components to overall dietary management,"*Prog Cardiovasc Dis* 41(6)(1999):451-460.

8.   LJ Appel LJ, "Nonpharmacologic therapies that reduce blood pressure: a fresh perspective," *Clin Cardiol* 22(7)(1999):III1-5.

9.   K Hermansen, "Diet, blood pressure and hypertension," Br J Nutr 83(Suppl 1)(2000):S113-119.

10. P Pietinen, A Aro, "The role of nutrition in the prevention and treatment of hypertension," *Adv Nutr Res* 8(1990):35-78.

11. FX Pi-Sunyer, "Medical hazards of obesity," *Ann Intern Med* 119 (7 PT 2)(1993):655-660.

12. PK Whelton, MJ Klag, "Hypertension as a risk factor for renal disease. Review of clinical and epidemiological evidence," *Hypertension* 13(Suppl 5)(1989):I19-27.

13. JL Zozaya, "Nutritional factors in high blood pressure," J Hum Hypertens 14 (Suppl 1)(2000)1:S100-104.

14. DA McCarron DA, "Diet and blood pressure--the paradigm shift," *Science* 281(5379)(1998):933-934.

15. JJ Dinicolantonio, AK Niazi, R Sadaf, OK JH, SC Lucan, CJ Lavie, "Dietary sodium restriction: take it with a grain of salt," *Am J Med* 126(11)(2013):951-955.

16. RA Dickey, JJ Janick, "Lifestyle modifications in the prevention and treatment of hypertension," *Endocr Pract* 7(5) (2001):392-399.

17. LJ Beilin, "Lifestyle and hypertension--an overview," *Clin Exp Hypertens* 21(5-6)(1999):749-762.

18. RM Krauss, RH Eckel, B Howard, LJ Appel, SR Daniels, RJ Deckelbaum, et al., "AHA Dietary Guidelines: revision 2000: A statement for healthcare professionals from the Nutrition Committee of the American Heart Association," *Circulation* 102(18) (2000):2284-2299.

19. S Oparil, "Antihypertensive therapy in the era of evidence based medical practice: what to do until the facts are in," *Curr Opin Nephrol Hypertens* 5(2)(1996):159-161.

20. W Barrie, "Cost-effective therapy for hypertension," *West J Med* 164(4)(1996):303-309.

21. TG Pickering, "Predicting the response to nonpharmacologic treatment in mild hypertension," *JAMA* 267(9)(1992):1256-1257.

22. JE Dimsdale, "Reflections on the impact of antihypertensive medications on mood, sedation, and neuropsychologic functioning," *Arch Intern Med* 152(1)(1992):35-39.

23. IL Rouse, BK Armstrong, LJ Beilin, "The relationship of blood pressure to diet and lifestyle in two religious populations," *J Hypertens* 1(1)(1983):65-71.

24. LJ Beilin,"Vegetarian approach to hypertension," *Can J Physiol Pharmacol* 84(6)(1986):852-855.

25. IW Webster, GK Rawson, "Health status of Seventh-Day Adventists," *Med J Aust* 1(10)(1979):417-420.

26. CL Melby, ML Toohey, J Cebrick, "Blood pressure and blood lipids among vegetarian, semivegetarian, and nonvegetarian African Americans," *Am J Clin Nutr* 59(1)(1994):103-109.

27. O Ophir, G Peer, J Gilad, M Blum, A Aviram, "Low blood pressure in vegetarians: the possible role of potassium," *Am J Clin Nutr* 37(5)(1983):755-762.

28. SE Sciarrone, MT Strahan, LJ Beilin, V Burke, P Rogers, IR Rouse, "Ambulatory blood pressure and heart rate responses to

vegetarian meals," *J Hypertens* 11(3)(1993):277-285.

29.   P Burstyn, "Effect of meat pm BP," *JAMA* 248(1)(1982):29-30.

30.   BM Margetts, LJ Beilin, BK Armstrong, R Vandongen, "Vegetarian diet in the treatment of mild hypertension: a random-ized controlled trial," *J Hypertens Suppl* 3(3)(1985):S429-431.

31.   O Lindahl, L Lindwall, A Spangberg, A Stenram, PA Ockerman, "A vegan regimen with reduced medication in the treat-ment of hypertension," *Br J Nutr* 52(1)(1984):11-20.

32.   J McDougall, K Litzau, E Haver, V Saunders, GA Spiller, "Rapid reduction of serum cholesterol and blood pressure by a twelve-day, very low fat, strictly vegetarian diet," *J Am Coll Nutr* 14(5)(1995):491-496.

33.   D Ornish, SE Brown, LW Scherwitz, JH Billings, WT Armstrong, TA Ports, et al., "Can lifestyle changes reverse coronary heart disease? The Lifestyle Heart Trial," *Lancet* 336(8708)(1990):129-133.

34.   LJ Beilin, V Burke, "Vegetarian diet components, protein and blood pressure: which nutrients are important?" *Clin Exp Pharmacol Physiol* 22(3)(1995):195-198.

35.   LJ Beilin, BK Armstrong, BM Margetts, IL Rouse, R Vandongen, "Vegetarian diet and blood pressure," *Nephron* 47(Suppl 1)(1987):37-41.

36.   ND Barnard, AR Scialli, G Turner-McGrievy, AJ Lanou, "Acceptability of a low-fat vegan diet compares favorably to a step II diet in a randomized, controlled trial," *J Cardiopulm Rehabil* 24(4)(2004):229-235.

37.   OY Hung, NL Keenan, J Fang, "Physicians' health habits are associated with lifestyle counseling for hypertensive pa-tients," *Am J Hypertens* 26(2)(2013):201-208.

Heather Shenkman

1.   John McEvoy, "Statins and risk of incident diabetes," *Lancet* 373(9716)(Feb. 27 2010): 735-742. doi:10.1016/S0140-6736(10)60985-3

2.   Aleesa A. Carter, Tara Gomes, Ximena Camacho, David N. Juurlink et al., "Risk of incident diabetes among patients treated with statins: population based study," *BMJ* 346(f2610)(2013). doi: http://dx.doi.org/10.1136/bmj.f2610.

Baxter Montgomery

1.   World Health Organization, "Obesity and Overweight Fact Sheet," (Mar. 2013) accessed November 4, 2013, http://www.who.int/mediacentre/factsheets/fs311/en/.

2.   World Health Organization, "The World Health Report 2002," accessed Nov. 4, 2013, http://www.who.int/whr/2002/en/.

3.   Judith Mackay and George Mensah, "The World Health Organization: Atlas of Heart Disease and Stroke," (last modified 2004), accessed Nov. 4, 2013, http://www.who.int/cardiovascular_diseases/resources/atlas/en/.

4.   E. Krieger, L. D. Youngaman, and T. C. Campbell, "The Modulation of Aflatoxin (AFBI) Induced Preneoplastic Lesions by Dietary Protein and Voluntary Exercise in Fisher 344 Rats," *The FASEB Journal* 2(1988): 3304 Abs.

5.   W. J. Craig and A. R. Mangels, "Position of the American Dietetic Association: Vegetarian Diets," *Journal of the American Dietetic Association* 109 (2009): 1266-1282.

6.   A. Ismail and W. Y. Lee, "Influence of Cooking Practice on Antioxidant Properties and Phenolic Content of Selected Veg-etables," *Asia Pacific Journal of Clinical Nutrition* 13(suppl.) 2004: S 162; L. Barros, P. Baptista, D. Correia, et al., "Effects of Conservation Treatment and Cooking on the Chemical Composition and Antioxidant Activity of Portuguese Wild Edible Mushrooms," *Journal of Agriculture and Food Chemistry* 55(12) (2007): 4781-4788; and, L. B. Link and J. D. Potter, "Raw Versus Cooked Vegetables and Cancer Risk," *Cancer Epidemiology, Biomarkers & Prevention* 13(9) (2004): 1422-35.

7.   Garnett Cheney, M.D., "Rapid Healing of Peptic Ulcers in Patients Receiving Fresh Cabbage Juice," *California Medicine* 70(1) (Jan. 1949): 10-15.

8.   N. W. Walker, *Raw Vegetable Juices* (New York: Pyramid Books, 1972).

9.   American Heart Association, "Cardiovascular Disease Statistics," 2007, accessed Nov. 4, 2013, http://americanheart.org/presenter.jhtml?identifier=4478.

Chapter 7

1.   JM Chan, MJ Stampfer, J Ma, PH Gann, JM Gaziano, E Giovannucci, "Dairy products, calcium, and prostate cancer risk in the Physicians' Health Study," *Am J Clin Nutr.* 74(4)(2001):549-554.

Joel Kahn

1.   CP Forest, Nathan H. Padma, HR Liker, "Efficacy and safety of pomegranate juice on improvement of erectile dysfunction in male patients with mild to moderate erectile dysfunction: a randomized, placebo-controlled, double-bind, crossover study," *Int J Impot Res*, 19(6)(Nov-Dec. 2007): 564-7.

2.   F. Giugliano, MI Maiorino, G. Bellastella, R. Autorino, M DeSio, D. Giugliano, K.
Esposito, "Adherence to Mediterranean diet and erectile dysfunction in men with type 2 diabetes," *J Sex Med* 7(5)(2010): 1911-7. doi: 10.1111/j.1743-6109.2010.01713.x.

3.   M. Aldemir, E. Okulu, S. Neselioglu, O Erel, O. Kayigil, "Pistachio diet improves erectile function parameters and serum lipid profiles in patients with erectile dysfunction," *Int J Impot Res* 23(1)(Jan.-Feb.-2011):32-8. doi:10.1038/ijir.2010.33.

4.   G. Rayipati, JA McClung, WS Aronow, SJ Peterson, WH Frishman, "Type 5 phosphodiesterase inhibitors in the treatment of erectile dysfunction and cardiovascular disease," *Cardiol Rev* 15(2)(Mar-Apr 2007):76-86.

Lawrence Derbes

1.   S.D. Chung, YK Chen, HC Lin, "Increased risk of stroke among men with erectile dysfunction: a nationwide population-based study," *J Sex Med* 8(1) 2011: 240-246.

2.   BA Inman, JL Sauver, DJ Jacobson et al., "A population-based, longitudinal study of erectile dysfunction and future coro-nary artery disease," *Mayo Clin Proc* 84(2)(2009):108-113.

3.   B Gupta, "The effect of lifestyle modification and cardiovascular risk factor reduction on erectile dysfunction," *Arch*

Intern Med 171(20)(2011): 1797-1803.

4. D. Trivedi et al., "Can simvastatin improve erectile function and health-related quality of life in men aged ≥ 40 years with erectile dysfunction? Results of the Erectile Dysfunction and Statins Trial," *BJU Int* 111(2)(2013):324-33.

5. RR Wing, RC Rosen, JL Fava et al., "Effects of weight-loss intervention on erectile function in older men with type 2 diabetes in the Look AHEAD trial," *J Sex Med* 7(1 pt 1)(2010):156-165.

Ron Allison

1. T Huang, B Yang, J Zheng, G Li, ML Wahlgvist, "Cardiovascular disease mortality and cancer incidence in vegetarians: a meta-analysis and systematic review," *Ann Nutr Metab* 60(4)(2012):233-40. doi:10.1159/0000337301.

2. GE Fraser, DJ Shavlik, "Ten years of life: is it a matter of choice?" *Arch Intern Med* 161(13)(2001):1645-52.

Gordon Saxe

1. American Cancer Society, *Cancer Facts & Figures 2008,* (Atlanta: American Cancer Society. 2008).

2. A Jemal, R Siegel, E Ward, T Murray, J Xu, and MJ Thun, "Cancer Statistics, 2007," *CA Cancer J Clin* 57(2007):43–66.

3. DV Makarov and HB Cartera, "The Discovery of Prostate Specific Antigen as a Biomarker for the Early Detection of Adenocarcinoma of the Prostate," *J Urol* 176(6)(2006): 2383-5.

4. L Sun, K Gancarczyk, and EL Paquette, "Introduction to Department of Defense

5. Center for Prostate Disease Research Multicenter National Prostate Cancer Database and Analysis of Changes in the PSA-era," *Urol Oncol* 6(2001):203-9.

6. CR Pound, AW Partin, MA Eisenberger, DW Chan, JD Pearson, and PC Walsh, "Natural history of progression after PSA elevation following radical prostatectomy," *JAMA* 281(17)(1999):1591-7.

7. JF Ward, ML Blute, J Slezak, EJ Bergstralh, and H Zincke, "The long-term clinical impact of biochemical recurrence of prostate cancer 5 or more years after radical prostatectomy," *J Urol* 170(2003):1872-6.

8. D Heber, WR Fair, and D Ornish, *Nutrition and prostate cancer: a monograph from the CaPCure Nutrition Project, 2nd Edition*, (Santa Monica, 1998).

9. DM Parkin, SL Whelan, J Ferlay, L Raymond, and J Young, "Cancer incidence in five continents," *Scientific Publications* XII: 143.

10. H Shimuzu, RK Ross, L Bernstein, R Yatani, BE Henderson, and TM Mack, "Cancers of the prostate and breast among Japanese and white immigrants to Los Angeles County," *Br J Cancer*, 63(1991): 963-6.

11. CS Muir, J Nectoux, and J Staszewski, "The epidemiology of prostatic cancer: Geographical distributions and time-trends," *Acta Oncol* 30(1991):133-40.

12. WR Fair, NE Fleshner, and WD Heston, "Cancer of the prostate: A nutritional disease?" *Urology* 50(1997): 840-8.

13. K Pienta and P Esper, "Risk factors for prostate cancer," *Ann Intern Med* 118(1993):793-803.

14. Amy Nomura and LN Kolonel, "Prostate cancer: A current perspective," *Am J Epidemiol* 13(1991): 200-27.

15. K Hickey, K-A Do, and A Green, "Smoking and prostate cancer," *Epidemiol Rev* 23(1)(2001): 115-25.

16. I-M Lee, HD Sesso, J-J Chen, and RS Paffenberger, "Does physical activity play a role in the prevention of prostate cancer?" *Epidemiol Rev* 23(1)(2001): 132-7.

17. HD Strickler and JJ Goedert, "Sexual behavior and evidence for an infectious cause of prostate cancer," *Epidemiol Rev* 23(1)(2001):144-51.

18. JS Mandel and LM Schuman, "Sexual factors and prostatic cancer," *J Gerontol* 42(1987): 259-64.

19. K Oishi, K Okada, O Yoshida, et al., "A case-control study of prostatic cancer in Kyoto, Japan: Sexual risk factors," *Prostate* 17(1990): 269-79.

20. JT Herbert, JD Birkhoff, PM Feorino, et al, "Herpes Simplex Type 2 and cancer of the prostate," *J Urology* 116(1976):611-2.

21. LH Baker, WK Mebust, TD Chin, et al., "The relationship of Herpesvirus to carcinoma of the prostate," J Urology 125(1981):370-4.

22. E Giovannucci, "Medical history and etiology of prostate cancer," *Epidemiol Rev* 23(1)(2001): 159-62.

23. M-E Parent and J Siemiatycki, "Occupation and prostate cancer," *Epidemiol Rev* 23(1)(2001):138-43.

24. LN Kolonel, "Fat, meat, and prostate cancer," *Epidemiol Rev* 23(1)(2001):72-81.

25. JM Chan and EL Giovannucci, "Dairy products, calcium, and vitamin D and risk of prostate cancer," *Epidemiol Rev* 23(1) (2001): 87-92.

26. DS Michaud, K Augustsson, EB Rimm, MJ Stampfer, WC Willett, and E Giovannucci, "A prospective study on intake of animal products and risk of prostate cancer," *Cancer Causes Control* 12(6)(2002):557-67.

27. E Giovannucci, EB Rimm, A Wolk, et al., "Calcium and fructose intake in relation to risk of prostate cancer," *Cancer Res* 58(1998): 442-7.

28. M Huncharek, J Muscat, and B Kupelnick, "Dairy products, dietary calcium and vitamin D intake as risk factors for prostate cancer: A meta-analysis of 26,769 cases from 45 observational studies,' *Nutr Cancer* 60(4)(2008):421-41.

29. World Cancer Research Fund/ American Institute for Cancer Research, *Food, Nutrition, Physical Activity, and the Prevention of Cancer: A Global Perspective*, (Washington DC: AICR, 2007.)

30. J Ghosh and CE Myers, "Arachidonic acid stimulates prostate cancer cell growth: Critical role of 5-lipoxygenase," *Biochem Biophys Res Commun* 233(1997):418-23.

31. J Ghosh and CE Myers, "Inhibition of arachidonate 5-lipoxygenase triggers massive apoptosis in human prostate cancer cells," *Proc Natl Acad Sci* 95(22)(1998):13182-7.

32. BR Konety and RH Getzenberg, "Vitamin D and prostate cancer," *Urol Clin North Amer* 29(1)(2002): 95-106.

33. J Chan and EL Giovannucci, "Vegetables, fruits, associated micronutrients, and risk of prostate cancer," *Epidemiol Rev* 23(1)(2001): 82-6.

34. JH Cohen, AR Kristal, and JL Stanford, "Fruit and vegetable intake and prostate cancer risk," *JNCI* 92(2000):61-8.

35. JD Brooks, VG Paton, and G Vidanes, "Potent induction of phase 2 enzymes in human prostate cancer cells by sulfora-

phane," *Cancer Epidemiol Biomarkers Prev* 10(9)(2001): 949-54.

36. SR Chinni, Y Li, S Upadhyay, PK Koppolu, and FH Sarkar, "Indole-3-carbinol (I3C) induced cell growth inhibition, G1 cell cycle arrest and apoptosis in prostate cancer cells," *Oncogene* 20(2001): 2927-36.

37. T Brody, *Vitamin A* In: Nutritional Biochemistry, (Boston: Academic Press, 1999):554-65.

38. E Giovannucci, "Tomatoes, tomato-based products, lycopene, and cancer: review of the epidemiological literature," *JNCI* 91(1999): 317-31.

39. J Chan and EL Giovannucci, "Vegetables, fruits, associated micronutrients, and risk of prostate cancer," *Epidemiol Rev* 23(1)(2001): 82-6.

40. DS Michaud, K Augustsson, EB Rimm, MJ Stampfer, WC Willett, and E Giovannucci, "A prospective study on intake of animal products and risk of prostate cancer," Cancer Causes Control 12(6)(2002): 557-67.

41. PH Gann, J Ma, E Giovannucci, et al, "Lower prostate cancer risk in men with elevated plasma lycopene levels: Results of a prospective analysis," *Cancer Res* 59(1999): 1225-30.

42. M Eichholzer, HB Stahelin, KF Gey, et al, "Predictions of male cancer mortality by plasma levels of interacting vitamins: 17-Year follow-up of the prospective Basel Study," *Int J Cancer* 66(1996):145-50.

43. JM Chan, MJ Stampfer, J Ma, et al, "Supplemental vitamin E intake and prostate cancer risk in a large cohort of men in the United States," *Cancer Epidemiol Biomarkers Prev* 8(1999):893-9.

44. NE Fleshner, "Vitamin E and prostate cancer," *Urol Clin North Amer* 29(1)(2002): 107-13.

45. JP Carter, GA Saxe, V Newbold, CE Peres, RJ Campeau, and L Bernal-Green, "Hypothesis: Dietary management may improve survival from nutritionally linked cancers based on analysis of representative cases," *J Amer Coll Nutr* 12(3)(1993): 209-226.

46. J Satia-About, RE Patterson, RN Schiller, and AR Kristal, "Energy from fat is associated with obesity in U.S. men: Results from the Prostate Cancer Prevention Trial," *Prev Med* 34(5)(2002): 493-501.

47. Amy Nomura, "Body size and prostate cancer," *Epidemiol Rev* 23(1)(2001):126-31.

48. P Cohen, DM Peehl, and RG Rosenfeld, "The IGF axis in the prostate," *Horm Metab Res* 26(1994):81-4.

49. CL Amling, RH Riffenburgh, L Sun, JW Moul, RS Lance, et al., "Pathologic variables and recurrence rates as related to obesity and race in men with prostate cancer undergoing radical prostatectomy," *J Clin Oncol* 22(3)(2004):439-45.

50. SJ Freedland, WJ Aronson, CJ Kane, JC Presti Jr, CL Amling, D Elashoff, and MK Terris, "Impact of obesity on biochemical control after radical prostatectomy for clinically localized prostate cancer: A report by the shared equal access regional cancer hospital database study group," *J Clin Oncol* 22(3)(2004): 446-53.

51. SJ Freedland, WB Isaacs, LA Mangold LA, et al., "Stronger association between obesity and biochemical progression after radical prostatectomy among men treated in the last 10 years," *Clin Cancer Res* 11(2005):2883–8.

52. CE Joshu, AM Mondul, A Menke, C Meinhold, et al., "Weight gain is associated with an increased risk of prostate cancer recurrence after prostatectomy in the PSA era," *Cancer Prev Res* 4(2011):544-51.

53. D Palma, T Pickles, and S Tyldesley, "Obesity as a predictor of biochemical recurrence and survival after radiation therapy for prostate cancer," *BJU Int* 100(2007):315–9.

54. American Cancer Society, Cancer Facts & Figures 2008, (Atlanta: American

55. Cancer Society. 2008).

56. A Jemal, R Siegel, E Ward, T Murray, J Xu, and MJ Thun, "Cancer Statistics, 2007," *CA Cancer J Clin* 57(2007):43–66.

57. DV Makarov and HB Cartera, "The Discovery of Prostate Specific Antigen as a Biomarker for the Early Detection of Adenocarcinoma of the Prostate," *J Urol* 176(6)(2006): 2383-5.

58. L Sun, K Gancarczyk, and EL Paquette, "Introduction to Department of Defense

59. Center for Prostate Disease Research Multicenter National Prostate Cancer

60. Database and Analysis of Changes in the PSA-era," *Urol Oncol* 6(2001):203-9.

61. CR Pound, AW Partin, MA Eisenberger, DW Chan, JD Pearson, and PC Walsh, "Natural history of progression after PSA elevation following radical prostatectomy," *JAMA* 281(17)(1999):1591-7.

62. JP Carter, GA Saxe, V Newbold, CE Peres, RJ Campeau, and L Bernal-Green, "Hypothesis: Dietary management may improve survival from nutritionally linked cancers based on analysis of representative cases," *J Amer Coll Nutr* 12(3)(1993): 209-226.

63. GA Saxe, JM Major, JY Nguyen, KM Freeman, TM Downs, and CE Salem, "Potential attenuation of disease progression in recurrent prostate cancer with plant-based diet and stress reduction," *Integr Cancer Ther* 5(3)(2006):206-13.

64. D Ornish, G Weidner, WR Fair, R Marlin, EB Pettengill, et al., "Intensive lifestyle changes may affect the progression of prostate cancer," *J Urol* 174(3)(2005):1065-9.

65. GA Saxe, JR Hebert, JF Carmody, J Kabat-Zinn, PH Rosenzweig, et al., "Can diet in conjunction with stress reduction affect the rate of increase in prostate specific antigen after biochemical recurrence of prostate cancer?" *J Urol* 166(12)(2001):2202-7.

66. D Spentzos, C Mantzoros, MM Regan, ME Morrissey, et al., "Minimal effect of a low-fat/high soy diet for asymptomatic, hormonally naive prostate cancer patients," *Clin Cancer Res* 15;9(9)(2003):3282-7.

Chapter 8

1. Guy Fagherazzi et al., "Dietary acid load and risk of type 2 diabetes: the E3N-EPIC cohort study," *Diabetologia*, (November 2013).

Eddie Ramirez

1. Ramzi S. Contran, Vinay Kumar, and Tucker Collins, "Chapter 20: The Pancreas" in *Robbins Pathologic Basis of Disease*, 6th ed. (Saunders, 1999), 917.

2. C. Patterson, G. Dahlquist, G. Soltész, and A. Green, "Is Childhood-Onset Type I Diabetes a Wealth-Related Disease? An Ecological Analysis of European Incidence Rates," *Diabetologia* 44(suppl 3) (2001): B9-B16.

3. R. B. Elliott, D. P. Harris, J. P. Hill, et al., "Type I (Insulin-Dependent) Diabetes Mellitus and Cow Milk: Casein Variant Consumption," *Diabetologia* 42(3) (1999): 292-296.

4. J. Karjalainen, J. M. Martin, M. Knip, et al., "A Bovine Albumin Peptide as a Possible Trigger of Insulin-Dependent Diabetes Mellitus," *The New England Journal of Medicine* 327(5) (1992): 302-307.

5. "Infant Feeding Practices and Their Possible Relationship to the Etiology of Diabetes Mellitus. American Academy of Pediatrics Work Group on Cow's Milk Protein and Diabetes Mellitus," *Pediatrics* 94(5) (1994): 752-754.

6. Frank D. Roylance, "Marshall Islands Stagger from Ravages of U.S. Control Struggle: U.S. Nuclear Tests and Westernization Have Crippled the Marshall Islands, Which have Contracted with the University of Maryland, Baltimore, to Recommend Reforms," *The Baltimore Sun* (Oct. 26, 1997), accessed Oct. 24, 2013, http://articles.baltimoresun.com/1997-10-26/news/1997299021_1_marshall-islands-majuro-two-islands.

7. K. M. Narayan, James P. Boyle, Theodore J. Thompson, Stephen W. Sorensen, and David F. Williamson, "Lifetime Risk for Diabetes Mellitus in the United States," *JAMA: The Journal of the American Medical Association* 290(14) (2003): 1884-1890.

8. Charmaine E. Lok, Matthew J. Oliver, Deanna M. Rothwell, and Janet E. Hux, "The Growing Volume of Diabetes-Related Dialysis: A Population Based Study," *Nephrology Dialysis Transplantation* 19(12) (2004): 3098-3103.

9. Scott D. Ramsey, Katherine Newton, David, Blough, David K. McCulloch, Nirmala Sandhu, Gaylee Reiber, and Edward H. Wagner, "Incidence, Outcomes, and Cost of Foot Ulcers in Patients with Diabetes," *Diabetes Care* 22(3) (1999): 382-387.

10. Maria Mota, C. Panu , E. Mota, Veronica Sfredel, A. Patra cu, Luminita Vanghelie, and Eva Toma, "Hand Abnormalities of the Patients with Diabetes Mellitus," *Romanian Journal of Internal Medicine* 38 (2000): 89.

11. Agnes Flöel, "tDCS-Enhanced Motor and Cognitive Function in Neurological Diseases," *Neuroimage* (2013).

12. Emma Kabakov, Clara Norymberg, Esther Osher, Michael Koffler, Karen Tordjman, Yona Greenman, and Naftali Stern, "Prevalence of Hypertension in Type 2 Diabetes Mellitus: Impact of the Tightening Definition of High Blood Pressure and Association with Confounding Risk Factors," *Journal of the Cardiometabolic Syndrome* 1(2) (2006): 95-101.

13. Gang Hu, Cinzia Sarti, Pekka Jousilahti, Markku Peltonen, Qing Qiao, Riitta Antikainen, and Jaakko Tuomilehto, "The Impact of History of Hypertension and Type 2 Diabetes at Baseline on the Incidence of Stroke and Stroke Mortality," *Stroke* 36(12) (2005): 2538-2543.

14. Alan S. Go, Dariush Mozaffarian, Véronique L. Roger, Emelia J. Benjamin, Jarett D. Berry, William B. Borden, Dawn M. Bravata, et al., "Executive Summary: Heart Disease and Stroke Statistics—2013 Update: A Report from the American Heart Association," *Circulation* 127(1) (2013): 143-152.

15. R. Klein, B. E. K. Klein, "Vision Disorders in Diabetes," in *Diabetes in America*, 2nd ed., ed. National Diabetes Data Group (Washington, DC: U.S. Department of Health and Human Services, National Institutes of Health, National Institute of Diabetes and Digestive and Kidney Diseases, 1995), 293, 336, NIH Publication No. 95-1468.

16. Saul Genuth, "Insights from the Diabetes Control and Complications Trial/Epidemiology of Diabetes Interventions and Complications Study on the Use of Intensive Glycemic Treatment to Reduce the Risk of Complications of Type 1 Diabetes," *Endocrine Practice* 12 (2006): 34-41.

17. "Diabetes - Know the Basics," *Ethnicity & Disease* 3 (2012).

18. Saul Genuth, K. G. Alberti, Peter Bennett, John Buse, Ralph Defronzo, Richard Kahn, J. Kitzmiller, et al., "Follow-Up Report on the Diagnosis of Diabetes Mellitus," *Diabetes Care* 26(11) (2003): 3160.

19. J. McDaniel and R. E. Roger Hernández, "Chapter 3: Spanish Influence," in *The Food Of Mexico* (Jan. 2003).

20. M. P. McMurry, M. T. Cerqueira, S. L. Connor, and W. E. Connor, "Changes in Lipid and Lipoprotein Levels and Body Weight in Tarahumara Indians After Consumption of an Affluent Diet," *The New England Journal Of Medicine* 325(24) (1991): 1704-1708.

21. Salim Yusuf, Srinath Reddy, Stephanie Ôunpuu, and Sonia Anand, "Global Burden of Cardiovascular Diseases Part I: General Considerations, the Epidemiologic Transition, Risk Factors, and Impact of Urbanization," *Circulation* 104(22) (2001): 2746-2753.

22. Nadia M. Bastide, Fabrice H. Pierre, and Denis E. Corpet, "Heme Iron from Meat and Risk of Colorectal Cancer: A Meta-Analysis and a Review of the Mechanisms Involved," *Cancer Prevention Research (Philadelphia, Pa.)* 4 (2) (2011): 177-184.

23. John J. O'Shea and Peter J. Murray, "Cytokine Signaling Modules in Inflammatory Responses," *Immunity* 28(4) (2008): 477-487.

24. An Pan, Qi Sun, Adam M Bernstein, et al., "Changes in Red Meat Consumption and Subsequent Risk of Type 2 Diabetes Mellitus: Three Cohorts of US Men and Women," *JAMA Internal Medicine* 173(14) (2013): 1328-1335.

25. Lei Chen, Dianna J. Magliano, and Paul Z. Zimmet, "The Worldwide Epidemiology of Type 2 Diabetes Mellitus--Present and Future Perspectives," *Nat Rev Endocrinol* 8(4) (2011): 228-236.

26. Ahmad Aljada, Priya Mohanty, Husam Ghanim, et al., "Increase in Intranuclear Nuclear Factor b and Decrease in Inhibitor b in Mononuclear Cells After a Mixed Meal: Evidence for a Proinflammatory Effect," *The American Journal of Clinical Nutrition* 79(4) (2004): 682-690.

27. G. E. Fraser and D. J. Shavlik, "Ten Years of Life: Is It a Matter of Choice?" *Archives of Internal Medicine* 161(13) (2001): 1645-1652.

28. Walter Willett, JoAnn Manson, and Simin Liu, "Glycemic Index, Glycemic Load, and Risk of Type 2 Diabetes," *The American Journal of Clinical Nutrition* 76(1) (2002): 274S-280S.

29. Robert Ross, John Rissanen, Heather Pedwell, Jennifer Clifford, and Peter Shragge, "Influence of Diet and Exercise on Skeletal Muscle and Visceral Adipose Tissue in Men," *Journal of Applied Physiology* 81(6) (1996): 2445-2455.

30. Frank B. Hu, JoAnn E. Manson, Meir J. Stampfer, Graham Colditz, Simin Liu, Caren G. Solomon, and Walter C. Willett, "Diet, Lifestyle, and the Risk of Type 2 Diabetes Mellitus in Women," *New England Journal of Medicine* 345(11) (2001): 790-797.

31. Frank B. Hu and Walter C. Willett, "Optimal Diets for Prevention of Coronary Heart Disease," *JAMA: The Journal of the American Medical Association* 288(20) (2002): 2569-2578.

32. Albert Sanchez, Richard W. Hubbard, Ellen Smit, and George F. Hilton, "Testing a Mechanism of Control in Human Cholesterol Metabolism: Relation of Arginine and Glycine to Insulin and Glucagon," *Atherosclerosis* 71(1) (1988): 87-92.

33. J. Stamler and R. Shekelle, "Dietary Cholesterol and Human Coronary Heart Disease. The Epidemiologic Evidence," *Archives of Pathology & Laboratory Medicine* 112(10) (1988): 1032-1040.

34. Ahmad Aljada, Priya Mohanty, Husam Ghanim, Toufic Abdo, Devjit Tripathy, Ajay Chaudhuri, and Paresh Dandona, "Increase in Intranuclear Nuclear Factor b and Decrease in Inhibitor Kb in Mononuclear Cells After a Mixed Meal: Evidence for a Proinflammatory Effect," *The American Journal of Clinical Nutrition* 79(4) (2004): 682-690.

35. Neal D. Barnard, Joshua Cohen, David J A Jenkins, Gabrielle Turner-McGrievy, Lise Gloede, Brent Jaster, Kim Seidl, Amber A Green, and Stanley Talpers, "A Low-Fat Vegan Diet Improves Glycemic Control and Cardiovascular Risk Factors in a Randomized Clinical Trial in Individuals with Type 2 Diabetes," *Diabetes Care* 29(8) (2006): 1777-1783.

36. Saul Genuth, K. G. Alberti, Peter Bennett, John Buse, Ralph Defronzo, Richard Kahn, J. Kitzmiller, et al., "Follow-Up Report on the Diagnosis of Diabetes Mellitus," *Diabetes Care* 26(11) (2003): 3160.

37. Alexandra E. Butler, Juliette Janson, Susan Bonner-Weir, Robert Ritzel, Robert A. Rizza, and Peter C. Butler, " -Cell Deficit and Increased -cell Apoptosis in Humans with Type 2 Diabetes," *Diabetes* 52(1) (2003): 102-110.

38. Neal D. Barnard, Joshua Cohen, David J A Jenkins, Gabrielle Turner-McGrievy, Lise Gloede, Brent Jaster, Kim Seidl, Amber A Green, and Stanley Talpers, "A Low-Fat Vegan Diet Improves Glycemic Control and Cardiovascular Risk Factors in a Randomized Clinical Trial in Individuals with Type 2 Diabetes," *Diabetes Care* 29(8) (2006): 1777-1783.

Veronika Powell

1. A Vang, PN Singh, JW Lee, EH Haddad, and CH Brinegar, "Meats, Processed Meats, Obesity, Weight Gain and Occurrence of Diabetes among Adults: Findings from Adventist Health Studies," *Annals of Nutrition and Metabolism* 52 (2)(2008): 96-104.

2. The InterAct Consortium, "Association between dietary meat consumption and incident type 2 diabetes: the EPIC-InterAct study," *Diabetologia* 56 (1)(2013): 47-59.

3. DI Phillips, S Caddy V Ilic, et al., "Intramuscular triglyceride and muscle insulin sensitivity: evidence for a relationship in nondiabetic subjects," *Metabolism* 45 (8)(1996): 947–50.

4. M. Krssak, K. Falk Petersen, A. Dresner, et al., "Intramyocellular lipid concentrations are correlated with insulin sensitivity in humans: a 1H NMR spectroscopy study," *Diabetologia*. 42 (1)(1999): 113–6.

5. KF. Petersen, S. Dufour, D. Befroy, et al., "Impaired mitochondrial activity in the insulin-resistant offspring of patients with type 2 diabetes," *New England Journal of Medicine* 350 (7)(2004): 664-71.

6. K Morino, K.F. Petersen, GI Shulman, "Molecular mechanisms of insulin resistance in humans and their potential links with mitochondrial dysfunction," *Diabetes* 55 (Suppl. 2)(2006): S9-S15.

7. J. Delarue, C Magnan, "Free fatty acids and insulin resistance," *Current Opinion in Clinical Nutrition and Metabolic Care* 10 (2)(2007): 142-8.

8. LM Sparks, H Xie, RA Koza, et al., "A high-fat diet coordinately downregulates genes required for mitochondrial oxidative phosphorylation in skeletal muscle," *Diabetes* 54 (7) (2005): 1926-33.

9. ND Barnard, Dr. Neal Barnard's program for reversing diabetes: the scientifically proven system for reversing diabetes without drugs.(New York: Rodale Inc, 2007).

10. J. Hoeks, NA van Herpen, M. Mensink, et al., "Prolonged fasting identifies skeletal muscle mitochondrial dysfunction as consequence rather than cause of human insulin resistance," Diabetes. 59 (9)(201): 2117-25.

11. RJ. Barnard, L. Lattimore, RG. Holly, et al., "Response of non-insulin-dependent diabetic patients to an intensive program of diet and exercise," Diabetes care 5(1982):370-4.

12. RJ. Barnard, MR Massey, S Cherny, et al., "Long-term use of high-complex-carbohudrate, high-fiber, low-fat diet and exercise in the treatment of NIDDM patients," Diabetes Care 6(1983): 268-73.

13. RJ. Barnard, T. Jung, SB Inkeles, "Diet and exercise in the treatment of NIDDM: The need for early emphasis," Diabetes Care 17 (12)(1994): 1469-72.

14. ND. Barnard, J. Cohen, DJ Jenkins, et al., "A low-fat, vegan diet improves glycemic control and cardiovascular risk factors in a randomized clinical trial in individuals with type 2 diabetes," Diabetes Care 29 (8)(2006): 1777-83.

15. ND Barnard, 2007, see note 9.

16. ND. Barnard, J. Cohen, DJA Jenkins, et al., "A low-fat vegan diet and conventional diabetes diet in the treatment of type 2 diabetes: a randomized, controlled, 74-wk clinical trial," American Journal of Clinical Nutrition 89 (5)(2009): 1588S-96S.

17. MG Crane and C Sample, "Regression of diabetic neuropathy with total vegetarian (vegan) diet," Journal of Nutritional Medicine 4(1994): 431–9.

18. E Liu, NM McKeown, PK Newby, et al., "Cross-sectional association of dietary patterns with insulin-resistant phenotypes among adults without diabetes in the Framingham Offspring Study," The British Journal of Nutrition 102 (4)(2009): 576-83.

19. American Diabetes Association, "Standards of medical care in diabetes," Diabetes Care 33 (Suppl. 1)(2010): S11-S61.

20. EL. Knight, MJ Stampfer, SE Hankinson, et al., "The impact of protein intake on renal function decline in women with normal renal function or mild renal insufficiency," Annals of Internal Medicine 138 (6)(2003): 460-7.

21. A. Barclay, H. Gilbertson, K. Marsh, C. Smart, "Dietary management in diabetes," Australian Family Physician 39 (8)(2010): 579-83.

22. ND. Barnard, 2007, see note 9.

23. F. Andreelli, C. Amouyal, C Magnan, G. Mithieux, "What can bariatric surgery teach us about the pathophysiology of type 2 diabetes?," Diabetes & Metabolism 35 (6)(2009): 499-507.

Eric Slywitch

1. G. E. Fraser, "Associations between Diet and Cancer, Ischemic Heart Disease, and All-Cause Mortality in Non-Hispanic

White California Seventh-Day Adventists," *Am J Clin Nutr* 70(3 suppl.) (1999): 532S-538S.

2. T. T. Fung, M. Schulze, J. E. Manson, W. C. Willett, and F. B. Hu, "Dietary Patterns, Meat Intake, and the Risk of Type 2 Diabetes in Women," *Arch Intern Med* 164(20) (Nov. 8, 2004): 2235-40.
3. C. J. Hung, et al., "Taiwanese Vegetarians Have Higher Insulin Sensitivity Than Omnivores," *Br J Nutr* 95(1) (2006): 129-35.
4. M. Valachovicova, et al., "No Evidence of Insulin Resistance in Normal Weight Vegetarians. A Case Control Study," *Eur J Nutr* 45(1) (2006): 52-4.
5. C. S. Kuo, et al., "Insulin Sensitivity in Chinese Ovo-Lactovegetarians Compared with Omnivores," *Eur J Clin Nutr* 58(2) (2004): 312-6.
6. N. D. Barnard, et al., "The Effects of a Low-Fat, Plant-Based Dietary Intervention on Body Weight, Metabolism, and Insulin Sensitivity," *Am J Med* 118(9) (2005): 991-7.
7. H. Kahleova, et al., "Vegetarian Diet Improves Insulin Resistance and Oxidative Stress Markers More Than Conventional Diet in Subjects with Type 2 Diabetes," *Diabet Med* 28(5) (2011): 549-59.
8. S. Tonstad, et al., "Vegetarian Diets and Incidence of Diabetes in the Adventist Health Study-2," *Nutr Metab Cardiovasc Dis* (2011).
9. N. D. Barnard, et al., "A Low-Fat Vegan Diet Elicits Greater Macronutrient Changes, but Is Comparable in Adherence and Acceptability, Compared with a More Conventional Diabetes Diet among Individuals with Type 2 Diabetes," *J Am Diet Assoc* 109(2) (2009): 263-72.
10. N. D. Barnard, et al., "A Low-Fat Vegan Diet and a Conventional Diabetes Diet in the Treatment of Type 2 Diabetes: A Randomized, Controlled, 74-Wk Clinical Trial," *Am J Clin Nutr* 89(5) (2009): 1588S-1596S.
11. G. M. Turner-McGrievy, et al., "Changes in Nutrient Intake and Dietary Quality among Participants with Type 2 Diabetes Following a Low-Fat Vegan Diet or a Conventional Diabetes Diet for 22 Weeks," *J Am Diet Assoc* 108(10) (2008): 1636-45.
12. C. B. Trapp and N.D. Barnard, "Usefulness of Vegetarian and Vegan Diets for Treating Type 2 Diabetes," *Curr Diab Rep* 10(2) (2010): 152-8.
13. N. D. Barnard, et al., "Vegetarian and Vegan Diets in Type 2 Diabetes Management," *Nutr Rev* 67(5) (2009): 255-63.
14. A. Pan, et al., "Red Meat Consumption and Risk of Type 2 Diabetes: 3 Cohorts of US Adults and an Updated Meta-Analysis," *Am J Clin Nutr* 94(4) (2011): 1088-96.
15. N. S. Rizzo, et al., "Vegetarian Dietary Patterns Are Associated with a Lower Risk of Metabolic Syndrome: The Adventist Health Study 2," *Diabetes Care* 34(5) (2011): 1225-7.

Anteneh Roba

1. Yiqing Song et al., "A Prospective Study of Red Meat Consumption and Type 2 diabetes in Middle Aged and Elderly Women," Diabetes Care 27(9)(2004): 2108-15.
2. Rob M. van Dam, WC Willett, EB Rimm, MJ Stampfer, FB HU., "Dietary Fat and Meat Intake in Relation to Risk of Type 2 Diabetes in Men," *Diabetes Care* 25(3)(2002):417-24.
3. A Pan, Qui Sun, AM Bernstein et al., "Red Meat Consumption and Mortality: results from 2 prospective cohort studies," *Archives of Internal Medicine*, 172(7)(2012):555-63. doi.10.1001/archinternmed.2011.2287. A Mar. 12, 2012 peer-reviewed study of 121,342 people found that eating red meat was associated with an increased risk of death from cancer and cardiovascular disease.
4. Scott M. Grundy "Metabolic Syndrome Pandemic" Center for Human Nutrition, University of Texas Southwestern Medical Center.
5. JV Neel, "Update to 'The Study of Natural Selection in Primitive and Civilized Human Populations," *Human Biology* **61** (5–6)(1989): 811–23.
6. JV Neel, "The "thrifty genotype" in 1998," *Nutr. Rev* 57 (5 Pt 2)(May 1999): S2–9. doi.10.1111/j.1753-4887.1999.tb01782.x.
7. David JA Jenkins, Cyril WC Kendall, and Augustine Marchie, et al., "Type 2 Diabetes and the Vegetarian Diet," *American Journal of Clinical Nutrition*, 2003
8. Paul N. Appleby, Gwyneth K. Davey, and Timothy J. Key, "Hypertension and Blood Pressure Among Meat Eaters, Fish Eaters, Vegetarians and Vegans in EPIC- Oxford," *Public Health Nutrition* 5(5)(2002):645-54.
9. Hope Ferdwosian, Neal Bernard, "Effects of Plant-Based Diets on Plasma Lipids," *American Journal of Cardiology* 104 (7) (2009): 947-956.
10. Pramil N. Singh, Joan Sabaté, and Gary E Fraser, "Does Low Meat Consumption Increase Life Expectancy in Humans?" *American Journal of Clinical Nutrition*, 78(3)(Sept 2003):526S-532S.
11. A peer-reviewed July 9, 2001 study of Seventh-Day Adventists who were vegetarian (or ate very little meat) showed longevity increases of 7.28 years for men and 4.42 years for women.
12. Michael J. Orlich, et al., "Vegetarian Dietary Patterns and Mortality in Adventist Health Study 2," *JAMA Internal Medicine* 173(13)(June 3, 2013): 1230-8. doi: 10.1001/jamainternmed.2013.6473.

Nandita Shah

1. TNN, "In 30 years, Chennai shows tenfold rise in diabetes," *The Times of India*, August 31ˢᵗ, 2013. http://articles.timesofindia.indiatimes.com/2013-08-16/chennai/41417164_1_indiab-diabetes-mdrf.
2. TNN, See note 1.

Mohamed H. Ismail

1. K. Yasuda, E. Hines III, and A. E. Kitabchi, "Hypercortisolism and Insulin Resistance: Comparative Effects of Prednisone, Hydrocortisone, and Dexamethasone on Insulin Binding of Human Erythrocytes," *Journal of Clinical Endocrinology & Metabolism* 55(5) (1982): 910–915, doi:10.1210/jcem-55-5-910, PMID 6749880.
2. E. W. Kraegen, et al., "Development of Muscle Insulin Resistance After Liver Insulin Resistance in High-Fat-Fed Rats," *Diabetes* 40 (11) (1991): 1397–1403, doi:10.2337/diabetes.40.11.1397, PMID 1936601.
3. L. H. Storlien, et al., "Influence of Dietary Fat Composition on Development of Insulin Resistance in Rats," *Diabetes* 40 (2)

(1991): 280–289, doi:10.2337/diabetes.40.2.280, PMID 1991575.

4.   J. Lovejoy and M. DiGirolamo, "Habitual Dietary Intake and Insulin Sensitivity in Lean and Obese Adults," *American Journal of Clinical Nutrition* 55 (6) (1992): 1174–9, PMID 1317665.

5.   L. H. Storlien, et al., "Fish Oil Prevents Insulin Resistance Induced by High-Fat Feeding in Rats," *Science* 237 (4817) (1987): 885–888, doi:10.1126/science.3303333, PMID 3303333.

6.   Jennifer C Lovejoy, "Dietary Fatty Acids and Insulin Resistance," *Current Atherosclerosis Reports* (1999).

7.   D. S. Kelley, et al., "Flaxseed Oil Prevents Trans-10, Cis-12-Conjugated Linoleic Acid-Induced Insulin Resistance in Mice," *British Journal of Nutrition* 101 (2009): 701–708, http://naldc.nal.usda.gov/download/30297/pdf.

8.   Dariush Mozaffarian, et al., "Interplay between Different Polyunsaturated Fatty Acids and Risk of Coronary Heart Disease in Men," *Circulation* 111(2) (2004): 157–164, doi:10.1161/01.CIR.0000152099.87287.83, PMC 1201401, PMID 15630029.

9.   Paul Wilkinson, Clare Leach, Eric E. Ah-Sing, et al., "Influence of A-Linolenic Acid and Fish-Oil on Markers of Cardiovascular Risk in Subjects with an Atherogenic Lipoprotein Phenotype," *Atherosclerosis* 181(1) (July 2005): 115-124, http://www.atherosclerosis-journal.com/article/S0021-9150(05)00012-2/abstract.

10. P. S. MacLean, D. Zheng, J. P. Jones, et al., "Exercise-Induced Transcription of the Muscle Glucose Transporter (GLUT 4) Gene," *Biochemical and Biophysical Research Communications* 292(2) (2002): 409–414, doi:10.1006/bbrc.2002.6654, PMID 11906177.

11. S. Tonstad, K. Stewart, K. Oda, et al., "Vegetarian Diets and Incidence of Diabetes in the Adventist Health Study-2," *Nutr Metab Cardiovasc Dis* 23(4) (Apr. 2013): 292-9, doi:10.1016/j.numecd.2011.07.004, Epub Oct. 7, 2011.

12. M. J. Orlich, et al., "Vegetarian Dietary Patterns and Mortality in Adventist Health Study 2," *JAMA Intern Med* 173(13) (July 8, 2013): 1230-8, doi:10.1001/jamainternmed.2013.6473.

Chapter 9

1.   D Ornish, MJ Magbanua, G Weidner, V Weinberg, C Kemp et al., "Changes in prostate gene expression in men undergoing an intensive nutrition and lifestyle intervention," *Proc Natl Acad Sci USA* 105(24)(2008):8369-74. doi:10.1073/pnas.0803080105.

Mary J. (Clifton) Wendt

1.   "Foods Highest in Methionine," *SELF NutritionData*, Accessed Nov. 25th 2013, http://nutritiondata.self.com/foods-000084000000000000000-1.html.

2.   Charles A Dinarello, "Interleukin 1 and interleukin 18 as mediators of inflammation and the aging process," *American Journal of Clinical Nutrition* 83(2)(2006):447S-455S.

3.   Michael Greger, "Avoiding Cooked Meat Carcinogens," *NutritionFacts.org*, Accessed Nov. 25th 2013, http://nutritionfacts.org/2013/07/04/avoiding-cooked-meat-carcinogens/.

John Kelly

1.   Dean Ornish, Mark Jesus M. Magbanua, Gerdi Weidner, et al., "Changes in prostate gene expression in men undergoing an intensive nutrition and lifestyle intervention," *PNAS*. 105(24)(2008):8369-8374.

2.   Guo-Qing Chang, Valeriya Gaysinskaya, Olga Karatayev, and Sarah F. Leibowitz, "Maternal High-Fat Diet and Fetal Programming: Increased Proliferation of Hypothalamic Peptide-Producing Neurons That Increase Risk for Overeating and Obesity," *The Journal of Neuroscience* 28(46)(2008):12107-12119.

3.   George L. Wolff, Ralph L. Kodell, Stephen R. Moore, Craig A. Cooney, "Maternal epigenetics and methyl supplements affect agouti gene expression in Avy/a mice," *FASEB J* 12(1998):949-957.

4.   Andrew P. Feinberg, "Epigenetics at the Epicenter of Modern Medicine," *JAMA* 299(11)(2008):1345-1350.

Lisa Bazzett-Matabele

1.   T Minamoto, M Mai, Z Ronai, "Environmental factors as regulators and effectors of multistep carcinogenesis," *Carcinogenesis* 20(1999):519–527.

2.   American Cancer Society, *Cancer Facts & Figures 2013,* (Atlanta: American Cancer Society, 2013).

3.   President's Cancer Panel, "Promoting Healthy Lifestyles: Policy, Program, and Personal Recommendations for Reducing Cancer Risk, 2006-2007 Annual Report,"*National Cancer Institute, U.S. Department of Health and Human Services*, (August 2007).

4.   PH Lahmann, AE Cust, CM Friedenreich, et al., „Anthropometric measures and epithelial ovarian cancer risk in the European Prospective Investigation into Cancer and Nutrition," *Int J Cancer* 126(2010):2404-2415.

5.   SC Larsson, N Orsini, A Wolk, "Milk, milk products and lactose intake and ovarian cancer risk: A meta-analysis of epidemiological studies," *Int J Cancer* 118(2006):431–441.

6.   SC Larsson, L Bergkvist, A Wolk, "Milk and lactose intakes and ovarian cancer risk in the Swedish Mammography Cohort.," *Am J Clin Nutr* 80(2004):1353-1357.

7.   Y Park, PN Mitrou, V Kipnis, A Hollenbeck, A Schatzkin, MF Leitzmann, "Calcium, dairy foods, and risk of incident and fatal prostate cancer: The NIH-AARP Diet and Health Study," *Am J Epidemiol* 166(2007):1270-1279.

8.   E. Giovannucci, EB Rimm, A Wolk, et al., "Calcium and fructose intake in relation to risk of prostate cancer," *Cancer Res* 58(1998):442–447.

9.   JM Chan, MJ Stampfer, J Ma, PH Gann, JM Gaziano, E Giovannucci, "Dairy products, calcium, and prostate cancer risk in the Physicians' Health Study," *Am J Clin Nutr* 74(2001):549–554.

10. KA Workowski, SM Berman , "Sexually transmitted diseases treatment guidelines," *Centers for Disease Control and Prevention MMWR Recomm. Rep* 55(2006):1.

11. JD Wright, J Li, DS Gerhard, et al., "Human papillomavirus type and tobacco use as predictors of survival in early stage cervical carcinoma," *Gynecol Oncol* 98(1)(2005):84-91.

12. R Garcia–Closas, X Castellsague, X Bosch, CA Gonzalez, "The role of diet and nutrition in cervical carcinogenesis: a review of recent evidence," *Int J Cancer* 117(2005):629–637.
13. AH Wu, MC Yu, CC Tseng, MC Pike, "Epidemiology of soy exposures and breast cancer risk," *Br J Cancer* 98(2008):9-14.
14. XO Shu, Y Zheng, H Cai, et al., "Soy food intake and breast cancer survival," *JAMA* 302(2009):2437-2443.
15. N Guha, MI Kwan, CP Quesenberry Jr, EK Weltzien, AL Castillo, BJ Caan, "Soy isoflavones and risk of cancer recurrence in a cohort of breast cancer survivors: the Life After Cancer Epidemiology study," *Breast Cancer Res Treat* 118(2009):395-405.

Alberto Peribanez Gonzalez

1. M Crovetto and R Uauy, "Recommendations for Cancer Prevention of World Center Research Fund (WCRF): Situational Analysis for Chile," *Rev Med Chil* 141(5)(2013):626-636.
2. American Cancer Society, 2013
3. R Siegel, D. Naishadham, A. Jernal, "Cancer Statistics 2013," *CA Cancer J Clin* 63(1)(2013):11-30. doi: 10.3322/caac.21166
4. GL Hildenbrand, LC Hildenbrand, K Bradford, SW Cavin, "Five-Year Survival Rates of Melanoma Patients treated by Diet Therapy after the Manner of Gerson: A Retrospective Review," *Altern Ther Health Med* 1(4)(1995):29-37.
5. A.W. Taylor, "Association Between Nutrition and the Evolution of Multimorbidity: The Importance of Fruits and Vegetables and Whole Grain Products" *Clin Nutr* (13)(2013): S0261-5614. doi: 10.1016/j.clnu.2013.07.009.
6. Rick Jansen et al., "Fruit and Vegetable Consumption is Inversely Associated with Having Pancreatic Cancer," *Cancer Causes Control* 22(12)(2011):1613-1625.doi. 10.1007/s10552-011-9839-0.
7. S. Tsugane et al., "Fruit and vegetable intake and breast cancer risk defined by estrogen and progesterone receptor status: the Japan public health center-based prospective study," *Cancer Causes Control* 24(2013):2117-28.
8. M Gerson, "A Cancer Therapy: Results of Fifty Cases and the Cure of Advanced Cancer by Diet Therapy: a Summary of 30 Years of Clinical Experimentation," *Gerson Institute*, (1958).
9. S. Kroschel, "Dying to Have Known," *Cinedigm*, (2006).
10. KL Manchester, "Louis Pasteur, fermentation and a Rival," *South African Journal of Science* 103(2007).
11. M Blecker, "Blood Examination in Darkfield," *Semmelweis-Verlag* (1993).
12. A. Vigano et al., "Metabolic Nutritional and Inflammatory Characteristics in Elderly Women with Advanced Cancer," *J Geriatr Oncol* 4(2)(2013):183-189.
13. Gabriel Cousens, *There is a cure for Diabetes, revised edition: The 21-days +Holistic Recovery Program,* (Berkeley, California: North Atlantic Books, 2013).
14. WH Holzapfel and U Schillinger, "Introduction to pre-and probiotics," *Food Research International* 35(2002):109-116.
15. JI Gordon et al., "Characterizing a Model Human Gut Microbiota composed of members of its two dominant bacterial phyla," *Proc Natl Acad Sci* 106(14)(2009): 5859-64.doi. 10.1073/pnas.0901529106.
16. J.I. Gordon et al., "Gut microbiomes of Malawian twin pairs discordant for Kwashiorkor, Science, (2013).
17. J. Krakoff et al., "Energy balance- studies reveal associations between gut microbes, caloric load and nutrient absorption in humans," *Am J Clin Nutr* 94(1) (2011):48-65. doi: 10.3945/ajcn.110.010132.
18. Sk Mazmanian, JL Round and DL Kasper, "A Microbial Symbiosis factor prevents intestinal inflammatory disease," *Nature* 453(7195)(2008): 620-5. doi:10.1038/nature07008.
19. ES Chong, "A potential role of probiotics in colorectal cancer prevention: review of possible mechanisms of action world," *J Microbiol Biotechnol* (Sept 26th 2013).
20. RS Chapkin et al., "The microbiome and colorectal neoplasia: environmental modifiers of Dysbiosis," *Curr Gastroenterol Rep* (9)(2013):346. doi:10.1007/s11894-013-0346-0.
21. RF Schwabe, C Jobin, "The Microbiome and Cancer," *Nat. Rev. Cancer* (11)(2013):800-12. doi:10.1038/nrc3610.
22. Gabriel Cousens, *Rainbow Green Live-Food Cuisine*, (Berkeley, California: North Atlantic Books, 2003).
23. A. Costantini and Johann Friedrich Oberlin-Verlag, "Fungal bionics" *Cancer* 2,(1994).
24. DF Birt, GJ Phillips, "Diet, genes and microbes: complexities of colon cancer prevention," *Toxicol Pathol* (2013).
25. Z. Magic et al., "Epigenetics: a new link between nutrition and cancer," *Nutr Cancer* 65,(6)(2013):781-792.
26. KL Schalinske et al., "Nutritional Epigenomics: a portal to disease prevention," *Advanced Nutr* 4(5)(2013):530-2. doi:10.3945/an.113.004168.
27. JW Locasale et al., "Epigenetics and Cancer Metabolism," *Cancer Letters* 13,(2013):S0304-3835. doi:10.1016/j.canlet.2013.09.04.
28. TO Tollefsbol, "Dietary Epigenetics in Cancer and Aging," *Cancer Treat Res* (2014):257-267.
29. HE Sartori, "Nutrients and Cancer: an introduction to Cesium Therapy," *Pharmacol Biochem Behav* 21,(Suppl 1)(1984):7-10.
30. Gabriel Cousens, *Conscious Eating,* (Berkeley, California: North Atlantic Books, 2000).
31. R. Dahlke, *Peace Food: Wie der Verzicht auf Fleisch und Milch Korper und Seele Heilt,* (Grafe und Unzer Verlag,2011).
32. AL Gittelman, *Beyond Probiotics- The Revolutionary Discovery of a Missing Link in our Immune System,* (Connecticut: Keats Publishing, 1998).
33. TC Campbell, TM Campbell II, *The ChinaStudy,* (Ben Bella Books, 2006).
34. J Satavavivad et al., "Glyphosate induces human breast cancer cells growth via estrogen receptors," *Food Chem Toxicol* (2013).
35. EG Garcia, MA Bussacos, FM Fisher, "Harmonization and Toxicological classification of pesticides in 1992 in Brazil and the need to foresee the impacts from the forthcoming introduction of GHS," *Cien Saude Colet* (2008).
36. S. Koifman et al., "In utero pesticide exposure and leukemia in Brazilian children < 2 years of age," *Environ Health Perspect* 121(2)(2013):269-275.

Aurora T. Leon

1. American Cancer Society, accessed August 2013, www.cancer.org,

2.   Longo, Fauchi, Kasper, et al., *Harrisons Principles of Internal Medicine, 18th ed.* (McGraw Gill, 2012), 768-774.
3.   Nutritionfacts.org, accessed August 2013.
4.   The Endogenous Hormones and Breast Cancer Collaborative Group, T. J. Key, P. N. Appleby, G. K. Reeves, and A. W. Roddam, "Insulin-Like growth factor 1 (IGF1), IGF Binding Protein 3 (IGFBP3), and Breast Cancer Risk: Pooled Individual Data Analysis of 17 Prospective Studies," *Lancet Oncol* 11(6) (June 2010): 530–542.
5.   N. E Allen, P. N. Appleby and G.K. Davey, "The Associations of Diet with Serum Insulin-Like Growth Factor 1 and Oits Main Binding Protein in 292 Women Meat Eaters, Vegetarians, and Vegans," *Cancer Epidemiol Biomarkets Prev* 11(11) (Nov. 2002): 1441-8.
6.   L. R. Jacobs, "Fiber and Colon Cancer," *Gastroenterol Clin North Am* 17(4) (Dec. 1988): 747-60.
7.   John A. McDougall, *Dr. McDougall's Digestive Tune-Up* (Healthy Living Publications, 2008), 107-116.
8.   T. Colin Campbell, *Whole: Rethinking the Since of Nutrition* (BenBella Books, 2013), 7.
9.   Sabine Rohrmann, Kim Overvad, H. Bas Bueno-de-Mesquita, et al., "Meat Consumption and mortality- results from the European Prospective Investigation into Cancer and Nutrition," *BMC Med* 11 (2013): 63.
10. Yanlei Ma, Yongzhi Yang, Feng Wang, Peng Zhang, Chenzhang Shi, Yang Zou, and Huanlong Qin, "Obesity and risk of colorectal cancer: a systematic review of prospective studies," *PLoS One* 8(1) (2013): e53916.
11. Neil Murphy, Teresa Norat, Pietro Ferrari, Mazda Jenab, et al., "Dietary Fiber Intake and Risks of Cancers of the Colon and Rectum in the European Prospective Investigation into Cancer and Nutrition (EPIC)," *PLoS One* 7(6) (2012): e39361.
12. M. Thorogood, J. Mann, P. Appleby, and K. McPherson, "Risk of Death from Cancer and Ischemic Heart Disease in Meat and Non-Meat Eaters," *Brit Med J* 308 (1994): 1667-70.
13. W. C. Willet, M. J. Stampfer, G. A. Colditz, B. A. Rosner, and F. E. Speizer, "Relation of Meat, Fat, and Fiber Intake to the Risk of Colon Cancer in a Prospective Study among Women," *N Eng J Med* 323 (1990): 1664-72.
14. E. Giovannucci, E. B. Rimm, M. J. Stampfer, G. A. Colditz, A. Ascherio, and W. C. Willet, "Intake of Fat, Meat, and Fiber in Relation to Risk of Colon Cancer in Men," *Cancer Res* 54 (1994): 2390-7.
15. L. Ferrarini, N. Pellegrini, T. Mazzeo, C. Miglio, S. Galati, F. Milano, C. Rossi, and A. Buschini, "Anti-Proliferative Activity and Chemoprotective Effects Towards DNA Oxidative Damage of Fresh and Cooked Brassicaceae," *Br J Nutr* (Nov. 17, 2011): 1-9.
16. N. Annema, J. S. Heyworth, S. A. McNaughton, B. Iacopetta, and L. Fritschi, "Fruit and Vegetable Consumption and the Risk of Proximal Colon, Distal Colon, and Rectal Cancers in a Case-Control Study in Western Australia," *J Am Diet Assoc* 111(10) (2011 Oct): 1479-90.

Jacqueline Maier

1.   TC Campbell, TM Campbell II, The ChinaStudy, (Ben Bella Books, 2006).
2.   Young Park, Bioactive Components in Milk and Dairy Products, (Iowa: Wiley Blackwell, 2009):163.
3.   Joseph Keon, Whitewash, (Canada: New Society Publishers, 2010). The Dairy Council, "Lactose intolerance: prevalence, symptoms and diagnosis," 2013, http://www.milk.co.uk/page.aspx?intPageID=138.
4.   K. Milton, "A Hypothesis to Explain the Role of Meat-Eating in Human Evolution," *Evolutionary Anthropology* 8(1) (1999): 11-21. Juliet Gellately, "What is our natural diet? Are humans evolutionary adapted to eat animals, plants or both?" *Viva! Health* 2013, http://www.vegetarian.org.uk/features/display.php?pid=10.
5.   American Cancer Society, *Colorectal Cancer Facts & Figures 2011-2013*, (Atlanta: American Cancer Society, 2011). World Cancer Research Fund, *Food, nutrition, physical activity, and the prevention of cancer: A global perspective*, (American Institute of Cancer Research. Washington, DC:2007).

Andrea Lusser

1.   R. Beliveau and D. Gingras, *Cancer Cells Do Not Like Raspberries* (Goldmann, 2010).
2.   A. Hildmann, *Vegan for Fit* (BJVV 2012).
3.   A. Hildmann, *Vegan Forever Young* (BJVV 2013).
4.   J. Krebs Budwig, "The Problem and the Solution," *Sensei*, 6th ed. (2004).
5.   I. Riede, "The Cause of Lifestyle Diseases and Their Defense," *Natural Healing* 63 (2010): 59-61.
6.   Switzer J.(2012): Heilkräftige Wildkräuter-Vitalkost-Rezepte, Ayurveda Health &Beauty Verlag
7.   R. Brosius Wildkräuter, *My Lifesaver from Nature*, 2nd ed. (Startling, 2012).
8.   I. Riede, "Amanita phalloides Certified Riede (Green Knollenblätterpilz) HP Naturopathic," *The Free Doctor* 10/10: 18.
9.   I. Riede, "Remission of a Tumor with the Amanita Therapy," *Naturopathic Practice* 66 (2013): 65-67.
10. I. Riede "Switch the Tumor Off – From Genes to Amanita Therapy," *American Journal of Biomedical Research*, 1, 4(2013):93-107
11. A. Lusser, "Swing Yourself Happy and Healthy," *CO'MED Magazine* (2013).

Michele Dodman

1.   Eugenia Calle, Carmen Rodriguez, Kimberly Walker-Thurmond, and Michael Thun, "Overweight, obesity, and mortality from cancer in a prospective studied cohor of US Adults," *N Engl J Med* 348,(2003):1625-38. doi:10.1056/NEJMoa021423.
2.   DM Torres, CD Williams, SA Harrison, "Features diagnosis, and treatment of nonalcoholic fatty liver disease," *Clin Gastroenterology Hepatol* 10,(2012): 837.
3.   E. Hashimoto, S Yatsui, M Tobrari, et al., "Hepatocellular carcinoma in patients with nonalcoholic steatohepatitis," *J Gastroenterol* 44, (Suppl 19)(2009):89.
4.   S. Dam-Larsen, M. Franzmann, IB Andersen, et al., "Long term prognosis of fatty liver; risk of chronic liver disease and death," *Gut* 53(2004):750.
5.   LA Adams, S Sanderson, KD Lindor, P Angulo, "The histological course of nonalcoholic fatty liver disease: a longitudinal study of 103 patients with sequential liver biopsies," *J Hepatol* 42(2005):132.
6.   SH Caldwell, DM Crespo, "The spectrum expanded: cryptogenic cirrhosis and the natural history of non-alcoholic fatty

liver disease," *J Hepatol* 40(2004):578.

7. Joel Levine, Dennis Ahnen, "Adenomatous Polyps of the Colon," *N Engl J Med* 355, (2006):2551-2557. doi: 10.1056/NEJM-cp063038.

8. JB Bristol, PM Emmett, KW Heaton, RCN Willimson, "Sugar, fat and the risk of colorectal cancer," *BMJ* 291 (1985):1467-70.

9. EE Callee, C Rodriguez, K Walker-Thurmond, M Thun, "Overweight, obesity, and mortality from cancer in a prospectively studied cohort of U.S. adults," *N Engl J Med* 348 (2003):1625.

10. "The causes of cancer: quantitative estimates of avoidable risks of cancer in the United States today" *J Natl Cancer Inst* 66 (1981):1191-308.

11. M Lazo R Hernaez, S Bonekamp, et al., "Non-alcoholic fatty liver disease and mortality among US adults: prospective cohort study," *BMJ* 343(2011):d6891.

Luigi Mario Chiechi

1. DA Relman, "The human microbiome: ecosystem resilience and health," *Nutrition Reviews* 70, (Suppl.1)(2012): S2-9.

2. B Pięta, K Chmaj-Wierzchowska, T Opala, "Life style and risk of development of breast and ovarian cancer," *Annals of Agricultural and Environmental Medicine* 19(No 3)(2012): 379-84.

3. AIRTUM (Associazione Italiana Registri Tumori) Report (2012): 12.

4. D. M. Parkin, L. Boyd, and L. C. Walker, "The Fraction of Cancer Attributable to Lifestyle and Environmental Factors in the UK in 2010," *British Journal of Cancer* 105 (2011): S77-81.

5. Harvard School of Public Health (HSPH), "Healthy Eating Plate," HSPH website, http://www.hsph.harvard.edu/nutrition-source/healthy-eating-plate/.

6. H. Marini, A. Bitto, et al., "Breast Safety and Efficacy of Genistein Aglycone for Postmenopausal Bone Loss: A Follow-Up Study," *J Clin Endocrinol Metab* 93 (2008): 4787-96.

7. H. Adlercreutz, "Phytoestrogens and Cancer," *Lancet Oncol* 3 (2002): 364-73.

8. H. Adlercreutz and W. Mazur, "Phytoestrogens and Western Diseases," *Ann Med* 29(2) (1997): 95-120.

9. R. Baber, "Phytoestrogens and Postreproductive Health," *Maturitas* 66 (2010): 344-9.

10. K. Buck, A. K. Zaineddin, et al., "Estimated Enterolignans, Lignin-Rich Food, and Fibre in Relation to Survival After Post-menopausal Breast Cancer," *British Journal of Cancer* 105 (2011): 1151-7.

11. L. S. Velentzis, M. M. Cantwell, et al., "Lignans and Breast Cancer Risk in Pre- and Postmenopausal Women: Meta-Analyses of Observational Studies," *British Journal of Cancer* 100 (2003): 1492-8.

12. P. Guglielmini, A. Rubagotti, and F. Boccardo, "Serum Enterolactone Levels and Mortality Outcome in Women with Early Breast Cancer: A Retrospective Cohort Study," *Breast Cancer Res Treat* 132 (2012): 661-8.

13. K. Buck, A. K. Zaineddin, et al., "Estimated Enterolignans, Lignin-Rich Food, and Fibre in Relation to Survival After Post-menopausal Breast Cancer," *British Journal of Cancer* 105 (2011): 1151-7.

14. D. M. Minich and J. S. Bland, "Personalized Lifestyle Medicine: Relevance for Nutrition and Lifestyle Recommendations," *The Scientific World Journal* 2013 (2013), Article ID 129841.

15. J. Kaput, "Diet-Disease Interactions," *Nutrition* 20 (2004): 26-31.

16. L. M. Chiechi, G. Secreto, et al., "The Effects of a Soy Rich Diet on Serum Lipids: The Menfis Randomized Trial. Maturitas," 41 (2002): 97-104.

17. L. M. Chiechi, G. Secreto, et al., "Efficacy of a Soy Rich Diet in Preventing Postmenopausal Osteoporosis: The Menfis Randomized Trial," *Maturitas* 42 (2002): 295-300.

18. L. M. Chiechi, G. Putignano, et al., "The Effect of a Soy Rich Diet on the Vaginal Epithelium in Postmenopause: A Randomized Double Blind Trial," *Maturitas* 45(4) (2003): 241-6.

19. N. J. Oliberding, U. Lim, et al., "Legume, Soy, Tofu, and Isoflavone Intake and Endometrial Cancer Risk in Postmenopausal Women in the Multiethnic Cohort Study," *J Natl Cancer Inst* 104 (2012): 67-76.

20. E. R. Prossnitz and M. Barton, "The G Protein-Coupled Estrogen Receptor GPER in Health and Disease," *Nat Rev Endocrinol* 7(12) (2011): 715-26.

21. V. C. Jordan, "Chemioprevention of Breast Cancer with Selective Oestrogen-Receptor Modulators," *Nat Rev Cancer* 7 (2007): 46-53.

22. L. M. Chiechi, "Dietary Phytoestrogens in Preventing Osteoporosis in Postmenopausal Women: Italian Aspects," in *Nutrition and Diet in Menopause*, ed. Humana Press (2013).

23. http://www.care2.com/greenliving/harvard-declares-dairy-not-part-of-healthy-diet.html

24. BC Melnik, SM John, G Schmitz. Over-stimulation of insulin/IGF-1 signaling by western diet may promote diseases of civilization: lessons learnt from Laron syndrome. Nutrition & Metabolism. 2011; 8-41-4

25. "Harvard Declares Dairy NOT Part of Healthy Diet,"

26. http://www.care2.com/greenliving/harvard-declares-dairy-not-part-of-healthy-diet.html.

27. F. W. Danby, "Acne, Dairy and Cancer," *Dermato-Endocrinology* 1(1) (2009): 12-6.

28. D. Aune, E. De Stefani, et al., "Egg Consumption and the Risk of Cancer: A Multisite Case-Control Study in Uruguay," *Asian Pacific J Cancer Prev* 10 (2009): 869-76.

29. A. L. Ronco, E. De Stefani, et al., "Dietary Patterns and Risk of Ductal Carcinoma of the Breast: A Factor Analysis in Uruguay," *Asian Pac J Cancer Prev* 11(5) (2010): 1187-93.

30. H. Adlercreutz, "Phytoestrogens and Cancer," *Lancet Oncol* 3 (2002): 364-73.

Chapter 10

1. TC Campbell and TM Campbell II, *The China Study*, (Dallas, Texas, USA: BenBella Books, 2006).

Justine Butler

1. CDC, "Heart Disease Facts," accessed August 19, 2013, http://www.cdc.gov/heartdisease/facts.htm.

2. L. Story, JW Anderson, WJ Chen, D Karounos, and B Jefferson, "Adherence to high-carbohydrate, high-fiber diets: long-term

studies of non-obese diabetic men," *Journal of the American Dietetic Association* 85 (9)(1985): 1105-10.

3. FL Crowe, PN Appleby, RC Travis, TJ Key, "Risk of hospitalization or death from ischemic heart disease among British vegetarians and nonvegetarians: results from the EPIC-Oxford cohort study," *American Journal of Clinical Nutrition* 97 (3)(2013): 597-603.

4. Frank Hu et al., "Plant-Based Foods and Prevention of Cardiovascular Disease: an overview," *American Journal of Clinical Nutrition* 78(3) (2001):544S-551S.

5. D Ornish, SE Brown, LW Scherwitz, JH Billings, WT Armstrong et al., "Can lifestyle changes reverse coronary heart disease? The Lifestyle Heart Trial," *The Lancet* 336 (8708)(1990): 129-33.

6. TC Campbell and TM Campbell II, *The China Study,* (Dallas, Texas, USA: BenBella Books, 2006).

7. CB Esselstyn Jr., *Prevent and Reverse Heart Disease,* (New York: Avery. 2007).

8. SA Bingham, R Luben, A Welch, N Wareham, KT Khaw and N Day, "Are imprecise methods obscuring a relation between fat and breast cancer?" *The Lancet* 362 (9379)(2003): 212-4.

9. E Cho, D Spiegelman, DJ Hunter, WY Chen, et al., "Premenopausal Fat Intake and Risk of Breast Cancer," *Journal of the National Cancer Institute* 95 (14)(2003): 1079-1085.

10. S Sieri, V Krogh, P Ferrari, F Berrino, V Pala, et al., "Dietary fat and breast cancer risk in the European Prospective Investigation into Cancer and Nutrition, "*American Journal of Clinical Nutrition* 88 (5)(2008): 1304-1312.

11. CE Grosvenor, MF Picciano, and CR Baumrucker, "Hormones and growth factors in milk," *Endocrine Reviews* 14 (6) (1992): 710-28.

12. SS. Epstein, "Unlabeled milk from cows treated with biosynthetic growth hormones: a case of regulatory abdication," *International Journal of Health Services* 26 (1)(1996): 173-85.

13. NJ Young, C Metcalfe, D Gunnell, MA Rowlands, et al., "A cross-sectional analysis of the association between diet and insulin-like growth factor (IGF)-I, IGF-II, IGF-binding protein (IGFBP)-2, and IGFBP-3 in men in the United Kingdom," *Cancer Causes Control* 23 (6)(2012): 907-917.

14. JL Outwater, A Nicholson and N Barnard, "Dairy products and breast cancer: the IGF-I, estrogen, and bGH hypothesis," *Medical Hypotheses* 48 (6)(1997): 453-61.

15. TC Campbell, 2004, see note 6.

16. J. Plant, *Your life in your hands, understanding, preventing and overcoming breast cancer,* (London: Virgin Publishing Limited, 2007).

17. American Cancer Society, "What are the key statistics about breast cancer?", accessed July 15 2013, http://www.cancer.org/cancer/breastcancer/detailedguide/breast-cancer-key-statistics.

18. IE Willetts, M Dalzell, JW Puntis and MD Stringer, "Cow's milk enteropathy: surgical pitfalls," *Journal of Pediatric Surgery* 34 (10)(1999): 1486-8.

19. EE Ziegler, "Consumption of cow's milk as a cause of iron deficiency in infants and toddlers, *Nutrition Reviews* 69 (1) (2011):S37-S42.

20. FA Oski, *Don't Drink Your Milk,* (New York: TEACH Services Inc, 1996).

21. GA. Martinez, AS Ryan, and DJ Malec, "Nutrient intakes of American infants and children fed cow's milk or infant formula," *American Journal of Diseases in Children* 139 (10)(1985): 1010-8.

22. STEDDY Study Group, "The Environmental Determinants of Diabetes in the Young (TEDDY) Study," *Annals of the New York Academy of Sciences* 1150(2008): 1-13.

23. E Patelarou, C Girvalaki, H Brokalaki, A Patelarou, Z Androulaki and C Vardavas, "Current evidence on the associations of breastfeeding, infant formula, and cow's milk introduction with type 1 diabetes mellitus: a systematic review," *Nutrition Reviews* 70 (9)(2012): 509-519.

24. L Story, JW Anderson, WJ Chen, D Karounos, and B Jefferson, "Adherence to high-carbohydrate, high-fiber diets: long-term studies of non-obese diabetic men," *Journal of the American Dietetic Association* 85 (9)(1985): 1105-10.

25. JW Anderson, Dietary fiber in nutrition management of diabetes. *In:* G. Vahouny, V. and D. Kritchevsky (eds.), *Dietary fiber: Basic and Clinical Aspects (*New York: Plenum Press, 1986).

26. B Spock, and SJ Parker, *Baby and Child Care, the one essential parenting book,* (London: Simon and Schuster UK Limited, 1998).

27. D. Feskanich, WC Willett, MJ Stampfer and GA Colditz, "Milk, dietary calcium, and bone fractures in women: a 12-year prospective study," *The American Journal of Public Health* 87 (6)(1997): 992-7.

28. AJ. Lanou, "Bone health in children," *BMJ Clinical Research Edition 4* 333 (7572)(2004): 763-764.

29. WHO, "Vitamin and mineral requirements in human nutrition second edition," World Health Organization and Food and Agriculture Organization, 2004/ accessed July 16 2013. http://whqlibdoc.who.int/publications/2004/9241546123.pdf

Kerrie Saunders

1. R. A. Lawrence and R. M. Lawrence, *Breastfeeding: A Guide for the Medical Profession* (2011).

2. Wasileska, et al., "Cow's-Milk-Induced Infant Apnea with Increased Serum Content of Bovine β-casomorphin-5," *J Pediatr Gastroenterol Nutr* 52(6) (June 2011): 772-5.

3. R. B. Elliott, D. P. Harris, J. P. Hill, N. J. Bibby, and H. E. Wasmuth, "Type I (Insulin-Dependent) Diabetes Mellitus and Cow Milk: Casein Variant Consumption," *Diabetologia* 42(3) (Mar. 1999): 292-6.

4. S. Kamiński, A. Cieslińska, and E. Kostyra, "Polymorphism of Bovine Beta-Casein and Its Potential Effect on Human Health," *J Appl Genet* 48(3) (2007): 189-98.

5. M. Kurek, M. Czerwionka-Szaflarska, and G. Doroszewska, "Pseudoallergic Skin Reactions to Opiate Sequences of Bovine Casein in Healthy Children," *Rocz Akad Med Bialymst* 40(3) (1995): 480-5.

6. E. E. Ziegler, "Adverse Effects of Cow's Milk in Infants," *Nestle Nutr Workshop Ser Pediatric Program* 60 ((2007): 185-196.

7. I. Jakobsson and T. Lindberg, "Cow Milk As a Cause of Infantile Colic in Breast Fed Infants," *Lancet* (Aug. 1978): 312.

8. I. Jakobsson and T. Lindberg, "Cow's Milk Proteins Cause Infantile Colic in Breastfed Infants, a Double-Blind Crossover

Study," *Pediatrics* 71(2) (Feb. 1983): 268-71.

9. A. Walker, "Breastmilk As the Gold Standard for Protective Nutrients," *J Pediatrics* 156(2 suppl.) (Feb. 2010): S377.
10. F. Rosner, "Moses Maimonides' Treatise on Asthma," *Thorax* 36 (1981): 245-251.
11. J. Bartley and S. R. McGlashan, "Does Milk Increase Mucus Production?" *Medical Hypotheses* 74(4) (Oct. 2009).
12. N. Barnard, *Breaking the Food Seduction* (St. Martin's Griffin, reprint edition, Sept. 23, 2004).
13. G. Goldman, *Medical Veritas, The Journal of Medical Truth* (2005).
14. J. R. Ifland, et. al., "Refined Food Addiction, a Classic Substance Use Disorder," *Medical Hypotheses* 72 (May 2009): 518-526.
15. R. Corwin and P. Grigson, "Symposium Overview-Food Addiction: Fact or Fiction?" *J Nutr* 139(3) (Mar. 2009): 617–619.
16. A. N. Gearhardt, W. Corbin, and K. Brownell, "Preliminary Validation of the Yale Food Addiction Scale," *Appetite* 52 (2009): 430-436.
17. Wang, et al., "Brain Dopamine and Obesity," *The Lancet*, 357 (Feb. 2001): 357.
18. K. Saunders, *The Vegan Diet as Chronic Disease Prevention* (2003).

Gilbert Manso

1. John McDougall, "Marketing Milk and Disease," (June 2013).

David Ryde

1. TC Campbell and TM Campbell II, *The China Study*, (Dallas, Texas, USA: BenBella Books, 2006).
2. Physicians Committee for Responsible Medicine, "Preventing and Reversing Osteoporosis," accessed November 25th 2013, http://www.pcrm.org/health/health-topics/preventing-and-reversing-osteoporosis.

Chapter 11

1. Harvard School of Public Health, "Calcium and Milk: What's best for your bone health?" The Nutrition Source, (December 2013). http://www.hsph.harvard.edu/nutritionsource/calcium-full-story/.

Scott Stoll

1. RP Heaney, CM Weaver, "Calcium absorption from kale," *Am J Clin Nutr* 51(1990):656-7. CM Weaver, KL Plawecki KL, "Dietary calcium: adequacy of a vegetarian diet," *Am J Clin Nutr* 59(1994):1238S-41S.
2. J. Vormann and T Remer, "Dietary, metabolic, physiologic, and disease-related aspects of acid-base balance: foreword to the contributions of the Second International Acid-Base Symposium," *J Nutr* 138(2008): 413S–414S. L Frassetto, K Todd, RC Morris Jr., A Sebastian, "Estimation of net endogenous noncarbonic acid production in humans from dietary protein and potassium contents," *Am J Clin Nutr* 68(1998):576–83. SA New, "The role of the skeleton in acid-base homeostasis: the 2001 Nutrition Society Medal Lecture," *Proc Nutr Soc* 61(2002):151–64.
3. SF Vondracek, LB Hansen, MT McDermott, "Osteoporosis risk in premenopausal women," *Pharmacotherapy* 29(3) (2009):305-17. LK Massey, SJ Whiting, "Caffeine, urinary calcium, calcium metabolism and bone," *J. Nutr* 123 (9)(1992): 1611-14. De Sellmeyer and KL Stone, A Sebastian, SR Cummings, "A high ratio of dietary animal to vegetable protein increases the rate of bone loss and the risk of fracture in postmenopausal women," Study of Osteoporotic Fractures Research Group *Am J Clin Nutr* 73(1)(2001):118-22.
4. T Remer, F Manz, "Estimation of the renal net acid excretion by adults consuming diets containing variable amounts of protein," Am J Clin Nutr 59(1994):1356-61.
5. "Postgraduate Symposium: Positive influence of nutritional alkalinity on bone health," *Proc Nutr Soc* 69(1)(2010):166-73.
6. Critics often point to a few studies which suggest vegetarians and vegans have decreased bone density compared to omnivores. However, comprehensive studies of the latest relevant articles find the association is clinically insignificant.
7. CL Shen, V von Bergen, MC Chyu, MR Jenkins et al., "Fruits and dietary phytochemicals in bone protection," *Nutr Res* 32(12)(2012):897-910.
8. Ya-Ling Hsu, Jiunn-Kae Chang, Chu-Hung Tsai, Tzu-Tsung et. al., "Myricetin induces human osteoblast differentiation through bone morphogenetic protein-2/p38 mitogen-activated protein kinase pathway," *Biochemical Pharmacology* 73 (4)(2007): 504-514.
9. Swati Srivastava, Rohini Bankar, Partha Roy, "Assessment of the role of flavonoids for inducing osteoblast differentiation in isolated mouse bone marrow derived mesenchymal stem cells," *Phytomedicine* 20(8–9)(2013):683-690.
10. K Kuhn, DD D'Lima, S Hashimoto, M Lotz, "Cell death in cartilage," *Osteoarthritis Cartilage* 12(2004):1–16.
11. JC Karpie, CR Chu, "Lidocaine exhibits dose- and time-dependent cytotoxic effects on bovine articular chondrocytes in vitro," *Am J Sports Med* 35(2007):1621–1627.
12. F Boglarka et al., "Increased Chondrocyte Death after Steroid and Local Anesthetic Combination," *Clinical Orthopedics and Related Research* 468 (11)(2010): 3112-3120.
13. J Parvizi, B Orhan, K Bozic, C Peters, "Hip Arthroscopy may cause Chondrolysis," *J Bone Joint Surg Br* 93(III)(2011): 251.
14. M Flavia et al., "Rate of knee cartilage loss after partial meniscectomy," *The Journal of Rheumatology* 29(2002):1954-1956. M Englund, et al., "Impact of type of meniscal tear on radiographic symptomatic knee osteoarthritis. A sixteen-year follow-up of meniscectomy with matched controls," *Arthritis and Rheumatism* 48(2003):2178-2187.
15. A. *Hailu, SF Knutsen, GE Fraser, "Associations between meat consumption and the prevalence of degenerative* arthritis and soft tissue disorders in the Adventist Health Study, California, USA," *J Nut Health Aging*, 10(1)(2006):7-14.
16. W Grant, "The role of meat in the expression of rheumatoid arthritis," *British Journal of Nutrition* 84(2000): 589±595.
17. SL Garrett, LG Kennedy and A Calin, "Patient's perceptions of disease modulation by diet in inflammatory (rheumatoid arthritis/ankylosing spondylitis) and degenerative arthropathies," *British Journal of Rheumatology* 32 (Suppl. 2)(1993): 43.
18. J Kjeldsen-Kragh J, "Rheumatoid arthritis treated with vegetarian diets," *American Journal of Clinical Nutrition*

(1999):70594S-600S. J. Kjeldsen-Kragh, M. Haugen, CF Borchgrevink, & E F rre, "Vegetarian diet for patients with rheumatoid arthritis ± status: two years after introduction of the diet," *Clinical Rheumatology*13 (1994): 475-482. J Kjeldsen-Kragh, M Haugen , CF Borchgrevink, E Laerum, et al., "Controlled trial of fasting and one-year vegetarian diet in rheumatoid arthritis," *Lancet* 338 (1991): 899-902. J. Kjeldsen-Kragh, et al., "Changes in laboratory variables in rheumatoid arthritis patients during a trial of fasting and one-year vegetarian diet," *Scandinavian journal of rheumatology* 24.2 (1995): 85-93.

19. J McDoughall, et al., "Effects of a very low-fat, vegan diet in subjects with rheumatoid arthritis," *The Journal of Alternative & Complementary Medicine* 8.1 (2002): 71-75.

20. K Kaartinen, K Lammi, M Hypen, M Nenonen, et al., "Vegan diet alleviates fibromyalgia symptoms," *Scand J Rheumatol* 29(2000):308-313.

21. Michael S. Donaldson, Neal Speight, and Stephen Loomis, "Fibromyalgia syndrome improved using a mostly raw vegetarian diet: An observational study," *BMC complementary and alternative medicine* 1.1 (2001): 7.

22. T McAlindon, DT Felson, "Nutrition: Risk Factors for Osteoarthritis," *Ann Rheum Dis* 56(1997): 397-400.

23. SK Bai, SJ Lee, HJ Na, et al., "b-Carotene inhibits inflammatory gene expressionby suppressing the activation of the redox-sensitive transcription factor, NF-kB," *Exp Mol Med* 37 (2005): 323–334. L Flohe, R Brigelius-Flohe, C Saliou, et al., "Redox regulation of NF-kB activation," *Free Radic Biol Med* 22 (1997):1115–1126.

24. Roman-Blas, J. A., and S. A. Jimenez. "NF- B as a potential therapeutic target in osteoarthritis and rheumatoid arthritis." *Osteoarthritis and cartilage* 14.9 (2006): 839-848.

25. Szarc vel Szic, Katarzyna, et al. "Nature or nurture: let food be your epigenetic medicine in chronic inflammatory disorders." *Biochemical pharmacology* 80.12 (2010): 1816-1832.

26. David Evans, Julie B. Hirsch, and Slavik Dushenkov. "Phenolics, inflammation and nutrigenomics." *Journal of the Science of Food and Agriculture* 86.15 (2006): 2503-2509.

27. Fulvia Zanichelli, Stefania Capasso, Marilena Cipollaro, Eleonora Pagnotta, Maria Cartenì, Fiorina Casale, Renato Iori, Umberto Galderisi, "Dose-dependent effects of R-sulforaphane isothiocyanate on the biology of human mesenchymal stem cells, at dietary amounts, it promotes cell proliferation and reduces senescence and apoptosis, while at anti-cancer drug doses, it has cytotoxic effect," *Age (Dordr)* 34(2)(2012): 281–293.

28. Zanichelli, Fulvia, et al. "Low concentrations of isothiocyanates protect mesenchymal stem cells from oxidative injuries, while high concentrations exacerbate DNA damage." *Apoptosis* 17.9 (2012): 964-974.

Stefan Kreuzer

1.   TC Campbell and TM Campbell II, *The China Study,* (Dallas, Texas, USA: BenBella Books, 2006).
2.   Joseph Keon, Whitewash, (Canada: New Society Publishers, 2010).

Amy J. Lanou

1.   O Johnell O and JA Kanis, "An Estimate of the Worldwide Prevalence and Disability Associated with Osteoporotic Fractures," *Osteoporos Int* 17(2006):1726.
2.   LA Frassetto et al., "Worldwide Incidence of Hip Fracture in Elderly Women: Relation to Consumption of Animal and Vegetable Foods," *Journal of Gerontology: Medical Sciences* 55(2000):M585.
3.   AJ Lanou, et al., "Calcium, Dairy Products, and Bone Health in Children and Young Adults: A Re-Evaluation of the Evidence," *Pediatrics* 115(2005):736.
4.   CM Weaver, KL Plawecki *Am J Clin Nutr* 59(1994):1238S-41S. RP Heaney, CM Weaver CM, *Am J Clin Nutr* 51(1990):656-7.
5.   AJ Lanou, et al., *Building Bone Vitality: A Revolutionary Plan to Prevent Bone Loss and Reverse Osteoporosis*, (Mc Graw Hill,2009).

Dennis Gates

1.   Dan Longo, Anthony Fauci, Dennis Kasper, Stephen Hauser, J. Jameson, and Joseph Loscalzo, *Harrison's Principles of Internal Medicine*, 18th ed. (McGraw Hill, 2011).
2.   M. Sinaki, "Musculoskeletal Challenges of Osteoporosis," *Aging (Milano)* 10(3) (June 1998): 249-62.
3.   Mehmet Oz, *Columbia University Integrative Healthcare Symposium* (New York, NY).
4.   Neal Barnard, *Food for Life: How the New Four Food Groups Can Save Your Life* (Harmony, 1994)
5.   Neal Barnard, *Turn off the Fat Genes: The Revolutionary Guide to Losing Weight* (Harmony, reprint edition, 2001).
6.   Joel Fuhrman, *Eat for Health* (Gift of Health Press, revised single paperback edition, 2012).
7.   Dennis Gates, M.D., personal communication to author, 2007.
8.   M. Sinaki, "Effect of Physical Activity on Bone Mass," *Curr Opin Rheumatol* 8(4) (July 1996): 376-83.
9.   Andrew Weil, "The Anti-Inflammatory Diet," in *Healthy Aging: A Lifelong Guide to Your Physical and Spiritual Well-Being*, 1st ed. (Knopf, 2005).
10. Joel Fuhrman, *Super Immunity: The Essential Nutrition Guide for Boosting Your Body's Defenses to Live Longer, Stronger, and Disease Free*, 1st ed. (HarperOne, 2011).
11. Michael Roizen and Mehmet Oz, *YOU: On a Diet Revised Edition: The Owner's Manual for Waist Management* (Scribner, reissue edition, 2009).
12. Dennis Gates, M.D., "Orthowellness Training Manual," 1996.

Rick Weissenger

1.   Web M.D., "Most Common Types of Arthritis," Accessed July 18, 2013, http://www.webmd.com/rheumatoid-arthritis/guide/most-common-arthritis-types.
2.   T. Neogi and Y. Zhang, "Epidemiology of Osteoarthritis," *Rheum Dis Clin North Am* 39(1) (2013) :1-19.
3.   E. Myasoedova, et al., "Is the Incidence of Rheumatoid Arthritis Rising?: Results from Olmsted County, Minnesota, 1955-2007," *Arthritis Rheum* 62(6) (June 2010): 1576-82.
4.   F. Berenbaum, et al., "Osteoarthritis inflammation and obesity," *Curr Opin Rheumatol* 25(1) (Jan. 2013): 114-8.

5. H. L. Lopez, "Nutritional Interventions to Prevent and Treat Osteoarthritis. Part I: Focus on Fatty Acids and Macronutrients," *PM & R* 4 (5 Suppl) (May 2012): S145-54.

6. M. Attur, et al., "Prognostic Biomarkers in Osteoarthritis," *Curr Opin Rheumatol* 25(1) (Jan. 2013): 136-44.

7. R. S. et al., "The Benefits of Bariatric Surgery in Obese Patients with Hip and Knee Osteoarthritis: A Systematic Review," *Obes Rev* 12(12) (Dec. 2011): 1083-9.

8. J. J. Cao, and F. H. Nielsen, "Acid Diet (High-Meat Protein) Effects on Calcium Metabolism and Bone Health," *Curr Opin Clin Nutr Metab Care* 13(6) (Nov. 2010): 698-702.

9. S. Blüher, J. Kratzsch, and W. Kiess, "Insulin-Like Growth Factor I, Growth Hormone and Insulin in White Adipose Tissue," *Best Pract Res Clin Endocrinol Metab* 19(4) (Dec. 2005): 577-87.

10. J. Kim, Y. Li, and B. A. Watkins, "Endocannabinoid Signaling and Energy Metabolism: A Target for Dietary Intervention," 27(6) *Nutrition* (June 2011): 624-32.

11. P. G. Williams, et al., "Cereal Grains, Legumes, and Weight Management: A Comprehensive Review of the Scientific Evidence," *Nutr Rev* 66(4) (April 2008): 171-82.

12. T. A. Ledoux, "Relationship of Fruit and Vegetable Intake with Adiposity: A Systematic Review," *Obes Rev* 12(5) (May 2011): e143-50.

13. W. B. Grant, "The Role of Meat in the Expression of Rheumatoid Arthritis," *Br J Nutr* 84(5) (Nov. 2000): 589-95.

14. D. J. Pattison, "The Role of Diet in Susceptibility to Rheumatoid Arthritis: A Systematic Review," *J Rheumatol* 31(7) (July 2004): 1310-9.

15. E. Benito-Garcia, et al., "Protein, Iron, and Meat Consumption and Risk for Rheumatoid Arthritis: A Prospective Cohort Study," *Arthritis Res Ther* 9(1) (2007): R16.

16. J. D. Spence, "Dietary Cholesterol and Egg Yolks: Not for Patients at Risk of Vascular Disease," *Can J Cardiol* 26(9) (Nov. 2010) e336-9.

17. A. Otaegui-Arrazola, et al., "Oxysterols: A World to Explore," *Food Chem Toxicol* 48(12) (Dec. 2010): 3289-3303.

18. M. Krajcovicová-Kudlácková, et al., "Advanced Glycation End Products and Nutrition," *Physiol Res* 51(3) (2002): 313-6.

19. A, Muñoz and M. Costa, "Nutritionally Mediated Oxidative Stress and Inflammation," *Oxid Med Cell Longev* 2013 (2013), Article ID 610950.

20. M. J. James, et al., "Dietary Polyunsaturated Fatty Acids and Inflammatory Mediator Production," *Am J Clin Nutr* 71(1 Suppl) (Jan. 2000): S343-48.

21. C. A. Hitchon, "Oxidation in Rheumatoid Arthritis," *Arthritis Res Ther* 6(6) (2004): 265-78.

22. A. Odermatt, "The Western-Style Diet: A Major Risk Factor for Impaired Kidney Function and Chronic Kidney Disease," *Am J Physiol Renal Physiol* 301(5) (Nov. 2011): F919-31.

23. R. Loeser, "Aging and Osteoarthritis," *Curr Opin Rheumatol* 23(5)(Sept. 2011):492-496.

24. L. R. Silveira, et al., "Updating the Effects of Fatty Acids on Skeletal Muscle," *J Cell Physiol* 217(1) (Oct. 2008): 1-12.

25. H. L. Lopez, "Nutritional Interventions to Prevent and Treat Osteoarthritis. Part II: Focus on Micronutrients and Supportive Nutraceuticals," *PM&R* 4(5 Suppl) (May 2012): S155-168.

26. P. L. van Lent, et al.,"NADPH-Oxidase-Driven Oxygen Radical Production Determines Chondrocyte Death and Partly Regulates Metalloproteinase-Mediated Cartilage Matrix Degradation During Interferon-Gamma-Stimulated Immune Complex Arthritis," *Arthritis Res Ther* 7(4) (2005): R885-95.

27. J. J. Belch, "Evening Primrose Oil and Borage Oil in Rheumatologic Conditions," *Am J Clin Nutr* 71(1 Suppl) (Jan. 2000): S352-56.

28. S. Cicerale, et al., "Antimicrobial, Antioxidant and Anti-Inflammatory Phenolic Activities in Extra Virgin Olive Oil," *Curr Opin Biotechnol* 23(2) (Apr. 2012): 129-35.

29. W. B. Weglicki, "Hypomagnesemia and Inflammation: Clinical and Basic Aspects," *Annu Rev Nutr* 32 (Aug. 21, 2012): 55-71.

30. B. Qin, et al., "Association of Dietary Magnesium Intake with Radiographic Knee Osteoarthritis: Results from a Population-Based Study," *Arthritis Care Res* 64(9) (Sept. 2012): 1306-11.

31. R. Goggs, et al., "Nutraceutical Therapies for Degenerative Joint Diseases: A Critical Review," *Crit Rev Food Sci Nutr* 45(3) 2005: 145-64.

32. M. Lahiri, et al., "Modifiable Risk Factors for RA: Prevention, Better Than Cure?" *Rheumatology* 51(3) (Mar. 2012): 499-512.

33. S. Chen, "Natural Products Triggering Biological Targets--A Review of the Anti-Inflammatory Phytochemicals Targeting the Arachidonic Acid Pathway in Allergy Asthma and Rheumatoid Arthritis," *Curr Drug Targets* 12(3) (Mar. 2011): 288-301.

34. C. L. Shen, et al., "Dietary Polyphenols and Mechanisms of Osteoarthritis," *J Nutr Biochem* 23(11) (Nov. 2012): 1367-77.

35. K. Kawaguchi, et al., "Effects of Antioxidant Polyphenols on TNF-Alpha-Related Diseases," *Curr Top Med Chem* 11(14) (2011): 1767-79.

36. N. Yeoh, et al., "The Role of the Microbiome in Rheumatic Diseases," *Curr Rheumatol Rep* 15(3) (Mar. 2013): 314.

37. M. M. Newkirk, et al., "Distinct Bacterial Colonization Patterns of Escherichia Coli Subtypes Associate with Rheumatoid Factor Status in Early Inflammatory Arthritis," *Rheumatology* 49(7) (Jul. 2010): 1311-6.

38. J. Kjeldsen-Kragh, et al., "Inhibition of Growth of Proteus Mirabilis and Escherichia Coli in Urine in Response to Fasting and Vegetarian Diet," *APMIS* 103(11) (Nov. 1995): 818-22.

39. J. Kjeldsen-Kragh, et al., "Controlled Trial of Fasting and One-Year Vegetarian Diet in Rheumatoid Arthritis," *Lancet* 338(8772) (Oct. 1991): 899-902.

40. R. Peltonen, et al., "Faecal Microbial Flora and Disease Activity in Rheumatoid Arthritis During a Vegan Diet," *Br J Rheumatol* 36(1) (Jan. 1997): 64-8.

Chapter 12

Lauren Graf

1. National Kidney Foundation, http://www.kidney.org/kidneydisease/aboutckd.cfm.

2. R. A. Hamer, A. M. El Nahas, "The Burden of Chronic Kidney Disease," *BMJ* 332 (2006): 563-564.

3. "Kidney Disease up 16% in the US," *WebMD*, http://www.webmd.com/news/20070301/cdc-kidney-disease-up-16-percent-in-us.

4. Allon N. Freidman, "New Evidence for an Old Strategy to Help Delay the Need for Dialysis," *Am J Kidney Dis* (2007): 563-565.

5. J. Uribarri and M. Oh, "The Key to Halting the Progression of CKD Might Be in the Produce Market, not in the Pharmacy," *Kidney Int* 81 (2012): 7-9.

6. A. Bernstein, L. Treyzon, and L. Zhaoping, "Are High-Protein, Vegetable-Based Diets Safe for Kidney Function? A Review of the Literature," *J Am Diet Assoc* 107 (2007): 644-650.

7. The American Diabetes Association, "Create Your Plate," http://www.diabetes.org/food-and-fitness/food/planning-meals/create-your-plate/.

8. Neal Barnard, Joshua Cohen, David J. A. Jenkins, et al., "A Low-Fat Vegan Diet Improves Glycemic Control and Cardiovascular Risk Factors in a Randomized Clinical Trial in Individuals with Type 2 Diabetes," *Diabetes Care* (2006): 1777-83.

9. S. Tonstad, T. Butler, R. Yan, et al., "Types of Vegetarian Diet, Body Weight and Prevalence of Type 2 Diabetes," *Diabetes Care* 32 (2009): 791-796.

10. D. A. Snowden and R. L. Phillips, "Does a Vegetarian Diet Reduce the Occurrence of Diabetes?" *Am J Public Health* 75 (1985): 507-512.

11. A. Vang, P. N. Singh, J. W. Lee, et al., "Meats, Processed Meats, Obesity, Weight Gain and Occurrence of Diabetes Among Adults: Findings from Adventist Health Studies," *Ann Nutr Metab* 52 (2008): 96-104.

12. Allon N. Freidman, "High Protein Diets: Potential Effects on the Kidneys in Renal Health and Disease," *Am J Kidney Dis* (2004): 950-62.

13. M. Jibani, L. Bloodworth, E. Foden, K. Griffith, and O. Galpin, "Predominantly Vegetarian Diet in Patients with Incipient and Early Clinical Diabetic Nephropathy: Effects on Albumin Excretion Rate and Nutritional Status," *Diabet Med* 8 (1991): 949-953.

14. P. Kontessis, S. Jones, R. Dodds, et al., "Renal, Metabolic and Hormonal Responses to Ingestion of Animal and Vegetable Proteins," *Kidney Int* 38 (1990): 136-44.

15. P. A. Kontessis, I. Bossinakou, L. Sarika, et al., "Renal, Metabolic and Hormonal Responses to Proteins of Different Origin in Normotensive, Nonproteinuric Type I Diabetic Patients," *Diabetes Care* 18 (1995): 1233-1239.

16. G. Barsotti, E. Morelli, A. Cupisti, M. Meola, et al, "A Low-Nitrogen Low-Phosphorus Vegan Diet for Patients with Chronic Renal Failure," *Nephron* 74 (1996): 390-94.

17. L. Azadbakht and A. Esmaillzadeh, "Soy-Protein Consumption and Kidney Related Biomarkers among Type 2 Diabetics: A Crossover, Randomized Clinical Trial," *J Ren Nutr* 19 (2009): 479-86.

18. L. Azadbakht, R. Shakerhosseini, S. Atabak, et al. "Beneficiary Effect of Dietary Soy Protein on Lowering Plasma Levels of Lipid and Improving Kidney Function in Type II Diabetes with Nephropathy," *Eur J Clin Nutr* 57 (2003): 1292-4.

19. S. R. Teixeira, K. A. Tappenden, L. Carson et al. "Isolated Soy Protein Consumption Reduces Urinary Albumin Excretion and Improves the Serum Lipid Profile in Men with Type 2 Diabetes Mellitus and Nephropathy," *J Nutr* 134 (2004): 1874-80.

20. N. Soroka, D. S. Silverberg, M. Greemland, et al., "Comparison of a Vegetable-Based (Soya) and an Animal-Based Low Protein Diet in Predialysis Chronic Renal Failure Patients," *Nephron* 79 (1998): 173-80.

21. G. B. Piccoli, M. Ferraresi, M. C. Deagostini, et al., "Vegetarian Low-Protein Diets Supplemented With Keto Analogues: A Niche for the Few or an Option for Many?" *Nephrol Dial Transplant* (2013): 1-11.

22. F. Bergesio, G. Monzani, A. Guasparini, et al., "Cardiovascular Risk Factors in Severe Chronic Renal Failure: The Role of Dietary Treatment," *Clin Nephrol* (2005): 103-112.

23. M. Tonelli, N. Wiebe, B. Culleton, et al., "Chronic Kidney Disease and Mortality Risk: A Systemic Review," *J Am Soc Nephrol* 17 (2006): 2034-47.

24. M. J. Sarnak, A. S. Levy, A. Schoolwerth, et al., "Kidney Disease as a Risk Factor for Cardiovascular Disease," *Circulation* 108 (2003): 2154-69.

25. L. M. Oude Griep, H. Wang, Q. Chan, "Empirically-Derived Dietary Patterns, Diet Quality Scores and Markers of Inflammation and Endothelial Dysfunction," *Curr Nutr Rep* 2 (2013): 97-104.

26. A. Pan, Q. Sun, A. Bernstein, et al., "Red Meat Consumption and Mortality," *Arch Intern Med* 134 (2012): 555-563.

27. A. Nanri, M. A. Moore, and S. Kono, "Impact of C-Reactive Protein on Disease Risk and It's Relation to Dietary Factors," *Asan Pac J Cancer Prev* 8 (2007): 167-177.

28. S. Moe, M. Zidehsarai, and M. Chambers, "Vegetarian Compared with Meat Dietary Protein Sources and Phosphorus Homeostasis in Chronic Kidney Disease," *Clin J Am Soc Nephrol* 6 (2011): 257-264.

29. N. Noori, J. Sims, J. Kopple, et al., "Organic and Inorganic Dietary Phosphorus and Its Management in Chronic Kidney Disease," *Iran J Kidney Dis* 4 (2010): 89-100.

30. K. Kalantar-Zadeh, L. Gutekunst, R. Mehrotra, et al., "Understanding Sources of Dietary Phosphorus in the Treatment of Patients with Chronic Kidney Disease," *Clin J Am Soc Nephrol* 5 (2010): 519-530.

31. S. Moe, N. Chen, M. Seifert, et al., "A Rat Model of Chronic Kidney Disease-Mineral Bone Disorder," *Kidney Int* 75 (2009) 176-184.

32. P. Evenepoel and B. Meijers, "Dietary Fiber and Protein: Nutritional Therapy in Chronic Kidney Disease and Beyond," *Kidney Int* 81 (2012): 227-229.

33. V. M. Krishnamurthy, G. Wei, B. Baird, et al., "High Dietary Fiber Intake is Associated with Decreased Inflammation and All-Cause Mortality in Patients with Chronic Kidney Disease," *Kidney Int* 81 (2012): 300-306.

34. "KDOQI Clinical Practice Guideline for Nutrition in Children with CKD: 2008 Update," S48-S52, National Kidney Foundation website, http://www.kidney.org/professionals/kdoqi/guidelines_updates/pdf/CPGPedNutr2008.pdf.

35. J. Uribarri, "The Obsession with High Dietary Protein Intake in ESRD Patients on Dialysis: Is it Justified?" *Nephron* 86

(2000): 105-108.

36.   N. Goraya, J. Simoni, C. Jo, et al., "A Comparison of Treating Metabolic Acidosis in CKD Stage 4 Hypertensive Kidney Disease with Fruits and Vegetables or Sodium Bicarbonate," *Clin J Am Soc Nephrol* 8 (2013): 371-381.

37.   N. Goraya, J. Simoni, C. Jo, et al., "Dietary Acid Reduction with Fruits and Vegetables or Bicarbonate Attenuates Kidney Injury in Patients with a Moderately Reduced Glomerular Filtration Rate Due to Hypertensive Nephropathy," *Kidney Int* 81 (2012): 86-93.

38.   D. E. Wesson, T. Nathan, T. Rose, et al., "Dietary Protein Induces Endothelian-Mediated Kidney Injury through Enhanced Intrinsic Acid Production," *Kidney Int* 71 (2007): 210-217.

Phillip Tuso

1.   Koeth et al., "Intestinal microbiota metabolism of l-carnitine, a nutrient in red meat, promotes atherosclerosis," *Nature Medicine* 19(2013): 576–585.

2.   R. Zamora–Ros et al., "High concentrations of a urinary biomarker of polyphenol intake are associated with decreased mortality in older adults," The Journal of Nutrition 143(9)(2013): 1445-50.

3.   Orlich et al., "Vegetarian dietary patterns and mortality in Adventist health study 2," *JAMA Intern Med* 173(13) (2013):1230-8.

Lino Guedes-Pires

1.   AL Harte, MC Varma, G Tripathi, KC McGee et al., "High fat intake leads to acute postprandial exposure to circulating endotoxin in type 2 diabetic subjects," Diabetes Care 35(2)(2012):375-82. C. Erridge, "The capacity of foodstuffs to induce innate immune activation of human monocytes in vitro is dependent on food content of stimulating of Toll-like receptors 2 and 4," BR J Nutr 105(1)(2011):15-23. R. Deopurkar, H. Ghanim, J Friedman, S. Abuaysheh, et al., "Differential effects of cream, glucose, and orange juice on inflammation, endotoxin, and the expression of Toll-like receptor-2 and suppressor of cytokine signaling-2, Diabetes Care 33(5)(2010):991-7.

Ira Michaelson

1.   Jacob Schor, "The Downsides of Acid Blocking Drugs," (2007), http://www.denvernaturopathic.com/acidblockers.htm.

2.   Ryan Madanick, "Proton Pump Inhibitor Side Effects and Drug Interactions: Much Ado about Nothing?" *Cleveland Clinic Journal of Medicine* 78(1) (2011): 34-39.

3.   Y. T. Ghebremariam, et al., "Unexpected Effect of Proton Pump Inhibitors: Elevation of the Cardiovascular Risk Factor Asymmetric Dimethylarginine," *Circulation* 128(8) (2013): 845-853.

4.   W. H. Aldoori, et al., "A Prospective Study of Diet and the Risk of Symptomatic Diverticular Disease in Men," *The American Journal of Clinical Nutrition* 60(5) (1994): 757-764.

5.   Montana Office of Public Instruction, "Fiber Facts," available from: http://healthymeals.nal.usda.gov/hsmrs/Montana/ FiberFoodsList.pdf.

6.   "Introducing Our Next Epidemic, Fatty Liver Disease," *Johns Hopkins Medicine Inside Tract* (Summer 2011), http://www. hopkinsmedicine.org/news/publications/inside_tract/inside_tract_summer_2011introducing_our_next_epidemic_fatty_liver_disease.

7.   A. Gastaldelli, et al., "Relationship between Hepatic/Visceral Fat and Hepatic Insulin Resistance in Nondiabetic and Type 2 Diabetic Subjects," *Gastroenterology* 133(2) (2007): 496-506.

8.   "Nutrition Hotline Online," American Institute for Cancer Research website, http://www.aicr.org/reduce-your-cancer-risk/diet/reduce_diet_nutrition_hotline_qa.html.

9.   "High Fructose Corn Syrup Contaminated with Toxic Mercury, Says Research (Opinion)," *Natural News* website (Jan. 27, 2009), http://www.naturalnews.com/025442_HFCS_Corn_Refiners_Association.html#ixzz2iw11zFIj.

10.   Dufault, LeBlanc, Schnoll, et al., "Mercury from Chlor-Alkali Plants: Measured Concentrations in Food Product Sugar," *Environmental Health* 8 (2009): 2.

11.   Hansen, M., et al., "Sucrose, Glucose and Fructose Have Similar Genotoxicity in the Rat Colon and Affect the Metabolome," *Food Chem Toxicol* 46(2) (2008): 752-60.

12.   Aller, E.E.J.G., et al., "Starches, Sugars and Obesity," *Nutrients* 3(3) (2011): 341-369.

13.   K. L. Stanhope, et al., "Consuming Fructose-Sweetened, Not Glucose-Sweetened, Beverages Increases Visceral Adiposity and Lipids and Decreases Insulin Sensitivity in Overweight/Obese Humans," *The Journal of Clinical Investigation* 119(5) (2009): 1322.

14.   Dufault, LeBlanc, Schnoll, et al., "Mercury from Chlor-Alkali Plants: Measured Concentrations in Food Product Sugar," *Environmental Health* 8 (2009): 2.

15.   Mori, A., et al., "Capsaicin, a Component of Red Peppers, Inhibits the Growth of Androgen-Independent, p53 Mutant Prostate Cancer Cells," *Cancer Res* 66(6) (2006): 3222-9.

16.   Lewis H. Kuller, et al., "10-Year Follow-up of Subclinical Cardiovascular Disease and Risk of Coronary Heart Disease in the Cardiovascular Health Study, " *Archives of Internal Medicine* 166(1) (2006): 71-78.

17.   Goff, L.M., et al., "Veganism and Its Relationship with Insulin Resistance and Intramyocellular Lipid," *Eur J Clin Nutr* 59(2) (2005): 291-8.

Adam Weinstein

1.   D. Festi, E Scaioli, F Baldi, A Vestito, et al., "Body weight, lifestyle, dietary habits and gastroesophageal reflux disease," *World J Gastroenterol* 15(2009):1690–1701.

2.   M Shapiro, C Green, JM Bautista, R Dekel, et al., "Assessment of dietary nutrients that influence perception of intra-oesophageal acid reflux events in patients with gastro-oesophageal reflux disease,"*Aliment Pharmacol Ther* 25(2007):93–101.

3.   K Iwakiri, M Kobayashi, M Kotoyori, H Yamada, et al., "Relationship between postprandial esophageal acid exposure and meal volume and fat content," *Dig Dis Sci* 41(1996):926–930.

4.   RH Holloway, E Lyrenas, A Ireland, J Dent, "Effect of intraduodenal fat on lower oesophageal sphincter function and gastro-oesophageal reflux," *Gut* 40(1997):449–453.
5.   JH Meyer, A Lembo, JD Elashoff, R Fass, EA Mayer, "Duodenal fat intensifies the perception of heart-burn," *Gut* 49(2001):624–628.
6.   W.J. Craig, AR Mangels, "Position of the American Dietetic Association: Vegetarian Diets," *Journal of the American Dietetic Association*, 109(7)(2009):1266-1282.

Lilli Link

1.   A Ananthakrishnan, L. Higuchi, E. Huang, et al., "Aspirin, Nonsteroidal Anti-Inflammatory Drug Use, and Risk for Crohn Disease and Ulcerative Colitis: A Cohort Study," *Ann Intern Med* 156 (2012): 350-9.
2.   J. A. Cornish, E. Tan, C. Simillis, et al., "The Risk of Oral Contraceptives in the Etiology of Inflammatory Bowel Disease: A Meta-Analysis," *Am J Gastroenterol* 103 (2008): 2394-2400.
3.   K. O. Gradel, H. L. Nielsen, H. C. Schonheyder, et al., "Increased Short- and Long-Term Risk of Inflammatory Bowel Disease After Salmonella or Campylobacter Gastroenteritis," *Gastroenterology* 137 (2009): 495-501.
4.   E. V. Loftus, Jr., "Clinical Epidemiology of Inflammatory Bowel Disease: Incidence, Prevalence, and Environmental Influences," *Gastroenterology* 126 (2004): 1504-17. 5.
5.   L. Halme, P. Paavola-Sakki, U, Turunen, et al., "Family and Twin Studies in Inflammatory Bowel Disease," *World J Gastroenterol* 12 (2006): 3668-72.
6.   M. Arumugam, J. Raes, E. Pelletier, et al., "Enterotypes of the Human Gut Microbiome," *Nature* 473 (2011): 174-80.
7.   F. Guarner and J. R. Malagelada, "Gut Flora in Health and Disease," *Lancet* 361(2003): 512-9.
8.   C. T. Brown, A. G. Davis-Richardson, A. Giongo, et al., "Gut Microbiome Metagenomics Analysis Suggests a Functional Model for the Development of Autoimmunity for Type 1 Diabetes," *PLoS One* 6 (2011): e25792.
9.   F. Scaldaferri, V. Gerardi, L. R. Lopetuso, et al., "Gut Microbial Flora, Prebiotics, and Probiotics in IBD: Their Current Usage and Utility," *Biomed Res Int* (2013): 435268.
10. P. Jantchou, S. Morois, F. Clavel-Chapelon, et al., "Animal Protein Intake and Risk of Inflammatory Bowel Disease: The E3N Prospective Study," *Am J Gastroenterol* 105(2010): 2195-2201.
11. S. D'Souza, E. Levy, D. Mack, et al., "Dietary Patterns and Risk for Crohn's Disease in Children," *Inflamm Bowel Dis* 14 (2008): 367-73.
12. "A Case-Control Study of Ulcerative Colitis in Relation to Dietary and Other Factors in Japan. The Epidemiology Group of the Research Committee of Inflammatory Bowel Disease in Japan," *J Gastroenterol* 30 (Suppl 8) (1995): 9-12.
13. S. L. Jowett, C. J. Seal, M. S. Pearce, et al., "Influence of Dietary Factors on the Clinical Course of Ulcerative Colitis: A Prospective Cohort Study," *Gut* 53 (2004): 1479-84.
14. J. K. Hou, B. Abraham, and H. El-Serag, "Dietary Intake and Risk of Developing Inflammatory Bowel Disease: A Systematic Review of the Literature," *Am J Gastroenterol* 106 (2011): 563-73.
15. D. Turner, P. S. Shaw, A. H. Steinhart, et al., "Maintenance of Remission in Inflammatory Bowel Disease Using Omega-3 Fatty Acids (Fish Oil): A Systematic Review and Meta-Analyses," *Inflamm Bowel Dis* 17 (2010): 336-45.
16. S. L. Jowett, C. J. Seal, M. S. Pearce, et al., "Influence of Dietary Factors on the Clinical Course of Ulcerative Colitis: A Prospective Cohort Study," *Gut* 53 (2004): 1479-84.
17. J. K. Hou, B. Abraham, and H. El-Serag, "Dietary Intake and Risk of Developing Inflammatory Bowel Disease: A Systematic Review of the Literature," *Am J Gastroenterol* 106 (2011): 563-73.
18. V. Andersen, A. Olsen, F. Carbonnel, et al., "Diet and Risk of Inflammatory Bowel Disease," *Dig Liver Dis* 44 (2012): 185-94.

Thomas Sult

1.   Lidy Pelsser, Klaas Frankena, Jan Toorman, Huub Savelkoul, Rob Pereira, Jan Buitelaar, "A randomized controlled trail into the effects of food on ADHD," European Child and Adolescent Psychiatry 18(1)(January 2009): 12-19. Jim Stevenson, Edmund Sonuga-Barke, Donna McCann, Kate Grimshaw, Karen Parker, Matthew Rose-Zerilli, John Holloway, John Warner, "The role of histamine degradation gene polymorphisms in moderating the effects of food additives on children's ADHD symptoms," *Am J Psychiatry* 167(2010):1108-1115. doi:10.1176/appi.ajp.2010.0910529.
2.   S Zar, D Kumar, "Role of food hypersensitivity in irritable bowel syndrome," *Minerva Medical* 93(5)(2002):403-412. "Nutritional Strategies for treating Chronic Fatigue Syndrome," *Altern Med Rev* 5(2)(2000):93-108.
3.   BMJ Group, "Lowering blood homocysteine with folic acid based supplements: meta-analysis of randomized trails," *BMJ* 316(7135)(March 1998):894-898.
4.   JH Cummings, EW Pomare, WJ Branch, CP Naylor, GT Macfarlane, "Short chain fatty acids in human large intestine, portal, hepatic and venous blood," *Gut* 28 (1987):1221-1227. doi.10.1136/gut.28.10.1221.
5.   June Round and Sarkis Mazmanian, "The gut microbiota shapes intestinal immune responses during health and disease," *Nature Reviews Immunology* 9 (May 2009):313-323. doi:10.1038/nri2515. John Furness, Wolfgang Kunze, Nadine Clerc, "The intestine as a sensory organ: neural, endocrine, and immune responses," *American Journal of Physiology- Gastrointestinal and Liver Physiology* 277(1999):G922-G928.
6.   Dorette Verhoeven, Hans Verhagen, R Alexandra Goldbohm, Piet A van den Brandt, Geert van Poppel, "A review of mechanisms underlying anticarcinogenicity by brassica vegetables," *Chemico-Biological Interactions* 103(2)(1997):79-129.
7.   Andrea Tarozzi, Cristina Angeloni, Marco Malaguti, Fabiana Morroni, Silvana Hrelia and Patrizia Hrelia, "Sulforaphane as a potential protective phytochemical against neurodegenerative diseases," *Oxidative Medicine and Cellular Longevity* 2013 (2013): 415078-415088. doi.org/10.1155/2013/415078.

Chapter 13

Chelsea M. Clinton

1.   Chavarro, Willett, and Skerrett, "Fat, Carbs and the Science of Conception," Newsweek (Dec. 10, 2007).

2. J. E. Chavarro, J. W. Rich-Edwards, B. Rosner, and W. C. Willet, "A Prospective Study of Dairy Foods Intake and Anovulatory Infertility," *Hum Reprod*, advance access published on February 28, 2007.

3. J. P. Carter, T. Furman, and H. R. Hutcheson, "Preeclampsia and Reproductive Performance in a Community of Vegans," *South Med J*;80(6) (June 1987): 692-7.

4. C. Qiu, K. B. Coughlin, I. O. Frederick, T. K. Sorensen, and M. A. Williams, "Dietary Fiber Intake in Early Pregnancy and Risk of Subsequent Preeclampsia," *Am J Hypertens* 21(8) (Aug. 2008): 903-9, Epub July 17, 2008.

5. Institute of Medicine, Food and Nutrition Board, *Dietary Reference Intakes for Vitamin A, Vitamin K, Arsenic, Boron, Chromium, Copper, Iodine, Iron, Manganese, Molybdenum, Nickel, Silicon, Vanadium, and Zinc* (Washington, DC: National Academy Press, 2001).

6. E. H. Haddad, L. S. Berk, J. D. Kettering, R. W. Hubbard, and W. R. Peters, "Dietary Intake and Biochemical, Hematologic, and Immune Status of Vegans Compared with Nonvegetarians," *Am J Clin Nutr* 70(suppl) (1999): 586S-93S; R. Obeid, J. Geisel, H. Schorr, et al., "The Impact of Vegetarianism on Some Haematological Parameters," *Eur J Haematol* 69 (2002): 275-9.

7. Beth Vincent, MHS, "The Importance of DHA During Pregnancy and Breastfeeding," pregnancyandbaby.com website.

8. A few recommendations of vegan supplements are VegLife (www.veglife.com), DEVA (www.devanutrition.com), Freeda (www.freedavitamins.com), Country Life (www.country-life.com), Rainbow Light (www.rainbowlight.com), www.vegetarianvitamin.com, and www.veganessentials.com.

9. J. L. Outwater, A. Nicholson, and N. Barnard, "Dairy Products and Breast Cancer: The IGF-1, Estrogen, and bGH Hypothesis," *Med Hypothesis* 48 (1997): 453-461.

10. A. J. Baars, M. I. Bakker, R. A. Baumann, et al., "Dioxins, Dioxin-Like PCBs and Non-Dioxin-Like PCBs in Foodstuffs: Occurrence and Dietary Intake in the Netherlands," *Toxicol Lett* 151 (2004): 51-61.

11. J. Hergenrather, G. Hlady, B. Wallace, and E. Savage, "Pollutants in Breast Milk of Vegetarians (letter)," *N Engl J Med* 304 (1981): 792.

12. T. Saukkonen, S. M. Virtanen, M. Karppinen, et al., "Significance of Cow's Milk Protein Antibodies As Risk Factor for Childhood IDDM: Interaction with Dietary Cow's Milk Intake and HLA-DQB1 Genotype. Childhood Diabetes in Finland Study Group,"
Dibetologia 41 (1998): 72-78.

13. J. F. Ferrer , S. J. Kenyon , and P. Gupta, "Milk of Dairy Cows Frequently Contains a Leukemogenic Virus," *Science* 213 (1981): 1014; "Beware of the Cow," (Editorial) *Lancet* 2 (1974): 30.

14. Deborah Wilson, MD

15. S. Okolo, "Incidence, Aetiology and Epidemiology of Uterine Fibroids," *Best Pract Res Clin Obstet Gynaecol* 22(4) (Aug. 2008): 571-88, doi:10.1016/j.bpobgyn.2008.04.002, Epub June 4, 2008.

16. F. M. Biro, M. P. Galvez, L. C. Greenspan, et al., "Pubertal Assessment Method and Baseline Characteristics in a Mixed Longitudinal Study of Girls," *Pediatrics* (2010).

17. W. Zheng, L. H. Kushi, J. D. Potter, et al., "Dietary Intake of Energy and Animal Foods and Endometrial Cancer Incidence. The Iowa Women's Health Study," *Am J Epidemiol* 142 (1995): 388-394.

18. L. A. Cohen, "Dietary Fiber and Breast Cancer," *Anticancer Res* 19(5A) (Sept.-Oct. 1999); 3685-8.

19. Ovarian Cancer National Alliance, "Statistics," accessed November 8th 2013, http://www.ovariancancer.org/about-ovarian-cancer/statistics/

20. C. M. Nagle, D. M. Purdie, P. M. Webb, A. Green, et al., "Dietary Influences on Survival after Ovarian Cancer," *International Journal of Cancer* 106(2) (2003).

Chapter 14

1. Center for Science in the Public Interest, "97% of Kids' meals flunk nutrition, as fried chicken fingers, burgers, fries, soda dominate at chain restaurants, (March 28th 2013), http://www.cspinet.org/new/201303281.html.

Yamileth Cazorla-Lancaster

1. Suyi Virtanen and Mikael Knip, "Nutritional risk predictors of cell autoimmunity and type 1 diabetes at a young age," *Am J Clin Nutr* 78(6)(2003):1053-1067. Mikael Knip, Suyi Virtanen, Hans Akerblom, "Infant feeding and the risk of type 1 diabetes," *Am J Clin Nutr* 91(5)(2010):1506S-1513S. doi:10.3945.ajcn.2010.28701C.

2. Joseph Keon, *Whitewash*, (Canada: New Society Publishers. 2010).

Joel Fuhrman

1. AL May, EV Kuklina, PW Yoon, "Prevalence of Cardiovascular disease risk factors among US adolescents, 1999-2008," *Pediatrics* 129(2012):1035. PW Franks, RL Hanson, WC Knowler, et al., "Childhood obesity, other cardiovascular risk factors, and premature death," *N Engl J Med* 362(2010):485-493. Joel Fuhrman, Disease-Proof Your Child, (New York: St. Martin's Press, 2005).

Divya-Devi Joshi

1. R Sinha et al. "Meat intake and mortality: a prospective study of over half a million people" *Arch Intern Med* 169(6) (2009):562-71.

2. M Ohrlich et al., "Vegetarian dietary patterns and mortality in Adventist Health Study 2" *JAMA Intern Med*, (June 3, 2013).

3. S Rohrmann et al., "Meat consumption and mortality- results from the European Prospective Investigation into Cancer and Nutrition," *BMC Medicine* 11(2013):63.

4. N Potischmann et al., "Invited commentary: are dietary intakes and other exposures in childhood and adolescence important for adult cancers?" *Am J Epidemiol* 178(2)(Jul 15 2013):184-9.

5. TT Mosby et al., "Nutrition in adult and childhood cancer: role of carcinogens and anti-carcinogens," *Anticancer Res* 32(10)(Oct 2012): 4171-92.

6. A Cross et al., "A prospective study of red and processed meat intake in relation to cancer risk," *Public Library of Science Medicine* 4 (2007):e325. DOI; 10.1371/journal.pmed.0040325.
7. JC van der Pols et al., "Childhood dairy intake and adult cancer risk: 65-year follow-up of the Boyd Orr cohort" *Am J Clin Nutr* 86(6)(Dec. 2007):1722-9.
8. M Maynard et al., "Fruit, vegetables, and antioxidants in childhood and risk of adult cancer: the Boyd Orr cohort," *J Epidemiol Community Health* 57(3)(Mar 2003):218-25.
9. JD Potter et al., "Vegetables, fruit and phytoestrogens as preventive agents" *IARC SCI Publ* (139)(1996):61-90.
10. KA Steinmetz et al., "Vegetables, fruit and cancer prevention: a review" *J Am Diet Assoc* 96(10)(Oct. 1996):1027-39.

Leila Masson

1. S Ip, M Chung, G Raman, TA Trikalinos, J Lau, "A summary of the Agency for Healthcare Research and Quality's evidence report on breastfeeding in developed countries," *Breastfeed Med* 4 (1)(Oct.2009):S17-30.

Marge Peppercorn

1. D. Feskanich, WC Willett, MJ Stampfer, WC, GA Colditz, "Milk and Dairy Calcium and Bone Fractures in 12 Year Prospective Study," *Am J Public Health* 87 (6)(1997): 992-7.
2. US Barzel, LK Massey, "Excess Dietary Protein Can Adversely Affect Bone," *J. Nutr* 128 (6)(1998): 1051-1053.
3. T. Colin Campbell PhD, Thomas Campbell II, *The China Project*, (Dallas: Ben Bell Books, 2004): 204-10.
4. WJ Craig, AR Mangels, "American Dietetic Association Position of the American Dietetic Association: Vegetarian Diets," *J Am Diet Assoc* 109 (7)(2009): 1266-82.
5. Benjamin Spock, *Dr. Spock's Baby and Child Care*, (Pocket Books, 2004).
6. T. Colin Campbell PhD, Thomas Campbell II, *The China Project*, (Dallas: Ben Bell Books, 2004): 158-160.
7. JM Chan, MJ Stampfer, J Mia J, et al., "Dairy Products, Calcium, and Prostate Cancer Risk in the Physician's Health Study," *Am J Clin Nutr* 74(2001): 549-54.
8. JE Torfadottir, L Steingrimsdottir, L Mucci, et al., "Milk in Early Life and Risk of Advanced Prostate Cancer," *Am J Epid* 175 (2)(2012): 144-53.
9. AD Anderson, JM Nelson, S Rossiter et al., "Public Health Consequences of Use of Antimicrobial Agents in Food Animals in US," *Microb Drug Resist* 9(4)(2003): 373-9.
10. GE. Fraser, "Associations between diet and cancer, ischemic heart diseae, and all cause mortality in non-Hispanic white California 7th Day Adventists," *Am J Clin Nutr* 70 (3)(1999): 532S-538S.

Chapter 15
Doug Lisle

1. Douglas Lisle, and Alan Goldhamer, *The Pleasure Trap: Mastering the Hidden Force that Undermines the Health and Happiness*, (Book Publishing Co, 2006).

Alan Goldhamer

1. Douglas Lisle, and Alan Goldhamer, *The Pleasure Trap: Mastering the Hidden Force that Undermines the Health and Happiness*, (Book Publishing Co, 2006).

David Musnick

1. J Uribarri, S Woodruff, S Goodman, W Cai, X Chen, et al., "Advanced glycation end products in foods and a practical guide to their reduction in the diet," *J Am Diet Assoc* 110(6)(Jun 2010):922-16. doi: 10.1016/j.jada.2010.03.018.

Chapter 16

1. AC Vergnaud, T Norat, D Romaguera, T Mouw, AM May et al., "Meat consumption and prospective weight change in participants of the EPIC-PANACEA study," *Am J Clin Nutr* 92(2)(2010):398-407. doi:10.3945/ajcn.2009.28713.

Garth Davis

1. Steven Malanga, "The Washington Diet," *City Journal* 21(2)(2011). Money Talks, *East-West Journal*, (1977), United States Congress Senate Selection Committee, "Nutrition and Human Needs: Dietary goals for the United States, (US Govt Print Office, 1977).
2. Food and Nutrition Board (FNB),"Dietary Reference Intakes for Energy, Carbohydrate, Fiber, Fat, Fatty Acids, Cholesterol, Protein, and Amino Acids (Macronutrients)" Institute of Medicine (IOM)(2002) *www.nap.edu/books/0309085373.html*
3. Dan Buettner, *The Blue Zones*, (Washington DC.: National Geographic Society, 2008)
4. Gary Fraser, David Shavlik, "Ten Years of Life: Is it a matter of choice?" *Arch Intern Med* 161(13)(2001):1645-1652. doi.10.1001/archinte.161.13.1645.
5. D. Feskanich, WC Willett, MJ Stampfer, GA Colditz, "Milk, dietary calcium, and bone fractures in women: a 12-year prospective study," *Am J Publ Health* 87(1997):992-7.
6. AC Vergnaud, T Norat, D Romaguera, T Mouw, AM May et al., "Meat consumption and prospective weight change in participants of the EPIC-PANACEA study," *Am J Clin Nutr* 92(2)(2010):398-407. doi:10.3945/ajcn.2009.28713.

Mary J. (Clifton) Wendt

1. Mary J. Clifton and Chelsea Clinton, *Waist Away, How to Joyfully Lose Weight and Supercharge your Life,* (Doctor Doctor Press, 2012).

Mark Berman

1. Boyd A. Swinburn, Gary Sacks, Kevin D Hall, et al., "Obesity 1: The Global Obesity Pandemic: Shaped by Global Drivers and Local Environments," *Lancet* 378 (2011): 804–14, http://flygxe.ua.edu/labmeeting_papers/paper%202-8.pdf.
2. Joanne Slavin, "Fiber and Prebiotics: Mechanisms and Health Benefits," *Nutrients* 5(4) (Apr. 2013): 1417–1435, http://

www.ncbi.nlm.nih.gov/pmc/articles/PMC3705355/; P. Koh-Banerjee and E. B. Rimm, "Whole Grain Consumption and Weight Gain: A Review of the Epidemiological Evidence, Potential Mechanisms and Opportunities for Future Research," *Proc Nutr Soc* 62(1) (Feb. 2003): 25-9, http://www.ncbi.nlm.nih.gov/pubmed/12740053?dopt=Abstract.

3. USDA, "Nutrient Content of the U.S. Food Supply, 1909-2000," U.S. *Department of Agriculture Center for Nutrition Policy and Promotion Home Economics Research Report* (Number 56) (November 2004), http://www.cnpp.usda.gov/publications/foodsupply/foodsupply1909-2000.pdf.

4. Judy Putnam, Jane Allshouse, and Linda Scott Kantor, "U.S. Per Capita Food Supply Trends: More Calories, Refined Carbohydrates, and Fats," *FoodReview*, 25, Issue 3 (Winter 2002), http://foodfarmsjobs.org/wp-content/uploads/2011/09/US-per-Capita-Food-Supply-Trends-More-Calories-Carbs-and-Fat.pdf.

5. M. F. Gregor and G. S. Hotamisligil, "Inflammatory Mechanisms in Obesity," *Annu Rev Immunol* 29 (2011): 415-45; Jin Chengcheng and Richard A. Flavell, "Innate Sensors of Pathogen and Stress: Linking Inflammation to Obesity," *J Allergy Clin Immunol* (Aug. 2013), http://download.journals.elsevierhealth.com/pdfs/journals/0091-6749/PIIS0091674913009901.pdf.

6. Jin Chengcheng and Richard Flavell, "Innate sensors of pathogen and stress: linking inflammation to obesity," *J Allergy Clin Immunol* 132(2)(2013), http://download.journals.elsevierhealth.com/pdfs/journals/0091-6749/PIIS0091674913009901.pdf

7. K. Liszt, J. Zwielehner, M. Handschur, et al., "Characterization of Bacteria, Clostridia and Bacteroides in Faeces of Vegetarians Using Qpcr and PCR-DGGE Fingerprinting," *Ann Nutr Metab* 54(4) (2009): 253-7, http://www.ncbi.nlm.nih.gov/pubmed/19641302; "Host-Gut Microbiota Metabolic Interactions," *Science 336(6086) (June 8, 2012)*: 1262-1267, doi:10.1126/science.1223813.

8. M. Rosell, "Weight Gain Over 5 Years" (see n. 5), http://www.ncbi.nlm.nih.gov/pubmed/?term=vegan%2C+BMI%2C+weight%2C+obesity%2C+EPIC.

9. USDA, "Nutrient Content of the U.S. Food Supply, 1909-2000," see note 3.

10. M. A. Marcello, A. C. Sampaio, B. Geloneze, et al., "Obesity and Excess Protein and Carbohydrate Consumption Are Risk Factors for Thyroid Cancer," *Nutr Cancer* 64(8) (2012): 1190-5, http://www.ncbi.nlm.nih.gov/pubmed/23163848.

11. U. Ericson, E. Sonestedt, B. Gullberg, et al., "High Intakes of Protein and Processed Meat Associate with Increased Incidence of Type 2 Diabetes," *Br J Nutr* 109(6) (Mar. 28, 2013): 1143-53, http://www.ncbi.nlm.nih.gov/pubmed/22850191.

12. Agnes N. Pedersen, Jens Kondrup, and Elisabet Børsheim, "Health Effects of Protein Intake in Healthy Adults: A Systematic Literature Review," *Food & Nutrition Research* 57 (2013): 21245, http://www.ncbi.nlm.nih.gov/pmc/articles/PMC3730112/pdf/FNR-57-21245.pdf.

13. E. Amy Janke and A. T. Kozak, "'The More Pain I Have, the More I Want to Eat': Obesity in the Context of Chronic Pain," *Obesity (Silver Spring)* 20(10) (Oct. 2012): 2027-34, http://www.ncbi.nlm.nih.gov/pubmed/22334258; S. K. Tanamas, A. E. Wluka, M. Davies-Tuck, et al., "Association of Weight Gain with Incident Knee Pain, Stiffness, and Functional Difficulties: A Longitudinal Study," *Arthritis Care Res (Hoboken)* 65(1) (Jan. 2013): 34-43, http://www.ncbi.nlm.nih.gov/pubmed/22674832; and E. R. Chasens, "Obstructive Sleep Apnea, Daytime Sleepiness, and Type 2 Diabetes," *Diabetes Educ* 33(3) (May-June 2007): 475-82, http://www.ncbi.nlm.nih.gov/pubmed/17570878.

14. "2013 Food and Health Survey: Consumer Attitudes Toward Food Safety, Nutrition and Health," *International Food Information Council Foundation* (May 2013).

15. Laura Dwyer-Lindgren, Greg Freedman, Rebecca E Engell, et al., "Prevalence of Physical Activity and Obesity in US Counties, 2001–2011: A Road Map for Action," *Popul Health Metr* 11 (2013): 7, http://www.ncbi.nlm.nih.gov/pmc/articles/PMC3718620/.

Racheal Whitaker

1. Joel Fuhrman, *Eat To Live 2ⁿᵈ Edition* (New York: Little, Brown and Company, 2011), 12-14.

2. National Cancer Institute, "Obesity and Cancer Risks," accessed July 21ˢᵗ, 2013, http://www.cancer.gov/cancertopics/factsheet/Risk/obesity.

3. American Congress of Obstetricians and Gynecologists (ACOG), "Breast cancer screening. Practice Bulletin No. 122.," *Obstet Gynecol* 118(2011): 372 – 82.

4. American Cancer Society, "Breast Cancer Facts & Figures: 2010," accessed July 2st, 2013, http://www.cancer.org/acs/groups/content/@nho/documents/.

5. American Congress of Obstetricians and Gynecologists ACOG, "Management of Endometrial Cancer Practice Bulletin No. 65.," *Obstet Gynecol* 106(2005):413–25.

Magda Robinson

1. J. W. Anderson, K. M. Randles, C. W. Kendall, et al., "Carbohydrate and Fiber Recommendations for Individuals with Diabetes: A Quantitative Assessment and Meta-Analysis of the Evidence," *Journal of the American College of Nutrition* 23(1) (2004): 5-17.

2. T. J. Stephenson, "Therapeutic Benefits of a Soya Protein Rich Diet in the Prevention and Treatment of Nephropathy in Young Persons with Type 1, Insulin-Dependent, Diabetes Mellitus" (PhD dissertation, University of Kentucky, Lexington, 2001), 1-238.

3. C. S. Hoyt and F. A. Billson, "Low-Carbohydrate Diet Optic Neuropathy," *Med J Aust* 1(3) (1977): 65-66. C. S. Hoyt and F. A. Billson, "Optic Neuropathy in Ketogenic Diet," *British Journal of Opthalmology* 63 (1979): 191-194.

4. S. A. Bingham, T. Norat, A. Moskal, et al., "Is the Association with Fiber from Foods in Colorectal Cancer Confounded by Folate Intake?" *Cancer Epidemiol Biomarkers Prev* 14(6) (2005): 1552-6.

5. R. J. Wurtman, J. J. Wurtman, M. M. Regan, et al., "Effects of Normal Meals Rich in Carbohydrates or Proteins on Plasma Tryptophan and Tyrosine Ratios," *Am J Clin Nutr* 77 (2003): 128-32.

6. G. D. Brinkworth, J. D. Buckley, M. Noakes, et al., "Long Term Effects of a Very Low-Carbohydrate Diet and a Low-Fat Diet

on Mood and Cognitive Function," *Arch Intern Med* 169(20) (2009): 1873-1880.

7.   S. E. Berkow and N. Barnard, "Vegetarian Diets and Weight Status," *Nutrition Reviews* 64(4) (2006): 175-88.

8.   G. E. Fraser, "Vegetarian Diets: What Do We Know of Their Effects on Common Chronic Diseases?" *Am J Clin Nutr* 89(suppl) (2009): 1607S-1612S.

9.   M. Bes-Rastrollo, A. Sanchez-Villegas, E. Gomez-Gracia, et al., "Predictors of Weight Gain in a Mediterranean Cohort: The Suguimiento Universidad de Navarra Study 1," *Am J Clin Nutr* 83 (2006): 362-370.

10.   D. Mozaffarian, T. Hao, E. B. Rimm, et al., "Changes in Diet and Lifestyle and Long-Term Weight Gain in Women and Men," *N Engl J Med* 364 (2011): 2392-404.

11.   P. N. Appleby, M. Thorogood, J. I. Mann, et al., "Low Body Mass Index in Non-Meat Eaters: The Possible Roles of Animal Fat, Dietary Fibre and Alcohol," *Int J Obesity Relat Metab Disord* 22(5) (1998): 454-460. W. C. Miller, M. G. Niederpruem, J. P. Wallace, et al., "Dietary Fat, Sugar, and Fiber Predict Body Fat Content," *J Am Diet Assoc* 94(6) (1994): 612-615.

12.   National Institute of Health and Nutrition, "Outline for the Results of the National Health and Nutrition Survey Japan, 2007" (2007), accessed Feb. 17, 2012, http://www.nih.go.jp/eiken/english/research/pdf/nhns2007.pdf.

13.   National Institute of Health and Nutrition, "Outline for the Results of the National Health and Nutrition Survey Japan, 2007" (2007), accessed Feb. 17, 2012, http://www.nih.go.jp/eiken/english/research/pdf/nhns2007.pdf. M. Center, J. Ahmedin, and E. Ward, "International Trends in Colorectal Cancer Incidence Rates," *Cancer Epidemiol Biomarkers Prev* 18(6) (2009): 1688.

Joseph Gonzales

1.   DL Katz, "Unfattening our children: forks over feet," *Int J Obes* 35(2001):33-37.

2.   BS Metcalf, J Hosking, AN Jeffery, LD Voss, W Henley, TJ Wilkin, "Fatness leads to inactivity, but inactivity does not lead to fatness: a longitudinal study in children,"*Arch Dis Child* (June 23, 2010). doi: 10.1136/adc.2009.175927.

3.   BA Swinburn, G Sacks, E Ravussin, "Increased energy intake alone virtually explains all the increase in body weight in the United States from the 1970s to the 2000s," *Obesity Facts* 2(2)(2009):6.

4.   BA Swinburn, G Sacks, SK Lo, et al., "Estimating the changes in energy flux that characterize the rise in obesity prevalence," *Am J Clin Nutr* 89(2009):1723-1728.

5.   Y Vorwerg, D Petroff, W Kiess, S Blüher, "Physical activity in 3-6 year old children measured by SenseWear Pro® direct accelerometry in the course of the week and relation to weight status, media consumption, and socioeconomic factors," *PLoS One* 8(2013):e60619.

6.   S Mishra, J Xu, U Agarwal, J Gonzales, S Levin, ND Barnard, "A multicenter randomized controlled trial of a plant-based nutrition program to reduce body weight and cardiovascular risk in the corporate setting: the GEICO study," *Eur J Clin Nutr* 67(7)(2013):718-24.

7.   GM Turner- McGrievy, ND Barnard, AR Scialli, "A two-year randomized weight loss trial comparing a vegan diet to a more moderate low-fat diet," *Obesity* (Silver Spring),15(9)(2007):2276-81.

Chapter 17

1.   Rebecca Adams, "Why its More Expensive to be a Woman," *Huffington Post*, (September 23, 2013).

2.   Joseph Keon, *Whitewash*, (Canada, New Society Publishers, 2010).

Michael Klaper

1.   CM Raynaud, L Sabatier, O Philipot, KA Olaussen, JC Soria, "Telomere length, telomeric proteins and genomic instability during the multistep carcinogenic process," *Crit Rev Oncol Hematol* 66(2)(2008):99-117. doi.10.1016/j.critrev-onc.2007.11.006.

2.   D Ornish, J Lin, JM Chan, E Epel, C Kemp et al., "Effect of comprehensive lifestyle changes on telomerase activity and telomere length in men with biopsy-proven low-risk prostate cancer: 5-year follow-up of a descriptive pilot study," *Lancet Oncol* 14(11)(2013): 1112-20. doi. 10.1016/S1470(13)70366-8.

3.   BC Melnik, "Evidence for acne-promoting effects of milk and other insulinotropic dairy products," Nestle Nutr Workshop Ser Pediatric Program 67(2011):131-45. T. Simonart, "Acne and whey protein supplementation among bodybuilders," *Dermatology* 225(3)(2012):256-8. doi.10.1159/000345102.

4.   B Melnik, "Dietary intervention in acne: attenuation of increased m TORC1 signaling promoted by western diet," *Dermatoendocrinol* 4(1)(2012):20-32. doi:10.4161/derm.19828.

5.   T Tanaka, K Kouda, M Kotani, "Vegetarian diet amerliorates sysmptoms of atopic dermatitis through reduction of the number of peripheral eosinophils and of PGE2 synthesis by monocytes," *J Physiol Anthropol Appl Human Sci* 20(6)(2001): 353-61.

6.   M Wolters, "Diet and psoriasis: experimental data and clinical evidence," *Br J Dermatol* 153(4)(2005):706-14.

Clayton Moliver

1.   Ananya Mandal, "Collagen, What is Collagen," *News Medical*, accessed November 25th 2013, http://www.news-medical.net/health/Collagen-What-is-Collagen.aspx

R. Saravanan

1.   BC Melnik, G Schmitz, "Role of insulin, insulin-like growth factor-1, hyperglycaemic food and milk consumption in the pathogenesis of acne vulgaris," *Exp Dermatol* 18(2009):833-841.

2.   CA Adebamowo, D Spiegelman, CS Berkey, et al., "Milk consumption and acne in adolescent girls," Dermatol Online J 12(4)(2006):1. http://www.ncbi.nlm.nih.gov/pubmed/15692464.

3.   CA Adebamowo, D Spiegelman, CS Berkey et al., "Milk consumption and acne in teenaged boys," J Am Acad Dermatol 58(5)(2008):787-93. http://www.ncbi.nlm.nih.gov/pubmed/18194824.

4.   AP Oranje, A Wolkerstorfer, FB de Waard van der Spek, " Natural course of cow's milk allergy in childhood atopic eczema/

dermatitis syndrome," Ann Allergy Asthma Immunol 89(6)(2002):52-55.

5.   AP Oranje, A Wolkerstorfer, FB de Waard van der Spek, " Natural course of cow's milk allergy in childhood atopic eczema/dermatitis syndrome," Ann Allergy Asthma Immunol 89(6)(2002):52-55.

6.   Colette Bouchez, Vitamins, minerals, and other nutrients can give your skin the youthful glow of good health," *Nutrients for Healthy Skin: Inside and out,* accessed Oct. 2013, http://www.wholehealtheducation.com/news/pdfs/nutrients-for-healthy-skin.pdf.

7.   J Lademann, A Patzelt, S Schanzer, H Richter, et al., "Uptake of antioxidants by natural nutrition and supplementation: pros and cons from the dermatological point of view," *Skin Pharmacol Physiol* 24(5)(2011):269-73. doi: 10.1159/000328725.

8.   Colette Bouchez, Vitamins, minerals, and other nutrients can give your skin the youthful glow of good health," *Nutrients for Healthy Skin: Inside and out,* accessed Oct. 2013, http://www.wholehealtheducation.com/news/pdfs/nutrients-for-healthy-skin.pdf.

9.   Linda D Rhein and Joachim Fluhr, "Chapter 13: Nutrition and Skin Aging by Maeve Cosgrove and Gail Jenkins," *Aging Skin: Current and Future Therapeutic Strategies* (Illinois: Allured Business Media, 2010).

10.   Linda D Rhein and Joachim Fluhr, "Chapter 13: Nutrition and Skin Aging by Maeve Cosgrove and Gail Jenkins," *Aging Skin: Current and Future Therapeutic Strategies* (Illinois: Allured Business Media, 2010).

Chapter 18

1.   MC Morris, DA Evans, CC Tangney, JL Bienias, JA Schneider, RS Wilson, PA Scherr, "Dietary copper and high saturated and trans fat intakes associated with cognitive decline," *Arch Neurol* 63(8)(2006):1085-8.

Neal Barnard

1.   Neal Barnard, *Power Foods for the Brain: The Effective 3-step plan to protect your mind and strengthen your memory,* (New York: Hachette Book Group, 2013).

Physician's Committee for Responsible Medicine (PCRM)

1.   Physicians Committee for Responsible Medicine, "Dietary Guidelines for Alzheimer's Prevention," Accessed November 2013, http://www.pcrm.org/health/reports/dietary-guidelines-for-alzheimers-prevention.

Carol Tavani

1.   Physicians Committee for Responsible Medicine "Factsheet: Metals of Concern in Common Multivitamins: A report from PCRM", (Summer 2013)

2.   Centers for Disease Control and Prevention, "Dietary Supplement Use Among U.S. Adults Has Increased Since NHANES III (1988–1994), *NCHS Data Brief* (2011):61.

3.   Office of Dietary Supplements, "Dietary Supplement Fact Sheet: Multivitamin/mineral Supplements," *National Institutes of Health,* (2013).

4.   Copper, A Barnea, and M Vidal-Colombani, "A ligand specific action of chelated copper on hypothalamic neurons," *Proc Natl Acad Sci USA* 81(23)(1984):7656-7660.

5.   YH Hung, AI Bush, RA Cherny, "Copper in the Brain and Alzheimers Disease," *J Biol Inorg Che* 15 (1)(2010): 61-76.

6.   GJ Brewer, "The risks of copper toxicity contributing to cognitive decline in the aging population and to Alzheimer's disease," *J Am Coll Nutr* 28(2009):238-242.

7.   PK Lam, D Kritz-Silverstein, E Barrett Connor, et al., "Plasma trace elements and cognitive function in older men and women: the Rancho Bernardo study," *J Nutr Health Aging* 12(2008):22-27.

8.   MC Morris et al., "Dietary copper and high saturated and trans fat intakes associated with cognitive decline," *Arch Neurol* 63(2006):1085-8.

9.   University of Rochester Medical Center, "Copper damages protein that Defends Against Alzheimer's," *Science Daily* November 8th 2007, http://www.sciencedaily.com/releases/2007/11/071107074329.htm.

10.   JM Stankiewicz, SD Brass, "Role of iron in neurotoxicity: a cause for concern in the elderly?" *Curr Opin Clin Nutr Metab Care* 12(2009):22-29.

11.   EP Raven, PH Lu et al., "Increased Iron Levels and Decreased Tissue Integrity in Hippocampus of Alzheimer's Disease Detected in vivo with MRI,".*J. Alzheimer's Dis* 37: 127-136.

12.   USDA, "3-Nitro (Roxarsone) and Chicken US Food and Drug Administration Product Safety Information," (October 1 2013).

13.   G Bartzokis, et al., "In vivo evaluation of brain iron in Alzheimer's Disease using magnetic resonance imaging," *Arch Gen Psych* 57(2000):47-53.

14.   JB Giardina, et al, "Oxidized LDL enhances coronary vasoconstriction by increasing the activity of Protein Kinase Isoforms a and e," *Hypertension* 37(2001): 561-8.

15.   H Fillit, "Cardiovascular disease risk factors and cognitive impairment," *Am J Cardiol* 97(8)(2006):1262-5.

16.   N Scarmeas, et al., "Mediterranean diet, Alzheimer's Disease, and vascular mediation," *Arch Neurol* 63(2006): 1709-17.

17.   Martin et al., "Statin medications may prevent dementia and memory loss with longer use, while not posing any short-term cognition problems," Mayo Clinic Proceedings (October 2013). doi: 10.1016/j.mayocp.2013.07.013.

18.   P Gunter et al., "Cholesterol lowering drugs and Alzheimer's Disease," *Future Lipidology* 2 (4)(2007): 423-32.

19.   K Rockwood, S Kirkland, DB Hogan et al., "Use of lipid-lowering agents; indication bias, and the risk of dementia in community-dwelling elderly people," *Arch Neurol* 59(2002):223-227.

20.   B Wolozin, W Kellman, P Ruosseau et al., "Decreased prevalence of Alzheimer disease associated with 3-hydroxy-3-methylglutaryl coenzyme A reductase inhibitors," *Arch Neurol* 57(2000):1439-1443.

21.   Notkolal et al., "Serum total cholesterol, apolipoprotein e epsilon 4 allele, and Alzheimer's Disease," *Neuroepidemiology* 17(1998):14-20.

22. Neal Barnard, *Power Foods for the Brain: The Effective 3-step plan to protect your mind and strengthen your memory,* (New York: Hachette Book Group, 2013).

23. R Clarke, AD Smith, D Phil et al., "Folate, Vitamin B12, and serum total homocysteine levels in confirmed Alzheimer disease," *Arch Neurol* 55(1998):1449-1455.

24. F *Leblhuber,* J Walli, E Artner-Dworzak et al., "Hyperhomocysteinemia in dementia," *J Neural Transm* 107(2000):1469-1474.

25. P. Giem, WL Beeson, GE Fraser, "The incidence of dementia and intake of animal products: preliminary findings from the adventist health study," *Neuroepidemiology* 12(1993):28-36.

26. P. Giem, WI Beeson, GE Fraser, "The incidence of dementia and intake of animal products: preliminary findings from the Adventist Healthy Study," *Neuroepidemiology* 12(1993):28-36.

27. H Misonou, M Morishima-Kawashima, Y Ihara, "Oxidative stress induces intracellular accumulation of amyloid B-protein (AB) in human neuroblastoma cells," *Biochemistry* 39(2000):6951-6959.

28. R. Lethem and M Orrell, "Antioxidants and Dementia," *Lancet* 349(1997):1189-1190.

29. A. Colm, Kelleher, *Brain Trust: The Hidden Connection between Mad Cow and Misdiagnosed Alzheimer's Disease* (Paraview Pocket Books, a division of Simon and Schuster, Inc., 2004).

30. Humane Society of the United States, "FAQs About Mad Cow Disease in the U.S.," www.humanesociety.org.

31. Neal Nathanson, J Wilesmith, C. Griot, "Bovine Spongiform Encephalopathy (BSE): Causes and Consequences of a Common Source Epidemic," *American Journal of Epidemiology* 145 (1997): 959-69.

32. "Mad Cow Disease and US Meat Regulations," *Sound Consumer* (Apr. 2001), http://www.pccnaturalmarkets.com/sc/.

33. Tracy Hampton, "What Now, Mad Cow?" *JAMA* 291 (5) (2004): 543-9.

34. John McDougall, M.D., "Treating Multiple Sclerosis with Diet: Fact or Fraud?" Physicians Committee for Responsible Medicine website, http://www.pcrm.org.

35. "Dioxins in Beef," *Foods and Nutrition Digest,* Extension Foods and Nutrition, Cooperative Extension Service, Kansas State University (Nov./Dec. 1994).

36. EPA Endocrine Disruptor Research Initiative, "EDRI Federal Project Inventory: Dioxins in Beef, Milk and Forage," EPA website, www.epa.gov.

37. Linda Ly, "FDA Finally Bans Most Arsenic in Chicken Feed-- Oh, By the Way, There›s Arsenic in Your Chicken," KCET website, FOOD section, http://www.kcet.org/living/food (Oct. 9, 2013).

38. K. E. Nachman, et al., "Arsenic Species in Poultry Feather Meal," *Sci Total Environ* 417-8 (Feb. 15, 2012): 183-88.

39. US Centers for Disease Control, "Third National Report on Human Exposure to Environmental Chemicals: Organochlorine Pesticides."

40. M. Barichella, "Major Nutritional Issues in the Management of Parkinsons Disease," *Mov Disord* 24 (13) (Oct. 15, 2009): 1881-92.

41. X. Gao, et al., "Prospective Study of Dietary Patterns and Risk of Parkinsons Disease," *Am J Clin Nutr* 86(5) (Nov. 2007): 1486-94.

42. S. C. Larsson, et al., "Red Meat Consumption and Risk of Stroke in Swedish Men," *Am J Clin Nutr* 94 (2) (Aug. 2011): 417-21.

43. J. C. Chen, et al., "Red and Processed Meat Consumption and Risk of Stroke: A Meta-Analysis of Prospective Cohort Studies," *Eur J Clin Nutr* 67 (2013): 91-5.

44. Aedín Cassidy, et al., "Dietary Flavonoids and Risk of Stroke in Women," *Stroke* 43 (4) (Apr. 2012): 946-51.

45. D. Corella, et al., "Mediterranean Diet Reduces the Adverse Effect of the TCF7L2-rs7903146 Polymorphism on Cardiovascular Risk Factors and Stroke Incidence: A Randomized Controlled Trial in a High-Cardiovascular-Risk Population," *Diabetes Care* 36 (11) (Aug. 15, 2013): 3803-11.

46. Stephen Schoenthaler et al., "The Effect of Randomized Vitamin-Mineral Supplementation on Violent and Non-Violent Antisocial Behavior among Incarcerated Juveniles," *J Nutr and Envir Med* 7(4) (1997): 343-352.

47. C. M. Milte, N. Parletta, et al., "Increased Erythrocyte Eicosapentaenoic Acid and Docosahexaenoic Acid Are Associated with Improved Attention and Behavior in Children with ADHD in a Randomized Controlled Three Way Crossover Trial," *J Attention Disorders* (Nov. 8, 2013), Epub ahead of print.

48. "Mediterranean Diet May Fight Depression," Web MD website (Oct. 5, 2009), taken from *Archives of General Psychiatry.*

49. Bret Stetka, "The Best Foods for the Brain: An Update," Medscape website (Jan. 24, 2013).

50. A. Sanchez-Villegas, et al., "Mediterranean Diet and Depression," *Public Health Nutr* 9(8A) (Dec. 2006): 1104-9.

Luca Vannetiello

1. Claudia Soto, "Unfolding the role of protein misfolding in neurodegenerative diseases," *Nature Reviews Neuroscience* 4(January 2003): 49-60. doi: 10.1038/nrn1007.

William Simpson

1. National Institute on Aging, "Alzheimer's Disease Genetics fact sheet," October 25th 2013, http://www.nia.nih.gov/alzheimers/publication/alzheimers-disease-genetics-fact-sheet.

2. Neal Barnard, Power Foods for the Brain: The Effective 3-step plan to protect your mind and strengthen your memory, (New York: Hachette Book Group, 2013).

3. Martin Prince, Maelenn Guercher, Alzheimer's Disease International, "World Alzheimer Report 2013: Journey of Caring," *Alzheimer's Disease International* (London, September 2013). http://www.alz.co.uk/research/WorldAlzheimerReport2013.pdf

4. Deborah Barnes, Kristine Yaffe, "The projected effect of risk factor reduction on Alzheimer's disease prevalence," *The Lancet Neurology* 10(9)(2011):819-828. Raj Kalaria, Gladys Maestre, Piero Antuono, "Alzheimer's disease and vascular dementia in developing countries: prevalence, management, and risk factors," The Lancet Neurology 7(9)(2008):812-826.

Michael Greger

1. H Chen, E O'Reilly, ML McCullough, C Rodriguez, MA Schwarzschild, EE Calle, MJ Thun, A. Ascherio, "Consumption of dairy products and risk of Parkinson's disease," *Am J Epidemiol* 165(9)(2007):998-1006.
2. A Kyrozis, A Ghika, "Stathopoulos P, Vassilopoulos D, Trichopoulos D, Trichopoulou A. Dietary and lifestyle variables in relation to incidence of Parkinson's disease in Greece," *Eur J Epidemiol* 28(1)(2013):67-77.
3. T. Niwa, H. Yoshizumi, N. Takeda, A. Tatematsu, S. Matsuura, T. Nagatsu, "Detection of Tetrahydroisoquinoline, a Parkinsonism-Related Compound, in Parkinsonian Brains and Foods by Gas Chromatography-Mass Spectrometry," *Advances in Behavioral Biology* 38A (1990): 313-316.
4. R Astarloo, MA Mena, V Sanchez, L de la Vega, JG de Yebens, " Clinical and pharmacokinetic effects of a diet rich in insoluble fiber on Parkinson's disease," *Clin Neuropharmacol* 15(5)(1992):373-80.
5. L Baroni, C Banetto, F Tessan, D Goldin, L Cenci, P Magnanini, G Zuliani, "Pilot dietary study with normaproteic protein-redistributed plant-food diet and motor performance in patients with Parkinson's disease," *Nutr Neurosci* 14(1)(2011):1-9.

Chapter 19

1. D. Ornish, "Mostly plants," Am J Cardiol 104(7)(2009):957-958.
2. MH Carlsen, BL Halvorsen, K Holte, SK Bohn, S Dragland, et al., "The total antioxidant content of more than 3100 foods, beverages, spices, herbs and supplements used worldwide," Nutr J 9(2010):3.

Pamela Wible

1. National Cancer Institute, "Antioxidants and Cancer Prevention Fact Sheet," http://www.cancer.gov/cancertopics/fact-sheet/prevention/antioxidants. National Center for Complementary and Alternative Medicine, "Antioxidants and Health: An Introduction," (November 2013). http://nccam.nih.gov/health/antioxidants/introduction.htm#thinking.
2. American Cancer Society, "Essaic Tea," (October 2011). http://www.cancer.org/treatment/treatmentsandsideeffects/complementaryandalternativemedicine/herbsvitaminsandminerals/essiac-tea. SM Zick, A Sen, Y Feng, J Green, S Olatunde, H Boon, "Trial of Essiac to ascertain its effect in women with breast cancer (TEA-BC)," *J Altern Complement Med* 12(2006):971-980.
3. Brad Chase, "Flax Seeds and Cholesterol," *Progressive Health*, (2013). http://www.progressivehealth.com/flax-seed-can-help-lower-cholesterol-ldl.htm. Beth Orenstein, "Tiny Flaxseed has big benefits," *everyday health*, (Sept. 2012).
4. Harvard School of Public Health, "Antioxidants- Beyond the Hype," *The Nutrition Source*, (2013). http://www.hsph.harvard.edu/nutritionsource/antioxidants/
5. American Cancer Society, "Turmeric," (December 12th, 2012). YG Lin, AB Kunnumakkara, A Nair, et al., "Curcumin inhibits tumor growth and angiogenesis in ovarian carcinoma by targeting the nuclear factor-kappa B pathway," *Clin Cancer Res* 12(2007):3423-3430. Memorial Sloan-Kettering Cancer Center, "Turmeric," (December 7th, 2012), www.mskcc.org/cancer-care/herb/turmeric.
6. American Cancer Society, "Maitake Mushrooms," (November 1st, 2008). N. Kodama, K Komuta, H Nanba, "Can maitake MD-fraction aid cancer patients," Altern Med Rev, 7(2002):451. N Kodama, Y Murata, A Asakawa et al., "Maitake D-fraction enhances antitumor effects and reduces immunosuppression by mitomycin-C in tumor-bearing mice," Nutrition 21(2005):634-629.
7. Tamanna Jahangir, Sarwat Sultana, "Perillyl alcohol protects against Fe-NTA- induced nephrotoxicity and early tumor promotional events in rat experimental model," *Evid Based Complement Alternat Med* 4(4)(2007):439-445. Mark Brudnak, "Cancer-preventing properties of essential oil monoterpenes d-limonene and perillyl alcohol," *Positive Health Online* 53 (2000). http://www.positivehealth.com/article/cancer/cancer-preventing-properties-of-essential-oil-monoterpenes-d-limonene-and-perillyl-alcohol.

Michela de Petris

1. AICR and World Cancer Research Fund, *"Food, Nutrition, Physical Activity and the Prevention of Cancer: a Global Perspective," WCRF International (London, 2013).* http://www.dietandcancerreport.org/.
2. TC Campbell and TM Campbell II, *The China Study*, (Dallas, Texas, USA: BenBella Books, 2006).
3. TC Campbell and TM Campbell II, *The China Study*, (Dallas, Texas, USA: BenBella Books, 2006).

Richard Opppenlander

1. Rui Hai Liu, "Health benefits of fruit and vegetables are from additive and synergistic combinations of phytochemicals," *American Journal Clin Nutr* 78(3)(2003): 517S-520S.

Chapter 20

1. Bryan Walsh, "Getting Real About the High Price of Cheap Food", *Time Magazine*, (August 2009). Hennin Steinfeld, et al, "Livestock's Long Shadow", *Food and Agricultural Organization*, (Rome 2007).

Hope Ferdowsian

1. AH Mokdad, JS Marks, DF Stroup, JL Gerberding, "Actual Causes of Death in the United States: 2000," *JAMA* 291(2004):1238-1245.
2. Food and Agriculture Organization of the United Nations, "FAOSTAT," accessed August 4, 2013, http://faostat.fao.org/.
3. World Health Organization, *The World Health Report 2002: Reducing Risks, Promoting Healthy Life,* (Geneva: World Health Organization, 2002).
4. International Obesity Taskforce (IOTF), "The Global Epidemic," accessed August 4, 2013, http://www.iaso.org/ iotf/obesity/obesitytheglobalepidemic/.
5. World Health Organization, "The Atlas of Heart Disease and Stroke," (Geneva, Switzerland: World Health Organiza-

tion, 2004). http://www.who.int/cardiovascular_diseases/resources/atlas/en/.

6. KM Narayan, P Zhang, AM Kanaya, et al., "Diabetes: The Pandemic and Potential Solutions," In: Jamison DT, Breman JG, Measham AR, eds. *Disease Control Priorities in Developing Countries* 2nd edition. (Washington, DC: The World Bank Press and New York: Oxford University Press, 2006): 591-604.

7. S Wild, G Roglic, A Green, R Sicree, H King, "Global Prevalence of Diabetes: Estimates for 2000 and Projections for 2030," *Diabetes Care*, 27(2004):1047-1053.

8. B Zhou, "Diet and cardiovascular disease in China," In: Shetty P, Gopalan C, eds. *Diet, Nutrition and Chronic Disease: An Asian Perspective*, (Bedford, UK: Smith-Gordon,1998): 47–49.

9. A deGraft Aikins, N Unwin, C Agyemang, P Allotey, C Campbell, D Arhinful, "Tackling Africa's Chronic Disease Burden: From the Local to the Global," *Globalization and Health* 6(2010):5.

10. D Wesangula, J Wanja, "Kenya: Obesity Related to Increase in Diabetes Cases," *Daily Nation*, (September 12, 2009). http://allafrica.com/stories/200909140551.html.

11. DT Jamison, RG Feachem, MW Makgoba, et al., *Disease and Mortality in Sub-Saharan Africa 2nd ed.* (Washington, DC: World Bank, 2006).

12. DA Snowdon, RI Phillips, "Does a vegetarian diet reduce the occurrence of diabetes?" *Am J Public Health* 75(5)(1985):507-12.

13. SE Berkow, N Barnard, "Vegetarian diets and weight status," *Nutr Rev* 64(4)(2006):175-88.

14. V Richter, F Rassoul, B Hentschel, et al., „Age-dependence of lipid parameters in the general population and vegetarians," *Z Gerontol Geriatr* 37(3)(2004):207-13.

15. Cheng Harris, "Asia-Pacific Faces Diabetes Challenge," *The Lancet* 375(2010):2207-2210.

16. International Diabetes Federation (IDF), IDF Diabetes Atlas, 5th ed. (2012), accessed August 4th, 2013, http://www.idf.org/sites/default/files/5E_IDFAtlasPoster_2012_EN.pdf.

17. National Heart, Lung, and Blood Institute, *Clinical Guidelines on the Identification, Evaluation, and Treatment of Overweight and Obesity in Adults*, (Bethesda, MD: National Institutes of Health; 1998). http://www.nhlbi.nih.gov/guidelines/obesity/ob_gdlns.pdf.

18. International Diabetes Federation, *Diabetes Atlas*. 3rd edition, (Brussels, Belgium: International Diabetes Federation, 2006).

19. CD Mathers, D Loncar, "Projections of global mortality and burden of disease from 2002 to 2030," *PLoS Med* 3(11)(2006). doi:10.1371/journal.pmed.0030442.

Aysha Akhtar

1. A Akhtar, *Animals and Public Health: Why Treating Animals Better is Critical to Human Welfare*, (Hampshire, UK: Palgrave Macmillan, 2012).

2. Food and Agriculture Organization of the United States, *FAOSTAT*, 2009.

3. A Akhtar A, et al., "Health professional's role in animal agriculture, climate change and human health," *American Journal of Preventive Medicine* 36 (2)(2009): 182–187.

4. J Pearson, et al., "Global risks of infectious animal diseases," *Council for Agricultural Science and technology* 28(2005).

5. JSM Peiris, et al., "Avian influenza virus (H5N1): A threat to human health," *Clinical Microbiology Reviews* 20(2007): 243–267.

6. I Capua, DJ Alexander, "Animal and human health implications of avian influenza infections," *Bioscience Reports* 27(2007): 359–372.

7. V Bavinck V, et al., "The role of backyard flocks in the epidemic of highly pathogenic avian influenza virus (H7N7) in the Netherlands in 2003," *Preventive Veterinary Medicine* 88(2009): 247–254.

8. *JH Leibler, et al. "Industrial food animal production and global health risks: Exploring the ecosystems and economics of avian influenza" EcoHealth 6(2009): 58-70.*

9. CA Nidom,. et al, "Influenza A (H5N1) viruses from pigs, Indonesia," *Emerging Infectious Diseases* 16(10)(2010): 1515–1523.

10. A Akhtar, "The need to include animal protection in public health policies," *Journal of Public Health Policy* (2013). doi: 10.1057/jphp.2013.29.

11. World Health Organization, "Cumulative number of confirmed human cases of avian influenza A(H5N1) reported to WHO, (Dec. 2013). http://www.who.int/influenza/human_animal_interface/H5N1_cumulative_table_archives/en/.

Richard Oppenlander

1. Richard Oppenlander, Comfortably Unaware, (Minneapolis: Langdon Street Press, 2011). Hennin Steinfeld, et al, "Livestock's Long Shadow", *Food and Agricultural Organization*, (Rome 2007).

2. Hennin Steinfeld, et al, "Livestock's Long Shadow", *Food and Agricultural Organization*, (Rome 2007). Daniel Imhoff, *The CAFO Reader: Tragedy of Industrial Animal Production,* (Foundation for Deep Ecology, 2010).

3. Bryan Walsh, "Getting Real About the High Price of Cheap Food", *Time Magazine* (August 2009). Environmental Working Group, "Meat Eater's Guide to Climate Change and Health," (2011), http://www.ewg.org/meateatersguide/interactive-graphic/grazing/.

4. Richard Oppenlander, "Freshwater abuse and loss: where is it all going?" Forks Over Knives (May 2013), http://www.forksoverknives.com/freshwater-abuse-and-loss-where-is-it-all-going/.

Index

Made in the USA
San Bernardino, CA
08 March 2014